The Ortho-Perio Patient: Clinical Evidence & Therapeutic Guidelines

DEDICATION

To the memory of our fathers

Library of Congress Cataloging-in-Publication Data

Names: Eliades, Theodore, editor. | Katsaros, Christos, 1962- editor.
Title: The ortho-perio patient : clinical evidence & therapeutic guidelines / edited by Theodore Eliades, Christos Katsaros.
Description: Batavia, IL : Quintessence Publishing Co, Inc, [2018] | Includes bibliographical references and index.
Identifiers: LCCN 2018035730 | ISBN 9780867156799 (hardcover)
Subjects: | MESH: Malocclusion--therapy | Periodontal Diseases--therapy | Evidence-Based Dentistry
Classification: LCC RK523 | NLM WU 440 | DDC 617.6/43--dc23
LC record available at https://lccn.loc.gov/2018035730

QUINTESSENCE PUBLISHING
USA

Quintessence Publishing Co, Inc
411 N Raddant Road
Batavia, IL 60510
www.quintpub.com

5 4 3 2 1

Editor: Leah Huffman
Cover design: Angelina Schmelter
Design: Sue Zubek
Production: Kaye Clemens

Printed in China

The Ortho-Perio Patient
Clinical Evidence & Therapeutic Guidelines

Edited by

Theodore Eliades, DDS, MS, Dr Med Sci, PhD
Professor and Director
Clinic of Orthodontics and Pediatric Dentistry
Center of Dental Medicine
University of Zurich
Zurich, Switzerland

Christos Katsaros, DDS, Dr med dent, Odont Dr/PhD
Professor and Chair
Department of Orthodontics and Dentofacial Orthopedics
School of Dental Medicine
University of Bern
Bern, Switzerland

QUINTESSENCE PUBLISHING

Berlin, Barcelona, Chicago, Istanbul, London, Milan, Moscow, New Delhi,
Paris, Prague, São Paulo, Seoul, Singapore, Tokyo, Warsaw

CONTENTS

Preface *vi*

Contributors *vii*

SECTION I: FUNDAMENTALS OF ORAL PHYSIOLOGY

1 Bone Biology and Response to Loading in Adult Orthodontic Patients 3
Dimitrios Konstantonis

2 Microbial Colonization of Teeth and Orthodontic Appliances 27
Georgios N. Belibasakis • Anastasios Grigoriadis • Carlos Marcelo da Silva Figueredo

3 Changes in the Oral Microbiota During Orthodontic Treatment 33
William Papaioannou • Margarita Makou

4 Pellicle Organization and Plaque Accumulation on Biomaterials 43
George Eliades • Theodore Eliades

SECTION II: PERIODONTAL CONSIDERATIONS FOR THE ORTHODONTIC PATIENT

5 Periodontal Examination of the Orthodontic Patient 59
Giovanni E. Salvi • Christoph A. Ramseier

6 Etiology and Treatment of Gingival Recessions in Orthodontically Treated Patients 71
Raluca Cosgarea • Dimitrios Kloukos • Christos Katsaros • Anton Sculean

7 Soft Tissue Augmentation at Maxillary and Mandibular Incisors in Orthodontic Patients 93
Dimitrios Kloukos • Theodore Eliades • Anton Sculean • Christos Katsaros

8 Periodontal Considerations in Orthodontic and Orthopedic Expansion *99*
Andrew Dentino • T. Gerard Bradley

9 Surgical Lengthening of the Clinical Crown *107*
Spyridon I. Vassilopoulos • Phoebus N. Madianos • Ioannis Vrotsos

10 Management of Impacted Maxillary Canines *121*
Marianna Evans • Nipul K. Tanna • Chun-Hsi Chung

SECTION III: ORTHODONTIC CONSIDERATIONS FOR THE PERIODONTIC PATIENT

11 Clinical Evidence on the Effect of Orthodontic Treatment on the Periodontal Tissues *161*
Spyridon N. Papageorgiou • Theodore Eliades

12 Orthodontic Mechanics in Patients with Periodontal Disease *175*
Carlalberta Verna • Turi Bassarelli

13 Orthodontic Treatment in Patients with Severe Periodontal Disease *189*
Tali Chackartchi • Stella Chaushu • Ayala Stabholz

Index *211*

PREFACE

This book gathers the available evidence and offers a thorough and substantiated discussion of treatment for the ortho-perio patient. With contributions from leading scholars and clinicians all over the world, the book systematically analyzes the interaction of the two specialties from both scientific and clinical perspectives. It includes an introductory section where the fundamentals of oral physiology with relation to orthodontic-periodontic interactions are analyzed, including bone biology in adult patients and the basics of oral microbiota attachment and pellicle organization on materials. The subsequent section on periodontal considerations for the orthodontic patient covers the periodontal examination of the orthodontic patient, aspects of gingival recession and grafting, clinical attachment level, orthodontic-periodontic effects of expansion, surgical crown lengthening, and ectopic canine eruption. The last section on orthodontic considerations for the periodontic patient includes chapters on clinical attachment level, the biomechanics in compromised periodontal tissues, and principles of orthodontic treatment in periodontic patients.

The evidence provided in this book and the case series portraying the adjunct role of each specialty in the treatment planning of patients with periodontal or orthodontic needs furnish important theoretical and clinical information as well as practical guidelines to improve the treatment outcome of therapeutic protocols involving ortho-perio interventions. Thus, the book not only acts as a reference book on the topic but, more importantly, includes substantiated guidelines and validated treatment approaches, which aid the practicing clinician in individualized treatment planning. It is therefore appropriate for academics, clinicians, and postgraduate students in orthodontics and periodontology and could be used as an accompanying text for the standard seminar of specialty training in dental schools.

It may be worth noting that this book was conceived 7 years ago with an additional editor, the late Dr Vincent G. Kokich, who was instrumental in developing the scope of the text and undertook the contribution of several chapters. With his sudden and tragic passing in 2013, the project had to be re-formed, and chapters were assigned to leading clinicians and academics in the field. The editors, who were fortunate to get acquainted with his brilliant clinical expertise and visionary academic and research service, return only a fragment of the debt they owe him for the collaboration they enjoyed by acknowledging his legendary path in the field.

CONTRIBUTORS

Turi Bassarelli, MD, DDS, MSc
Senior Research and Teaching Fellow
Department of Orthodontics and Pediatric Dentistry
University Center for Dental Medicine
University of Basel
Basel, Switzerland

Georgios N. Belibasakis, DDS, MSc, PhD, FHEA
Professor and Head of Division of Oral Diseases
Department of Dental Medicine
Karolinska Institute
Solna, Sweden

T. Gerard Bradley, BDS, MS, Dr med dent
Dean and Professor of Orthodontics
School of Dentistry
University of Louisville
Louisville, Kentucky, USA

Tali Chackartchi, DMD
Senior Instructor
Department of Periodontology
Faculty of Dental Medicine
Hadassah and Hebrew University
Jerusalem, Israel

Stella Chaushu, DMD, PhD
Associate Professor and Chair
Department of Orthodontics
Faculty of Dental Medicine
Hadassah and Hebrew University
Jerusalem, Israel

Chun-Hsi Chung, BDS, DMD, MS
Associate Professor and Chair
Department of Orthodontics
School of Dental Medicine
University of Pennsylvania
Philadelphia, Pennsylvania, USA

Raluca Cosgarea, DDS, Dr med dent
Assistant Professor and Research Fellow
Department of Periodontology
Faculty of Medicine
Philipps University of Marburg
Marburg, Germany

Carlos Marcelo da Silva Figueredo, DDS, MDSc, PhD
Associate Professor
Department of Dentistry and Oral Health
School of Periodontology
Griffith University
Brisbane, Australia

Andrew Dentino, DDS, PhD
Professor and Director
Department of Periodontics
Marquette University
Milwaukee, Wisconsin, USA

George Eliades, DDS, DrDent
Professor and Head
Department of Dental Biomaterials
School of Dentistry
National and Kapodistrian University of Athens
Athens, Greece

Theodore Eliades, DDS, MS, Dr Med Sci, PhD
Professor and Director
Clinic of Orthodontics and Pediatric Dentistry
Center of Dental Medicine
University of Zurich
Zurich, Switzerland

Marianna Evans, DMD
Clinical Associate
Department of Orthodontics
School of Dental Medicine
University of Pennsylvania
Philadelphia, Pennsylvania, USA

Private Practice
Newtown Square, Pennsylvania, USA

Anastasios Grigoriadis, DDS, PhD
Lecturer and Senior Dentist
Department of Dental Medicine
Division of Oral Diagnostics and Rehabilitation
Karolinska Institute
Huddinge, Sweden

Christos Katsaros, DDS, Dr med dent, Odont Dr/PhD
Professor and Chair
Department of Orthodontics and Dentofacial Orthopedics
School of Dental Medicine
University of Bern
Bern, Switzerland

Dimitrios Kloukos, DDS, Dr med dent, MAS, MSc
Head of Orthodontic Department
General Hospital of Greek Air Force
Athens, Greece

Research Associate
Department of Orthodontics and Dentofacial Orthopedics
School of Dental Medicine
University of Bern
Bern, Switzerland

Dimitrios Konstantonis, DDS, MS, PhD
Research Associate
Department of Orthodontics
School of Dentistry
National and Kapodistrian University of Athens
Athens, Greece

Research Visiting Fellow
Clinic of Orthodontics and Pediatric Dentistry
Center of Dental Medicine
University of Zurich
Zurich, Switzerland

Phoebus N. Madianos, DDS, PhD
Professor
Department of Periodontology
School of Dentistry
National and Kapodistrian University of Athens
Athens, Greece

Margarita Makou, DDS, MS, DrDent
Professor Emeritus
Department of Orthodontics
School of Dentistry
National and Kapodistrian University of Athens
Athens, Greece

Spyridon N. Papageorgiou, DDS, Dr med dent
Senior Teaching and Research Assistant
Clinic of Orthodontics and Pediatric Dentistry
Center of Dental Medicine
University of Zurich
Zurich, Switzerland

William Papaioannou, DDS, MScD, PhD
Assistant Professor
Department of Preventative and Community Dentistry
National and Kapodistrian University of Athens
Athens, Greece

Christoph A. Ramseier, DDS, Dr med dent
Senior Lecturer
Department of Periodontology
School of Dental Medicine
University of Bern
Bern, Switzerland

Giovanni E. Salvi, DDS, Dr med dent
Associate Professor, Vice Chairman, and Graduate Program Director
Department of Periodontology
School of Dental Medicine
University of Bern
Bern, Switzerland

Anton Sculean, DDS, MS, Dr med dent, Dr hc
Professor and Chair
Department of Periodontology
School of Dental Medicine
University of Bern
Bern, Switzerland

Ayala Stabholz, DMD
Senior Dentist
Department of Periodontology
Faculty of Dental Medicine
Hadassah and Hebrew University
Jerusalem, Israel

Nipul K. Tanna, DMD
Assistant Professor
Department of Orthodontics
School of Dental Medicine
University of Pennsylvania
Philadelphia, Pennsylvania, USA

Spyridon I. Vassilopoulos, DDS, MSc, DrDent
Assistant Professor
Department of Periodontology
School of Dentistry
National and Kapodistrian University of Athens
Athens, Greece

Carlalberta Verna, DDS, Dr med dent, PhD
Professor and Head
Department of Orthodontics and Pediatric Dentistry
University Center for Dental Medicine
University of Basel
Basel, Switzerland

Ioannis Vrotsos, DDS, MSD, DrDent
Professor and Director
Department of Periodontology
School of Dentistry
National and Kapodistrian University of Athens
Athens, Greece

SECTION I

Fundamentals of Oral Physiology

CHAPTER 1

Bone Biology and Response to Loading in Adult Orthodontic Patients

Dimitrios Konstantonis

Orthodontic movement is achieved due to the ability of alveolar bone to remodel.[1–3] The bone-remodeling process is controlled by an equilibrium between bone formation in the areas of pressure and bone resorption in the areas of tension as the teeth respond to mechanical forces during treatment. The main mediators of mechanical stress to the alveolar bone are the cells of the periodontal ligament (PDL). The PDL consists of a heterogenous cell population comprised by nondifferentiated multipotent mesenchymal cells as well as fibroblasts. The periodontal fibroblasts have the capacity to differentiate into osteoblasts in response to various external mechanical stimuli. This feature of the PDL fibroblasts plays a key role in the regeneration of the alveolar bone and the acceleration of orthodontic movement.

Current research provides scientific data that elucidates the molecular response of the human PDL fibroblasts after mechanical stimulation.[4–6] Integrins at focal adhesions function both as cell-adhesion molecules and as intracellular signal receptors. Upon stress application, a series of biochemical responses expressed via signaling pathway cascades, involving GTPases (enzymes that bind and hydrolyze guanosine triphosphate [GTP]), mitogen-activated protein kinases (MAPKs), and transcription factors like activator protein 1 (AP-1) and runt-related transcription factor 2 (Runx2), stimulate DNA binding potential to specific genes, thus leading to osteoblast differentiation. Consecutively, the activation of cytokines like receptor activator of nuclear factor κB ligand (RANKL) and osteoprotegerin (OPG) regulates osteoclast activity. Despite the importance of these biologic phenomena, the number of reports on the molecular response of human periodontal fibroblasts after mechanical stimulation and on the subsequent activation of signaling pathways is limited.

Age has a considerable impact on the composition and integrity of the periodontal tissues and, according to clinical beliefs and research studies, plays a significant role in the rate of orthodontic tooth movement.[7–12] Apart from the observed cellular morphologic changes, the levels of proliferation and differentiation of alveolar bone and PDL cells also diminish with age. At a molecular level, aged human PDL fibroblasts show alterations in signal transduction pathways, leading to a catabolic phenotype displayed by a significantly decreased ability for osteoblastic differentiation, thus affecting tissue development and integrity.[13,14] Currently, the difference in molecular response to orthodontic load among different age groups is considered of utmost importance. Still, the clinical application of biologic modifiers to expedite or decrease the rate of orthodontic tooth movement is underway.

Biology of Tooth Movement

ALVEOLAR BONE

The alveolar bone is the thickened ridge of the jaw that contains the tooth sockets, in which the teeth are embedded. The alveolar process contains a region of compact bone adjacent to the PDL called the *lamina dura*.[15] When viewed on radiographs, it is the uniformly radiopaque part, and it is attached to the cementum of the roots by the PDL. Although the lamina dura is often described as a solid wall, it is in fact a perforated construction through which the compressed fluids of the PDL can be expressed. The permeability of the lamina dura varies depending on its position in the alveolar process and the age of the patient. Under the lamina dura lies the cancellous bone, which appears on radiographs as less bright. The tiny spicules of bone crisscrossing the cancellous bone are the trabeculae and make the bone look spongy. These trabeculae separate the cancellous bone into tiny compartments, which contain the blood-producing marrow.

The alveolar bone or process is divided into the alveolar bone proper and the supporting alveolar bone. Microscopically, both the alveolar bone proper and the supporting alveolar bone have the same components: fibers, cells, intercellular substances, nerves, blood vessels, and lymphatics. The alveolar bone is comprised of calcified organic extracellular matrix containing bone cells. The organic matrix is comprised of collagen fibers and ground substance. The collagen fibers are produced by osteoblasts and consist of 95% collagen type I and 5% collagen type III. The ground substance contains the collagen fibers, glycosaminoglycans, and other proteins. The noncalcified organic matrix is called *osteoid*. Calcification of the alveolar bone occurs by deposition of carbonated hydroxyapatite crystals around the osteoid and between the collagen fibers. Noncollagenous proteins like osteocalcin and osteonectin also participate in the calcification process.

The cells of the alveolar bone are divided into four types[16]:

- Osteoblasts: Specialized mesenchymal cells forming bone
- Osteoclasts: Multinucleated cells responsible for bone resorption
- Lining cells: Undifferentiated osteoblastic cells
- Osteocytes: Osteoblasts located within the compact bone

The alveolar bone is an extremely important part of the dentoalveolar device and is the final recipient of forces during mastication and orthodontic treatment. The reaction to these forces include bending of the alveolar socket and subsequent bone resorption and deposition, which depends on the time, magnitude, and duration of the force. Although the biologic mechanisms underlying these cellular changes are not fully known, it seems they resemble those of the body frame, where mechanical loading has osteogenic effects. Despite the similarities between the alveolar and compact bone, the different response to mechanical loading is attributed to the presence of the PDL, a tissue full of undifferentiated mesenchymal cells, which serves as the means through which the signal is transmitted to the alveolar bone.

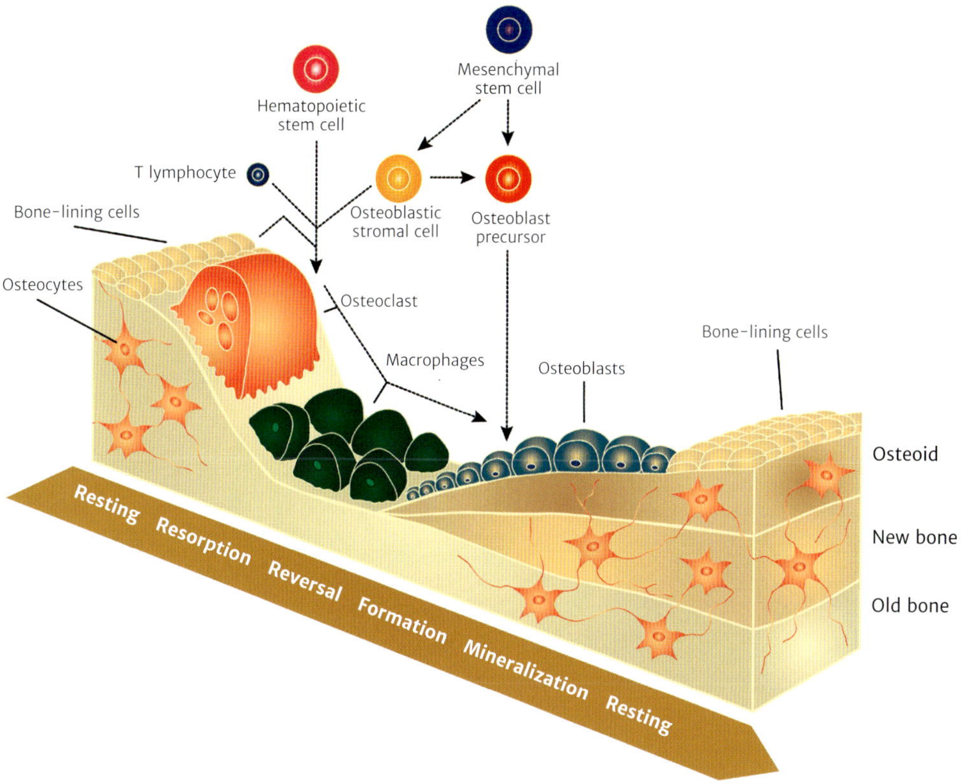

Fig 1-1 The basic multicellular unit. Cells are stimulated by a variety of signals in order to start bone remodeling. In the model suggested here, the hematopoietic precursors interact with cells of the osteoblast lineage and along with inflammatory cells (mainly T cells) trigger osteoclast activation. After osteoclast formation, a brief resorption phase followed by a reversal phase begins. In the reversal phase, the bone surface is covered by mononuclear cells. The formation phase lasts considerably longer and implicates the production of matrix by the osteoblasts. Subsequently, the osteoblasts become flat lining cells that are embedded in the bone as osteocytes or go through apoptosis. Through this mechanism, approximately 10% of the skeletal mass of an adult is remodeled each year.

CONTEMPORARY DATA ON BONE BIOLOGY

Recent studies report interesting findings on bone biology. Bone morphogenetic proteins (BMPs) are a group of growth factors, also known as *cytokines*, that act on undifferentiated mesenchymal cells to induce osteogenic cell lines and, with the mediation of growth and systemic factors, lead to cell proliferation, osteoblast and chondrocyte differentiation, and subsequently bone and cartilage production.[17] Osteoblasts derive from nonhematopoietic sites of bone marrow that contain groups of fibroblast cells, which have the potential to differentiate into bone-type cells known as *mesenchymal stem cells*, *skeletal stem cells derived from bone marrow*, *bone marrow stromal cells*, and *multipotent mesenchymal stromal cells*.[18]

Bone is constantly being created and replaced in a process known as *remodeling*. This ongoing turnover of bone is a process of resorption followed by replacement of bone that results in little change in shape. This is accomplished through osteoblasts and osteoclasts. Cells are stimulated by a variety of signals, and together they are referred to as a *remodeling unit*. Approximately 10% of the skeletal mass of an adult is remodeled each year.[19] The basic multicellular unit (BMU) is a wandering group of cells that dissolves a portion of the surface of the bone and then fills it by new bone deposition[20] (Fig 1-1).

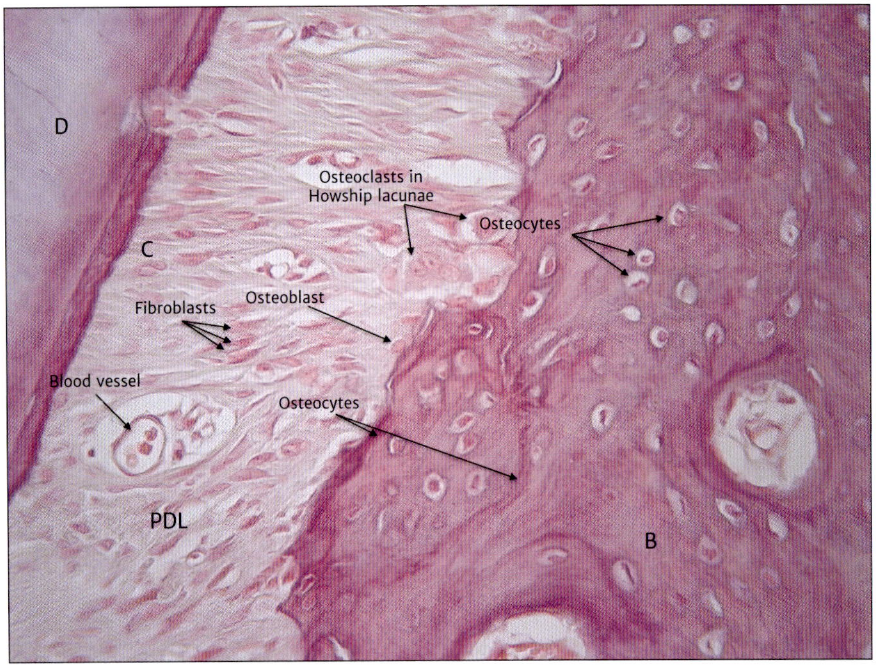

Fig 1-2 Histologic cross section through a PDL under mechanical load. D, dentin; C, cementum; B, alveolar bone. (Courtesy of Dr K. Tosios, National and Kapodistrian University of Athens, Greece.)

The osteoblasts are dominant elements of the basic skeletal anatomical structure of the BMU. The BMU consists of bone-forming cells (osteoblasts, osteocytes, and bone-lining cells), bone-resorbing cells (osteoclasts), and their precursor cells and associated cells (endothelial, nerve cells).

The bone is deposited by osteoblasts producing matrix (collagen) and two further noncollagenous proteins: osteocalcin and osteonectin. Activation of the bone resorption process is initiated by the preosteoclasts, which are induced and differentiated under the influence of cytokines and growth factors into active mature osteoclasts. Osteoclasts break down old bone and bring the end of the resorption process[21] (Fig 1-2).

The cycle of bone remodeling starts with the regulation of osteoblast growth and differentiation, which is accomplished through the osteogenic signaling pathways. A hierarchy of sequential expression of transcription factors results in the production of bone. Undifferentiated multipotent mesenchymal cells progressively differentiate into mature active osteoblasts expressing osteoblastic phenotypic genes and then transform into osteocytes within the bone matrix or undergo apoptosis.

The following three families of growth factors show a considerable impact on osteoblastic activity[22]:

- Transforming growth factor βs (TGF-βs)
- Insulinlike growth factors
- BMPs

Growth factors act primarily through specialized intracellular interactions and interactions with hormones or transcription factors. They also act in response to the activity of glucocorticoids, parathyroid hormone, prostaglandin, sex hormones, and more. The BMPs induce the production of bone in vivo by promoting the expression of Runx2 in mesenchymal osteoprogenitor and osteoblastic cells and the expression of Osterix in osteoblastic cells. The TGF-βs play a crucial role in osteoblast differentiation by promoting bone formation through the upregulation of Runx2 while simultaneously reducing the levels of transcription factors that lead the cells to adipogenesis.

Table 1-1 Clinical deformities resulting from transcription factor mutation

Transcription factor	*Deformity*
Parathyroid hormone–related protein (PTHrP)	Fatal chondroplasia
Sox5, Sox6, Sox9	Campomelic dysplasia
Fibroblast growth factor receptor 3 (FGFR3)	Achondroplasia
Runx2/3	Cleidocranial dysplasia

The absence or dysfunction of several transcription factors involved in bone metabolism leads to severe clinical deformities[23] (Table 1-1).

RUNX2 TRANSCRIPTION FACTOR

Runx2, also known as *core-binding factor subunit α1* (CBF-α1), is a protein that in humans is encoded by the *RUNX2* gene.[24] Runx2 is a key transcription factor associated with osteoblast differentiation. This protein is a member of the Runx family of transcription factors and has a Runt DNA-binding domain. It is essential for osteoblastic differentiation in both intramembranous and endochondral ossification and acts as a scaffold for nucleic acids and regulatory factors involved in skeletal gene expression. The protein can bind DNA either as a monomer or, with more affinity, as a subunit of a heterodimeric complex. Transcript variants of the gene that encode different protein isoforms result from the use of alternate promoters as well as alternate splicing. Differences in Runx2 are hypothesized to be the cause of the skeletal differences (eg, different skull shape and chest shape) between modern humans and early humans such as Neanderthals.[25]

Mutations in this gene in humans have been associated with the bone development disorder cleidocranial dysplasia[26,27] (Fig 1-3; see also Table 1-1). Other diseases associated with Runx2 include metaphyseal dysplasia with maxillary hypoplasia with or without brachydactyly. Among its related pathways are endochondral ossification and the fibroblast growth factor signaling pathway.[28] Deactivation of the gene in transgenic mice (*RUNX2-/-*) leads to complete lack of intramembranous and endochondral calcification due to lack of mature osteoblasts.[29] The mesenchymal cells in these animals retain the ability to further differentiate into adipocytes and chondrocytes.

PERIODONTAL LIGAMENT

The PDL is a dense fibrous connective tissue 0.15 to 0.40 mm thick that occupies the space between the root of the tooth and the alveolus.[16] The narrowest area of the PDL is at the midroot (fulcrum). The region at the alveolar crest is the widest area, followed by the apical region. The width is generally reduced in nonfunctional teeth and unerupted teeth, whereas it increases in teeth subjected to occlusal load within the physiologic limits and in primary teeth.

Histologically it presents a heterogenous, highly cellular structure comprised of a thick extracellular matrix with incorporated fibers arranged along the root[30] (Fig 1-4). The tooth does not come in direct contact with the alveolar bone but recedes into the alveolus, where it is retained by the PDL fibers.[31] These fibers act as shock absorbers and help the

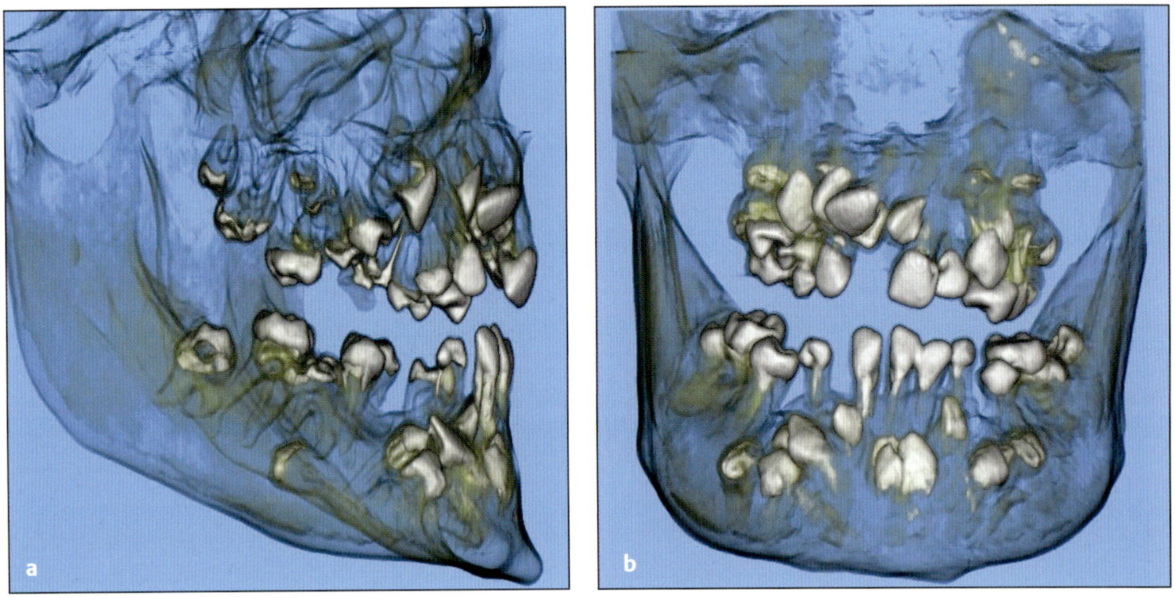

Fig 1-3 *(a and b)* Volume rendering image of cone beam computed tomography data of an adult male patient diagnosed with cleidocranial dysplasia.

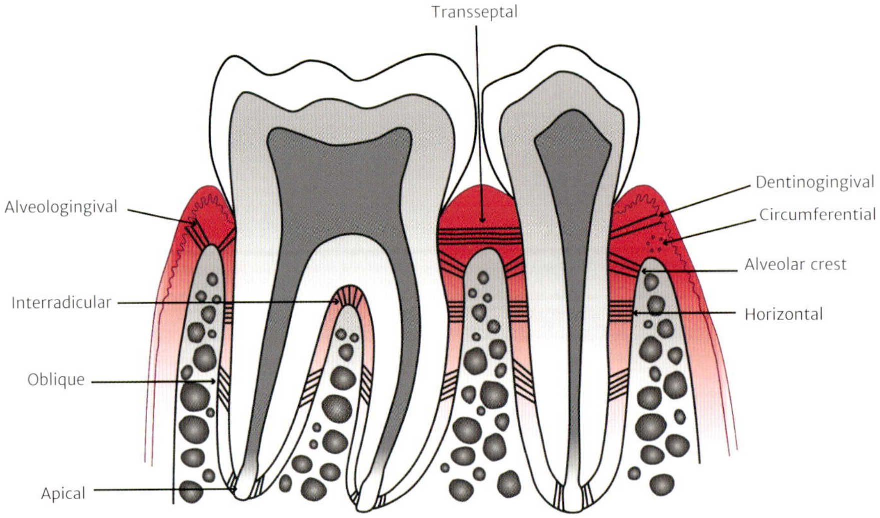

Fig 1-4 The PDL fibers are primarily composed of bundles of type I collagen fibrils. Their classification into several groups is made on the basis of their anatomical location. The principal fiber groups of the PDL are depicted here.

tooth withstand mastication forces and also respond to orthodontic load.

Like any other connective tissue, the PDL is composed of cells and extracellular components. The PDL cells comprise mainly fibroblasts (65%), which derive from undifferentiated mesenchymal cells with the ability to differentiate to preosteoblasts and cementoblasts; they produce collagen types I, II, and V. Additionally, they show similar characteristics to osteoblasts, like production of alkaline phosphatase (ALP) and osteocalcin, and response to 1,25 dihydroxyvitamin D3.

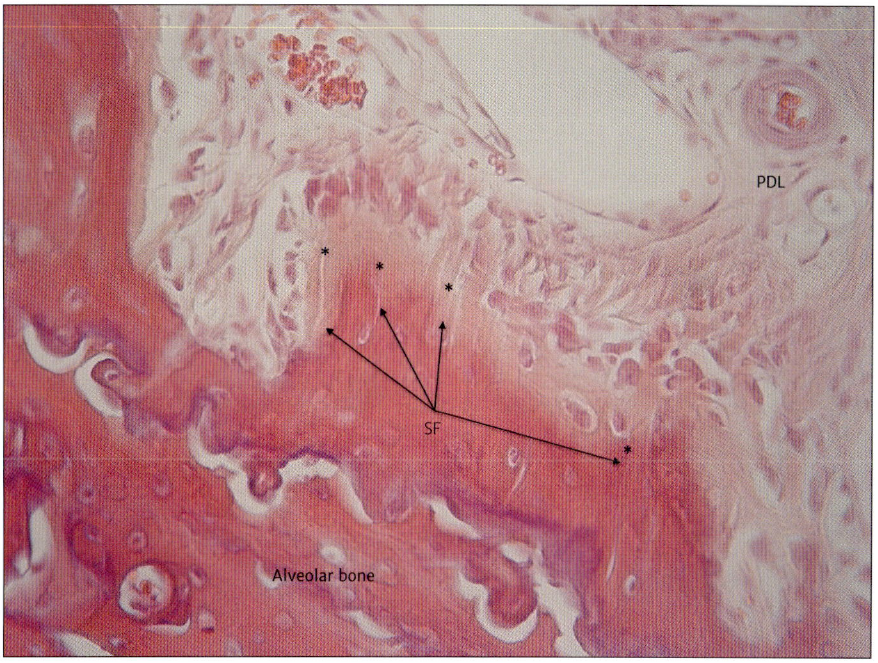

Fig 1-5 Higher magnification of the junction of the PDL with the bone. Sharpey fibers, which are the mineralized part of the thick fiber bundles (marked with an *), originate in the PDL and help anchor the tooth to the bone. In this histologic section, the mineralized bone (including the Sharpey fibers) appears magenta as compared to the purple color of the nonmineralized portions of the fibers. (Courtesy of Dr K. Tosios, National and Kapodistrian University of Athens, Greece.)

The possibility of differentiation of the PDL fibroblasts to preosteoblasts upon the application of orthodontic force plays an important role in bone remodeling.[32] Recent investigations report that the PDL is a major source of multipotent mesenchymal stromal cells that could be used for in vivo tissue regeneration such as cementum and the PDL itself.[33–37] The potential transplant of these cells, which may be detached with relative ease and then proliferate ex vivo, has significant therapeutic use on the restoration of periodontal breakdown in periodontic patients.

The rest of the PDL cells include cementoblasts, osteoblasts, osteoclasts, undifferentiated mesenchymal cells, and the epithelial rest cells of Malassez. The PDL cells play synthetic, resorptive, and defensive roles. They are also progenitor cells. The ground substance is a gel-like matrix that accounts for 65% of the PDL volume and comprises glycoproteins and proteoglycans. It contains 70% water and has a significant effect on the tooth's ability to sustain load. Cellular components like the collagen fibers are embedded within this matrix. The collagen fibers according to their location are divided into transseptal, alveolar crest, horizontal, interradicular, oblique, and apical. The PDL supports and protects the teeth within the alveolus with simultaneous sensory, nutritive, and formative functions.[31] The teeth are anchored into the alveolar process by Sharpey fibers, which are the terminal ends of the principal PDL fibers that insert into the cementum and the periosteum of the alveolar bone (Fig 1-5).

The integrity of the alveolar bone is also associated with the presence of the PDL. In extraction sites or in ankylosed teeth, the PDL is destroyed, and progressive absorption of the alveolar ridge occurs (Fig 1-6). The imbalance between osteoblasts and osteoclasts leads to degenerative bone activity. This is due to the reduction in the number of osteoblasts and the simultaneous increase in osteoclasts. In the continuous cycle of bone remodeling that takes place around the tooth alveolus, the PDL has a role of a continuous source of osteoblasts.

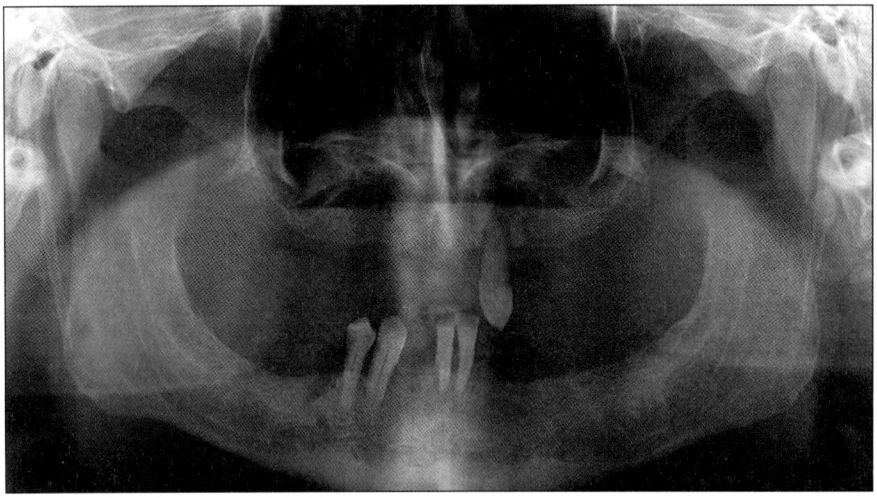

Fig 1-6 Panoramic radiograph of a 70-year-old man with excessive bone resorption in the edentulous areas.

Orthodontic Tooth Movement at the Molecular Level

Orthodontic movement is possible because of the bone remodeling of alveolar bone.[1–3] The forces exerted by the wires on the teeth are transduced to the PDL, provoking cellular and extracellular tissue response. The theories of orthodontic tooth movement have shifted from the tissue and cellular levels to the molecular level. Bone remodeling is regulated by a balanced system of two types of cells—osteoblasts and osteoclasts—and includes a complex network of interactions between cells and extracellular matrix in the presence of hormones, cytokines, growth factors, and mechanical loading. Bone resorption and formation constitutes a single process leading to skeleton renewal while maintaining its structural integrity.

Orthodontic and orthopedic theory and practice have a lot in common. The biology of bone remodeling is the subject of both disciplines and requires an understanding of the mechanism of mechanical stress and the response of different types of cells present in and around the bones. However, in tooth movement there is involvement of the PDL, which differs from the bone in composition and remodeling properties. Upon normal activities such as moving, the physical skeleton is under periodic stress. The alveolar bone is under similar periodic stress during mastication, which during orthodontic treatment becomes continuous, resulting in its bend, remodeling, and consequently tooth displacement. Regarding the body frame, the stress-remodeling mechanism is not fully clarified, yet it appears that stress application is a primary factor of bone regeneration.[38,39] The osteogenic response is attributed to the activation of the "calm" lining cells of the periosteum that do not require any kind of previous resorption phase.[40–42] On the other hand, upon orthodontic movement, alveolar bone undergoes significant resorption and apposition, the degree of which is directly correlated to the volume, direction, and duration of the force applied. Clinical orthodontists taking advantage of this well-organized system of bone remodeling exert biologic forces to achieve tooth movements.

The study of the molecular mechanisms involved with mechanical loading of the PDL through the signal transduction pathways is of outmost importance. Studies related to the investigation of the mechanical properties of the PDL can be classified according to the characteristics and condition of the tissue (age, presence of disease) and the type of the applied force (direction, magnitude, rate, duration). The duration and the rate of the mechanical load, however, constitute the major distinguishing factor

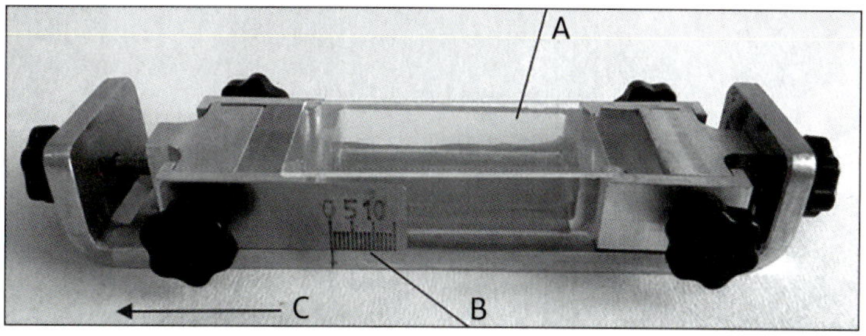

Fig 1-7 Static model of mechanical stimulation. A, flexible rectangular silicone dish; B, calibrated plate indicating the applied deformation of the silicone dish; C, direction of applied force.

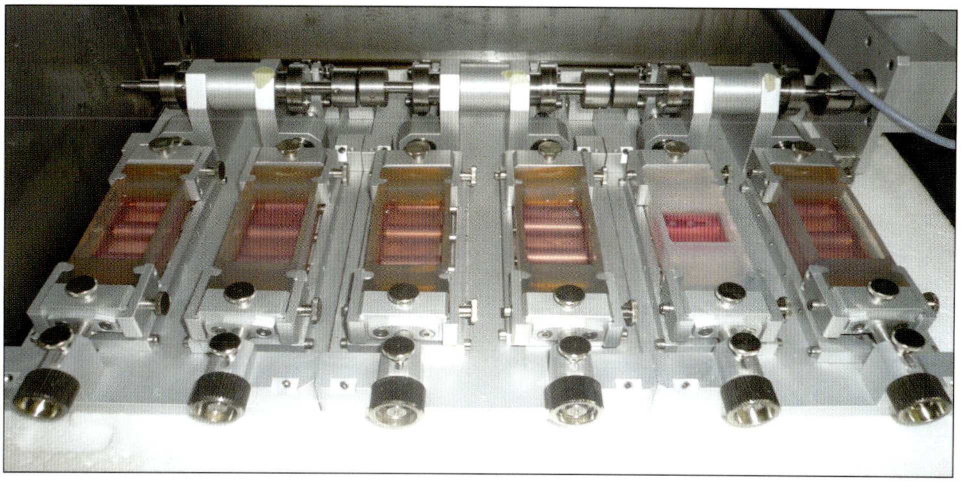

Fig 1-8 Dynamic model of mechanical stimulation. The purpose of the device is the mechanical stress transfer to cells attached to the bottom of flexible silicone culture dishes. The device is driven by an electric motor and generates cyclic mechanical stress to the specially designed silicone plates. Thereby, the mechanical stress is transferred to the adherent human PDL cells. The effect of the cyclic mechanical stimulation on cells is further studied by Western blot analysis and quantitative real-time polymerase chain reaction, allowing the researcher to analyze the effects of mechanical stress on the cells.

in the classification of research because of the direct clinical interest: Relatively short-duration forces are considered to take place in a sound system, whereas long-term forces represent parafunctional impact as in orthodontic movement.

The effect of mechanical stimulation of periodontal fibroblasts has been studied with different experimental models. These models are necessary to mimic clinical conditions either under mechanical stimulation (such as during orthodontic movement) or under the impact of physiologic functions (chewing, muscle and tongue movements, etc). In the static model, fibroblasts are cultured in collagen substrates that can be stressed or are placed on petri dishes with a flexible membrane on the bottom and then positioned on top of a convex surface (Fig 1-7). In the latter model, stretch application can vary, being more intense at the center of the dish than at the periphery.[4–6,24,43–45] Furthermore, a dynamic model is employed to investigate the fibroblasts' response to cyclic mechanical stress (Fig 1-8). A special device is driven by an electric motor generating cyclic stress. A piston on which flexible silicone culture dishes are attached moves at desired frequencies. The output stress is transferred to the adherent fibroblasts, the properties of which are subsequently investigated.[46]

Early research on the signaling pathways showed that an immediate result of the mechanical stress to the cells was the production of prostaglandins and secondary messengers cyclic adenosine monophosphate[47,48] and inositol phosphates.[49] Additionally, other authors reported changes in intracellular calcium (Ca^{2+}) after activation-stretching of ion channels.[50,51]

SIGNAL TRANSDUCTION PATHWAYS

Bone formation

In recent years, the investigation of bone-specific mechanical load-related signaling pathways has attracted researchers' attention. Cells inside the tissues as well as in cell cultures are connected with the extracellular matrix or their substrate by specialized sites of cell attachments called *focal adhesions*.[52] Through specialized proteins called *integrins*, the actin-associated cytoskeletal proteins are linked to the extracellular matrix.[53] Integrins are composed of structurally distinct subunits (α and β) that in combination form heterodimeric receptors with unique binding properties for collagen, vitronectin, laminin, etc. In the focal adhesions, integrins link the actin-associated proteins (talin, vanculin, α-actinin) and signaling molecules such as focal adhesion kinase and paxillin to the structural molecules of the extracellular matrix as well as to the outer surfaces of adjacent cells. Actions that cause disturbances in this link generate cellular responses associated with migration, proliferation, and differentiation.[54,55] Consequently, integrins function as cell adhesion molecules and intracellular signal receptors.

Mechanical load applied to cells causes perturbation of the cell-to-cell and to cell-to–extracellular matrix attachment, acting as a signal to initiate further biochemical responses of the cell. Integrins serve as mechanoreceptors, and the stress fibers are necessary for the transduction of applied forces.[56] Scientific data provide evidence that changes in cell signaling in response to mechanical stimulation are downstream of events mediated by integrins at focal adhesions.[57–59]

Once the cells recognize mechanical perturbation, they start transmitting the signal intracellularly through the cytoskeleton, mechanosensitive ion channels, phospholipids, and G-protein coupled receptors in the cell membrane. The low–molecular weight, small GTP-binding proteins of Ras-related GTPases, Rab and Rho, as well as the MAPK subtypes that are components of integrin-mediated signaling have been shown to be altered in mechanically stretched PDL fibroblasts.[5,6,60,61] Research data have shown that signaling through the MAPKs is essential for the early stages of osteoblastic differentiation. To this end, there is evidence that low levels of continuous mechanical stress of human PDL cells induce rapidly the principal constituents of the transcription factor AP-1, c-Jun and c-Fos.[24,61–63] Activation of the transcription factor AP-1 via extracellular signal-related kinase (ERK)/c-Jun N-terminal kinase (JNK) signaling enhances its DNA-binding activity on osteoblast-specific genes, hence moderating their expression rate. As a result, a shift toward differentiation occurs, marking the onset of the osteoblast phenotype.

Bone is formed by osteoblasts, which derive from undifferentiated mesenchymal cells. It has been postulated recently that the main regulator of osteoblastic differentiation is transcription factor CBF-α1 or Runx2, a member of the Runx transcription family. Runx2 binds to the osteoblast-specific cis-acting element 2 (OSE2), which is found in the promoter regions of all the major osteoblast-specific genes (ie, osteocalcin, osteopontin, bone sialoprotein, collagen type I, alkaline phosphatase, and collagenase-3) and controls their expression. Apart from this key role in osteoblast differentiation and skeletogenesis, Runx2 was also found to be a fundamental sensor of mechanical stimulation applied to PDL fibroblasts. Direct upregulation of the expression and binding activity of Runx2 occurs after low-level mechanical stretching of the PDL cells.[24,63] This effect is mediated by stretched-triggered induction of ERK-MAPK, as this kinase was found to physically interact and phosphorylate endogenous Runx2 in vivo, ultimately potentiating this transcription factor. These data provide a link between mechanical stress and osteoblast differentiation.

Recent research suggests that another transcription factor, polycystin-1 (PC1), may play an important role in skeletogenesis through regulation of the bone-specific transcription factor

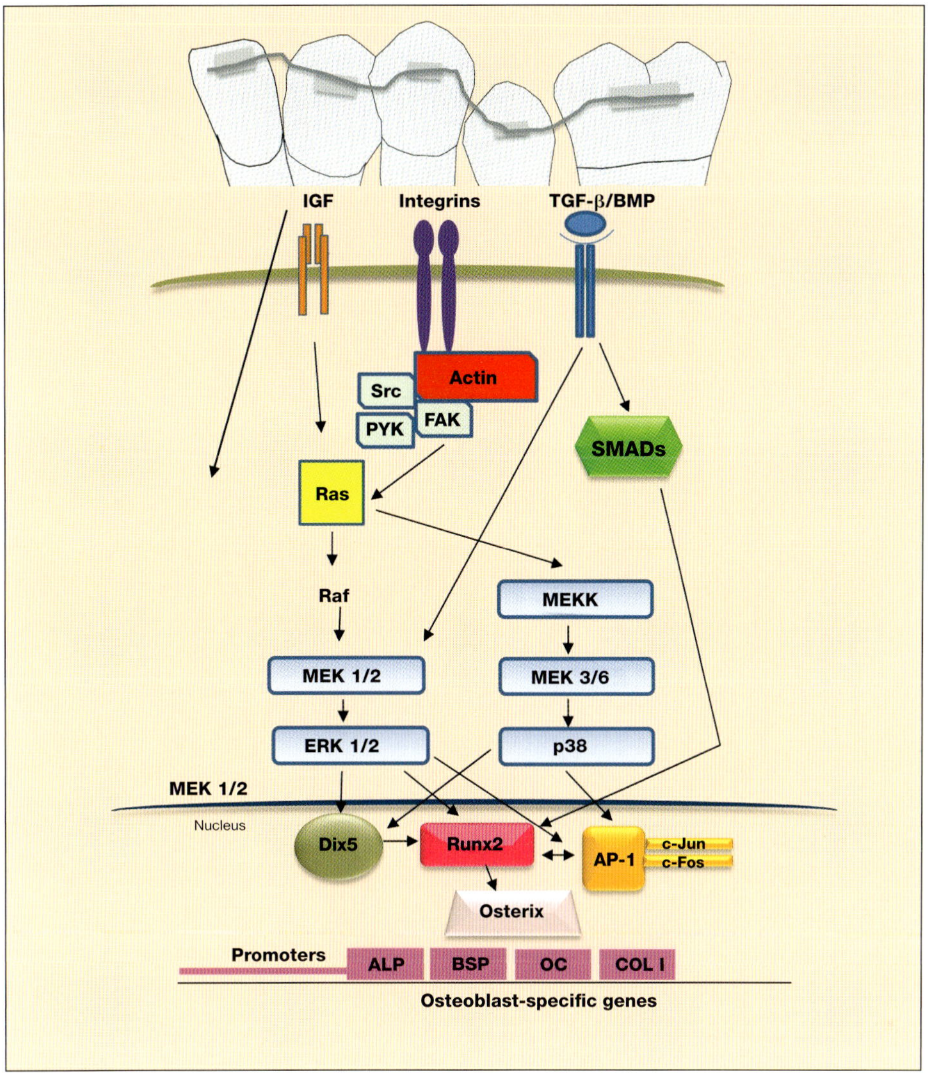

Fig 1-9 Signal transduction pathways under mechanical stress exerted by orthodontic archwires.

Runx2. Furthermore, PC1 colocalizes with the calcium channel polycystin-2 (PC2) in primary cilia of MC3T3-E1 osteoblasts.[64,65] These findings indicate that PC1 regulates osteoblast function through intracellular calcium-dependent control of Runx2 expression. The overall function of the primary cilium-polycystin complex may be to sense and transduce environmental clues into signals regulating osteoblast differentiation and bone development. It is recently postulated that PC1 acts as the chief mechanosensing molecule that modulates osteoblastic gene transcription and hence bone-cell differentiation through the calcineurin/NFAT (nuclear factor of activated T cells) signaling cascade.[66,67]

The signaling pathway cascade activated after the application of mechanical stimuli in the undifferentiated mesenchymal PDL cells with the potential to differentiate to osteoblasts can be summarized as follows[4–6,24,60–63] (Fig 1-9):

1. Disturbances in cell attachment through integrins at focal adhesions.

2. Transmission to the cytoplasm via small GTPases (Rho and Rab).
3. Triggering of the MAPK (ERK/JNK) cascades.
4. Activation of bone-specific and bone-related factors Runx2, c-Jun, and c-Fos.
5. Binding of these transcription factors to the OSE2 at the promoter regions of all major osteoblastic genes (*OC*, *OPN*, *ALP*, *BSP*, *COL I*, *MMP13*), thus controlling their expression.

Ultimately these biochemical cascades result in changes to gene expression and reprogramming of the cells toward an osteoblast phenotype.

Bone resorption

The cycle of this orthodontic force-induced bone remodeling is maintained through the existence of the PDL. It is apparent that the PDL with its pluripotent cell population acts as a provider of undifferentiated cells, which under mechanical stress differentiate into osteoblasts. Then mature osteoblasts induce osteoclast differentiation and bone resorption activities by the production of cytokines (ie, RANKL and OPG). Furthermore, nitric oxide (NO), prostaglandins, and tumor necrosis factor-α (TNF-α) also induce osteoclast differentiation and bone resorption.[68–70] In vitro studies suggest that while certain cytokines produced by osteocytes activate osteoclast precursors in the PDL at the resorption site, NO inhibits osteoclast activity at the opposite site in rats.[71]

Actual bone resorption is preceded by degradation of the nonmineralized layer of the osteoid by the osteoblasts. Only after this layer is degraded through matrix metalloproteinase (MMP) activity can the differentiated osteoclasts attach to the bone surface.[72,73] This attachment is regulated by increased levels of osteopontin found at the resorption site, produced by osteoblasts and osteocytes.[74,75]

Cytokines are proteins produced by connective tissue cells such as fibroblasts and osteoblasts. These low-molecular weight proteins (<25 kDa) regulate or modify the action of other cells in an autocrine or paracrine mode. The synthesis and action of cytokines is controlled by systemic hormones and mechanical stimuli. Among the first recognized bone-related cytokines are interleukin-1 (IL-1) and TNF, both stimulating bone resorption in vitro.[76–78] It is evident that the study of their role will provide important information regarding remodeling procedures and will in particular clarify the interaction between osteoclasts and osteoblasts.

RANKL, which is a member of the membrane-associated TNF ligand family, is considered a cytokine of great importance, playing a vital role in osteoclast formation and function.[79,80] Osteoclast precursors and osteoclasts express the receptor of RANKL (ie, RANK) on which RANKL binds, inducing osteoclast differentiation. Other transcription factors involved in resorption activities such as parathyroid hormone, IL-1, IL-6, and TNF-α act by upregulating RANKL expression by osteoblast precursors and osteoblasts.

With regard to bone remodeling, a pivotal role is similarly attributed to OPG.[81] Also produced by osteoblast precursors and osteoblasts, OPG inhibits osteoclast formation by competing with RANKL for the membrane receptor RANK. The equilibrium between RANKL and OPG, while maintained for purposes of tissue homeostasis, is disturbed when an orthodontic force is applied to the fibroblasts of the PDL (Fig 1-10). Of these two competing transcription factors, the prevailing one occasionally shifts the pendulum toward osteoclast or osteoblast activity.

In rats with experimental periodontitis, it was shown that the systematic administration of human OPG-Fc fusion protein inhibited the alveolar bone resorption by inhibiting the RANKL receptor.[82] This may suggest an innovative therapeutic approach for the treatment of periodontitis in the future. Still, the local administration of OPG-Fc mesial to the first molars of Sprague-Dawley rats led to inhibited osteoclastogenesis and tooth movement at the targeted dental sites.[83] Recent scientific data suggest that the biochemical interplay and its regulation by these two cytokines will enlighten the signaling pathway of orthodontic-induced bone remodeling and will allow for pharmacologic intervention in the future.[84,85]

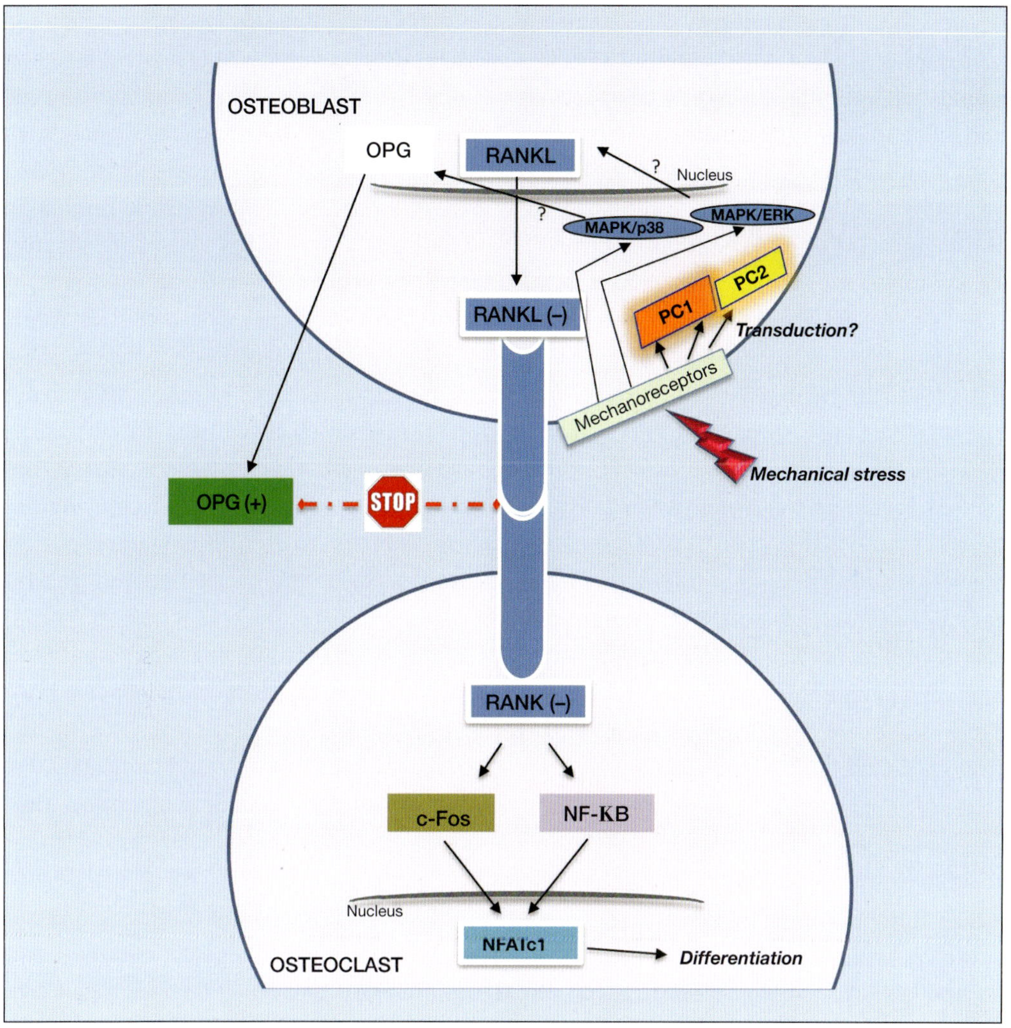

Fig 1-10 The equilibrium between RANKL and OPG plays a pivotal role in bone remodeling.

THE ROLE OF INFLAMMATION IN TOOTH MOVEMENT

The issue of inflammation as a cellular response of tissues involved in orthodontic tooth movement has recently attracted researchers' interest. Existing evidence showing that both cytokines (often referred to in the literature as *mediators of inflammation* or *proinflammatory cytokines*) and neurotransmitters such as calcitonin gene-related peptide and neuropeptide are involved in bone remodeling gave impetus to the theory that tooth movement is an inflammatory process.[86,87]

Research data show that mechanical stimulation in cells causes inflammatory responses similar to those caused by inflammation factors.[88] In particular, nuclear factor κB (NF-κB) is found in stimulated bone cells.[89] NF-κB is a transcription factor located in the cell nucleus that is present in all types of cells and involved in cellular responses to stimuli such as stress, cytokines, free radicals, ultraviolet radiation, and bacterial or viral antigens. In addition, NF-κB plays an important role in the immune response to infection and as a transcription factor in the regulation of genes involved in growth and development. Accordingly, erroneous regulation of

NF-κB is associated with carcinogenesis, inflammatory and autoimmune reactions, septic shock, viral infections, and inappropriate immune development. Inhibition of NF-κB has been recently suggested in the course of inflammation and cancer treatment.[90,91]

Because inflammation is a localized host response to microbial infection or to cell distraction, one could argue that when biologic forces are applied, tooth movement is an aseptic process. If any potential tissue damage occurs, it is due solely to the exaggerated magnitude of the exerted force. However, the description of the orthodontic movement as an inflammatory process gives the false impression that this may be a pathologic event. In attempting to describe in one sentence the response of tissues to orthodontic tooth movement, one could argue that it involves an exaggerated form of productive activity combined with foci of tissue repair, especially in loading and unloading zones adjacent to the PDL where bone and cementum remodel.

Effect of Age on Tissue Response and Remodeling

AGING AND BONE

All tissues, including bone, undergo changes in composition and morphology with age as well as changes at the cellular and molecular levels.[92] Cortical bone becomes more brittle, bone density and elasticity are reduced, and there is less resistance to mechanical loads.[93–96] Histomorphometric studies on human cadavers have suggested that with age, the region of osteoid covered by active osteoblasts is reduced along with the number of osteoclasts in bone-resorption surfaces. Also, it has been shown that age provokes degenerative morphologic changes in osteoblasts, which included size reduction and existence of pycnotic cores, while their ability to proliferate was diminished.[97] More recent studies corroborated that osteoblast and osteoclast differentiation decreases with age.[98,99]

The changes observed at the cellular and molecular levels in bone may be associated with decreased ability of cells to respond to mechanical stress, thus reducing the rate of bone remodeling.[100,101] At the molecular level, it is reported that aged osteoblasts show reduced levels of ALP expression, collagen type I, and osteocalcin.[102] Several studies on alveolar bone osteoblasts conclude that the levels of proliferation and differentiation are reduced with increasing age.[103] It was also reported that women present a reduced expression of the transcription factor Runx2 in bone marrow stromal cells, while RANKL levels are increased.[103] In an experimental study in bone cells of adult mice, the gene expression levels presented in the Wnt signaling pathway were decreased when compared with their young counterparts.[104]

Osteoporosis

Osteoporosis is the most common age-related metabolic bone disease with severe social and economic impact and high morbidity and mortality. It is characterized by a decrease in bone mass, disorder of the bone microarchitecture, decreased strength, and increased fracture rates (Fig 1-11). Bone loss occurs due to excessive osteoclast activity and decreased osteoblast activity. Recently it has been shown that osteoblastic activity may be promoted by mechanical stimulation of the osteoblasts. Osteoporosis is an established and well-defined disease that affects more than 75 million people in Europe, Japan, and the United States and causes more than 2.3 million fractures annually in Europe and the United States alone.[105]

Osteoporosis may be due to lower-than-normal peak bone mass and greater-than-normal bone loss. The deregulation of bone remodeling can be attributed to several factors like hormone levels, diet, physical status, and a number of diseases or treatments including alcoholism, anorexia, hyperthyroidism, surgical removal of the ovaries, and kidney diseases. Also, certain medications increase the rate of bone loss, including antiepileptic drugs, chemotherapy, and steroids.

Reduction of mechanical load on bone inhibits osteoblast-mediated bone formation and accelerates osteoclast-mediated bone resorption and leads

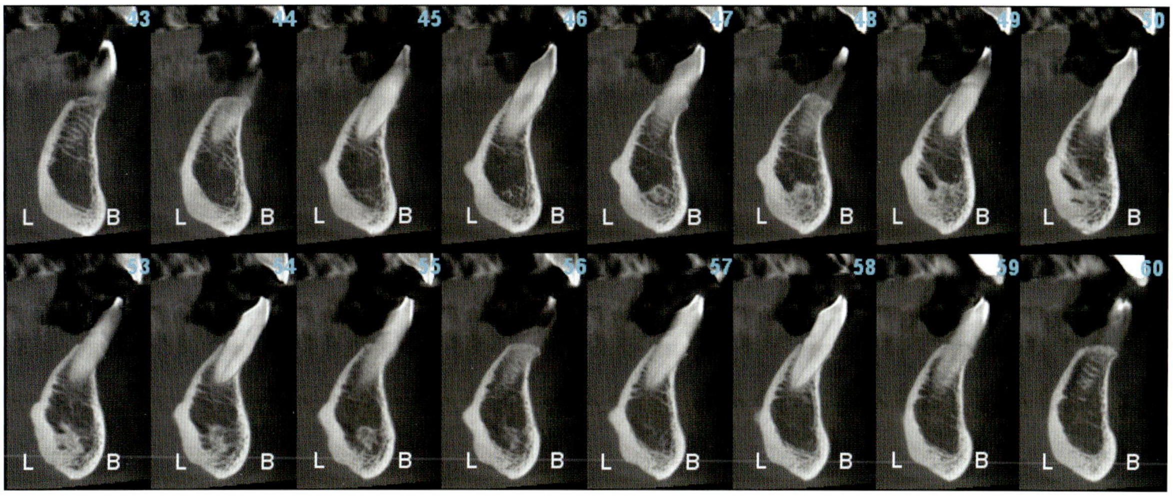

Fig 1-11 CBCT of the mandibular right lateral incisor area of a 55-year-old woman. The altered bone density and microarchitecture are due to osteoporosis. (Courtesy of Dr S. Petsaros.)

to what has been called *disuse osteoporosis*. Disuse osteoporosis is caused by lack of normal physical activity, immobilization, or long-term bed rest and affects an ever-increasing number of people around the world. Studies show that osteoblasts in disuse osteoporosis cannot proceed to normal-level bone synthesis after the osteoclast activity, thus resulting in significant bone loss.[106] Osteoporosis is clinically defined as a bone density 2.5 standard deviations below that of a young adult. This is typically measured by dual-energy x-ray absorptiometry at the hip.[105]

Recently it has been shown that women at menopause with osteoporosis present with statistically significantly higher periodontal index scores than those without osteoporosis. Gingival retraction was also significantly higher in women at menopause with osteoporosis than in the control group. There was thus reported a real correlation between bone mineral density (BMD) and periodontal index, while no correlation was shown between BMD and dental mobility.[107]

Altered mechanotransduction signaling pathways have been shown to result in deregulated bone remodeling in osteoporosis.[108] Reduced estrogen levels are known to play a pivotal role in age-related bone mass decrease and osteoporosis. Recent scientific data suggest the combined effects of estrogen receptor–related pathways and mechanotransduction signaling on bone loss. More specifically, an interaction between estrogen receptor and Wnt/β-catenin pathways has been observed. When mechanical load is applied, the estrogen receptor signaling in synchronization with mechanical signaling results in increased expression of prostaglandin E2 (PGE2), which in turn leads to decreased sclerostin production. As sclerostin is an endogenous Wnt signaling antagonist and a bone-synthesis inhibitor, the above signals result in increased bone formation.[109] When this signaling pathway is interrupted, as in age-related osteoporosis, reduced bone matrix synthesis is observed. Because of its properties, a decrease in sclerostin in combination with exercise has been proposed as a therapeutic strategy against bone loss at greater ages.[110]

The ERK1/2 mechanotransduction signaling was also found to be interrupted in research on the differentiating mesenchymal stem cells of aged animals. Decreased responsiveness to short and long periods of mechanical stimulation through ERK1/2 signaling as well as long periods of mechanical loading to NO pathways was observed. Furthermore, a

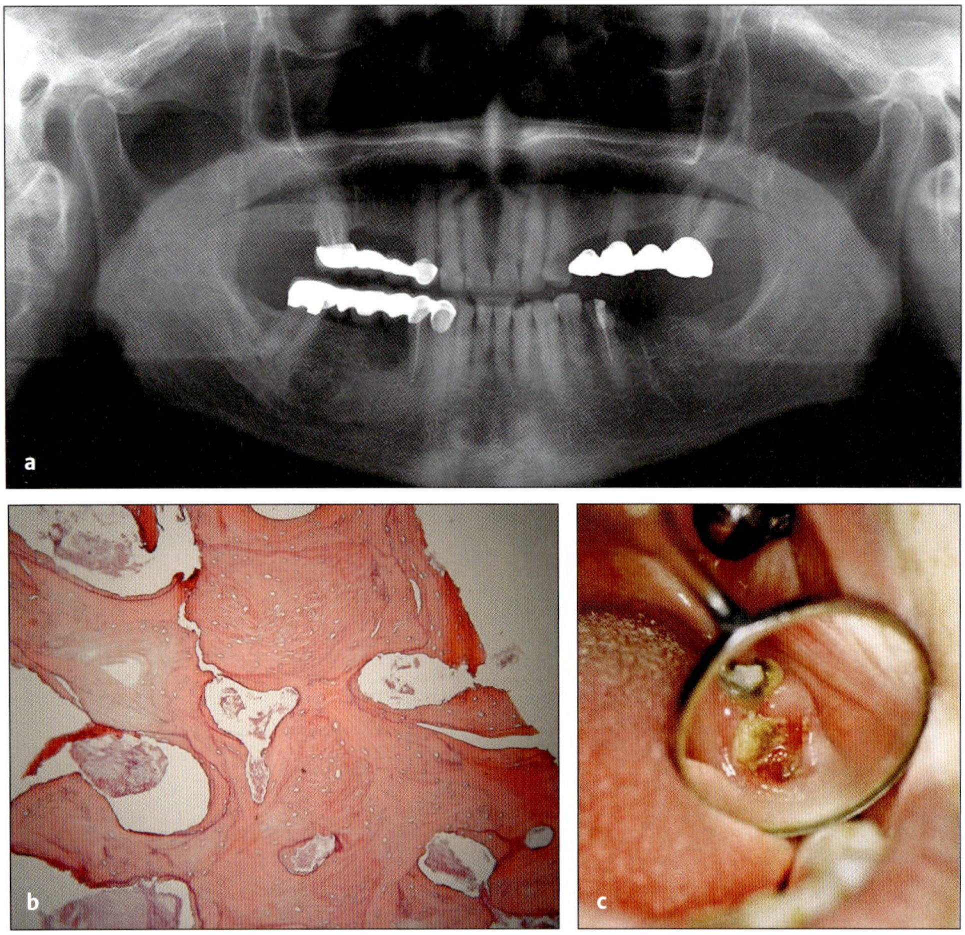

Fig 1-12 *(a to c)* Radiographic, histologic, and clinical images of a 65-year-old woman with mandibular osteonecrosis following extraction of the mandibular left first molar. The patient was undergoing treatment for osteoporosis with bisphosphonates. (Courtesy of Dr K. Tosios, National and Kapodistrian University of Athens, Greece.)

greater increase was observed in PGE2 signaling levels in mesenchymal stem cells from aged animals, most likely as a compensation for decreased ERK1/2 and NO signaling.[111]

Bisphosphonates are a synthetic class of pyrophosphate analogs that inhibit bone resorption by reducing osteoclast activity. They are commonly used as a medication for the prevention and therapy of osteoporosis and osteopenia but are also used to treat tumor diseases. Bisphosphonates have unique pharmacologic characteristics unlike those of any other drug group, and their half-life can be more than 10 years.[112] Because these drugs interfere with bone metabolism, they have a considerable impact on orthodontic treatment. The pharmacologic effects of these drugs, which can change bone physiology and interfere with osteoclastic resorption, could probably decrease the rate of orthodontic tooth movement and subsequently hinder treatment. Orthodontic treatment should begin after obtaining the patient's informed consent.[112] One important side effect is bisphosphonate-associated osteonecrosis of the jaws[113–118] (Fig 1-12). The severity of osteonecrosis is dependent on the type of bisphosphonate used as well as the dose, duration, and route of administration (intravenous or oral).

Recent studies report interesting results concerning the possible use of these drugs in the course of orthodontic treatment. Bisphosphonates have succeeded in reducing the amount of root resorption in experimental animal trials.[119,120] In clinical orthodontics, this could prove beneficial for patients. Additionally, possible local administration of bisphosphonates in the future could reinforce the anchorage sites, thus ensuring that orthodontic movement occurs in the desired direction. Enhanced retention has been obtained experimentally when bisphosphonates have been combined with mechanical retention after expansion treatment.[116,119,121,122] However, these results from various animal studies still need to be verified in human clinical trials.

MECHANOSTIMULATION

Apart from pharmaceutical treatments with antiresorptive agents, which has been the norm to achieve increased bone density, mechanical stimulation has been given considerable attention.[123] The trend to develop nonpharmaceutical treatments aims at the avoidance of the serious side effects these drugs may present. Numerous studies have demonstrated the role of mechanostimulation in acquiring a higher bone mass quantity, thus contributing to the restoration of bone integrity. It has been shown that low-intensity mechanical signals result in bone remodeling activation and increased bone mass and that following a period of time bestow regenerative abilities to bone tissues.[124] Also, mechanical stimulation of PDL cells and osteoblast cell lines leads to enhanced OPG expression and therefore RANK/RANKL signaling interruption, resulting in decreased osteoclastogenesis.[125,126] Furthermore, upon stimulation cyclo-oxygenase (COX) enzymes and prostaglandins both reduce RANKL production, thus blocking bone resorption in vitro.[127,128] Mechanical stimuli have also been proven to activate the Wnt/β-catenin pathway on osteoblasts, enhancing osteoblast differentiation and bone synthesis.[129] Studies on 3D models report that osteoblasts receiving dynamic application of mechanical pressure expressed elevated ALP, Runx2, and osteocalcin levels.[130,131] In cases of bone-implant integration, mechanostimulation moderated osteoblast differentiation through upregulation of Runx2 and osteocalcin levels.[132] Mechanostimulation already has a variety of applications in dentistry, orthopedics, craniofacial development, and treatment of bone fractures.

PERIODONTAL LIGAMENT

The PDL undergoes various changes with age, namely related to the composition of the matrix, cell populations, and metabolic activities, that are likely to alter the response to mechanical stimuli and especially orthodontic forces. These changes include decreased vascularity, cellularity, and thickness.

Experimental studies in animals showed a decrease in extracellular matrix, collagen, and the protein synthesis rate with age.[133–135] Aged human PDL cells present decreased proliferation along with additional disorganization, findings confirmed also under the application of orthodontic forces[136–138] (Fig 1-13).

Numerous studies have recently been conducted at a molecular level in order to clarify why aged PDL shows catabolic activity and reduced regenerative capacity, thus leading to a decrease in the bone-remodeling rate. Adult PDL fibroblasts show increased production of inflammatory mediators, exhibiting increased expression of COX2, IL-1β, and IL-6 both at rest and upon cyclic tension force.[139] Similar results with additional increase in PGE2 levels were reported under the application of mechanical load both in adult and senescent PDL cells.[140,141] Still, pronounced inflammatory responses leading to degradation of the matrix are shown by the increased activity of the plasminogen activator in senescent human PDL fibroblasts under load.[142]

Aged PDL cells show an inflammatory phenotype with predominantly catabolic activities as suggested by the elevated mRNA levels of IL-1, IL-6 cytokines, and osteonectin and the absence of c-Fos expression, which lead to a reduction in the proliferation rate. Additionally, an increase in OPG levels and reduced levels of RANKL indicate a decompensation of the catabolic activities.[143–145]

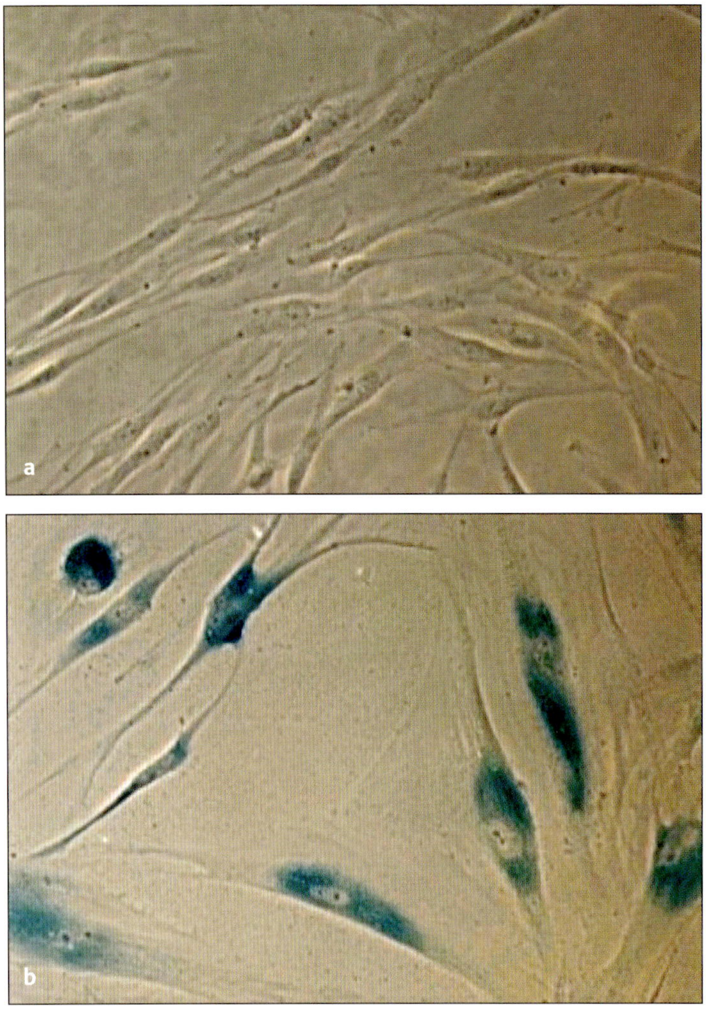

Fig 1-13 Young *(a)* and aged *(b)* human PDL fibroblasts stained with Sa-β-Gal staining, a classical marker of cellular senescence. Aged fibroblasts presented a typical flattened appearance. Photographs were taken under a phase-contrast microscope.

Increased catabolic activity manifestations in aged PDL include the elevation of MMP-2 and MMP-8, which degrade the extracellular matrix and also decrease the synthesis of collagen types I and III and the formation of mineral-like nodules.[146] In senescent PDL cells, increased expression of cathepsin and diminished activity of ALP, which is a basic osteoid index, is also observed.[147,148] Age-induced changes are also manifested by reduced levels of mRNA of integrin-α6 and integrin-β4, which indicate the changes in signaling pathways and altered interactions of PDL cells with their environment.[149]

Recent research studies investigated the effect of cellular senescence on human PDL fibroblasts that became senescent either after replicative exhaustion or after exposure to ionizing radiation. The results showed a decrease in collagen type I and an increase in MMP-2 expression, while Runx2 was downregulated in a p53-dependent manner. ALP gene expression and activity were also considerably decreased. Interestingly, cells from both types of senescence expressed similar characteristics, implying analogous functions in vivo. Replicative and ionizing senescent human PDL fibroblasts express a catabolic phenotype displaying a significantly decreased ability toward an osteoblastic differentiation, thus affecting tissue development and integrity.[13,14]

Conclusion

Age is considered an important biologic parameter and, according to clinical beliefs, plays a significant role in the rate of orthodontic tooth movement. However, the biologic truth behind this underlying conviction is the subject of recent investigations. The application of orthodontic force generates sequences of biochemical cascades leading to a series of cellular and molecular changes. The signal transduction of orthodontic force results in the activation of bone-specific genes that ultimately induce bone remodeling. Different age groups respond in various ways to mechanical stimuli. Additionally, osteoporosis of the jaws and its pharmaceutical treatment affects orthodontic treatment.

Decoding of the human genome along with new data from molecular biology will impact orthodontics in the future. Currently, an extensive series of pioneering research on bone biology is underway. Orthodontists have a paramount role in these investigations.

More than a century after the first publications on tooth movement,[150] an information superhighway has empowered the scientific community by elucidating bone-remodeling mechanisms at a molecular level. Nevertheless, a plethora of issues still remain unresolved and require further investigation. The ultimate goal is clinical manipulation of the transcription factors involved through pharmaceutical intervention. The scientific knowledge that constantly arises from multilevel research in orthodontics argues that the biology of the patient is an integral part of orthodontic diagnosis and treatment planning. Therefore, the implemented biomechanics and specific procedures should be ultimately planned in light of the biologic profile of each patient.

References

1. Verna C, Dalstra M, Melsen B. The rate and the type of orthodontic tooth movement is influenced by bone turnover in a rat model. Eur J Orthod 2000;22:343–352.
2. Reitan K. The initial tissue reaction incident to orthodontic tooth movement as related to the influence of function; an experimental histologic study on animal and human material. Acta Odontol Scand Suppl 1951;6:1–240.
3. Reitan K. Tissue rearrangement during retention of orthodontically rotated teeth. Angle Orthod 1959;29:105–113.
4. Basdra EK, Kohl A, Komposch G. Mechanical stretching of periodontal ligament fibroblasts—A study on cytoskeletal involvement. J Orofac Orthop 1996;57:24–30.
5. Basdra EK, Papavassiliou AG, Huber LA. Rab and rho GTPases are involved in specific response of periodontal ligament fibroblasts to mechanical stretching. Biochim Biophys Acta 1995;1268:209–213.
6. Basdra EK, Komposch G, Huber LA, Papavassiliou AG. Mechanically-stretched human periodontal ligament fibroblasts: Identifying components of the mechanotransduction cascade. In: Davidovitch Z, Norton LA (eds). Biological Mechanisms of Tooth Movement and Craniofacial Adaptation [Proceedings of the International Conference, 19–22 Oct 1995, Danvers, MA]. Boston: Harvard Society for the Advancement of Orthodontics, 1996:41–49.
7. Shimpo S, Horiguchi Y, Nakamura Y, et al. Compensatory bone formation in young and old rats during tooth movement. Eur J Orthod 2003;25:1–7.
8. Komatsu K, Kanazashi M, Shimada A, Shibata T, Viidik A, Chiba M. Effects of age on the stress-strain and stress-relaxation properties of the rat molar periodontal ligament. Arch Oral Biol 2004;49:817–824.
9. Komatsu K, Shibata T, Shimada A, Viidik A, Chiba M. Age-related and regional differences in the stress-strain and stress-relaxation behaviours of the rat incisor periodontal ligament. J Biomech 2004;37:1097–1106.
10. Ren Y, Kuijpers-Jagtman AM, Maltha JC. Immunohistochemical evaluation of osteoclast recruitment during experimental tooth movement in young and adult rats. Arch Oral Biol 2005;50:1032–1039.
11. Ren Y, Maltha JC, van't Hof MA, Kuijpers-Jagtman AM. Optimum force magnitude for orthodontic tooth movement: A mathematic model. Am J Orthod Dentofacial Orthop 2004;125:71–77.
12. Nakamoto N, Nagasaka H, Daimaruya T, Takahashi I, Sugawara J, Mitani H. Experimental tooth movement through mature and immature bone regenerates after distraction osteogenesis in dogs. Am J Orthod Dentofacial Orthop 2002;121:385–395.
13. Konstantonis D, Papadopoulou A, Makou M, Eliades T, Basdra E, Kletsas D. The role of cellular senescence on the cyclic stretching-mediated activation of MAPK and ALP expression and activity in human periodontal ligament fibroblasts. Exp Gerontol 2014;57:175–180.
14. Konstantonis D, Papadopoulou A, Makou M, Eliades T, Basdra EK, Kletsas D. Senescent human periodontal ligament fibroblasts after replicative exhaustion or ionizing radiation have a decreased capacity towards osteoblastic differentiation. Biogerontology 2013;14:741–751.
15. Hopewell-Smith A. The Histology and Patho-Histology of the Teeth and Associated Parts. London: Dental Manufacturing, 1903.
16. Lang NP, Lindhe J (eds). Clinical Periodontology and Implant Dentistry, ed 6. Ames, IA: Wiley, 2015.

17. Li X, Yi W, Jin A, Duan Y, Min S. Effects of sequentially released BMP-2 and BMP-7 from PELA microcapsule-based scaffolds on the bone regeneration. Am J Transl Res 2015;7:1417–1428.
18. Jiang Y, Jahagirdar BN, Reinhardt RL, et al. Pluripotency of mesenchymal stem cells derived from adult marrow. Nature 2002;418:41–49.
19. Manolagas SC. Birth and death of bone cells: Basic regulatory mechanisms and implications for the pathogenesis and treatment of osteoporosis. Endocr Rev 2000;21:115–137.
20. Krishnan V, Davidovitch Z (eds). Biological Mechanisms of Tooth Movement. Oxford: Blackwell, 2009.
21. Raggatt LJ, Partridge NC. Cellular and molecular mechanisms of bone remodeling. J Biol Chem 2010;285: 25103–25108.
22. Simpson AH, Mills L, Noble B. The role of growth factors and related agents in accelerating fracture healing. J Bone Joint Surg Br 2006;88:701–705.
23. Krakow D, Rimoin DL. The skeletal dysplasias. Genet Med 2010;12:327–341.
24. Ziros PG, Basdra EK, Papavassiliou AG. Runx2: Of bone and stretch. Int J Biochem Cell Biol 2008;40:1659–1663.
25. Green RE, Krause J, Briggs AW, et al. A draft sequence of the Neandertal genome. Science 2010;328:710–722.
26. Tanaka JL, Ono E, Filho EM, Castilho JC, Moraes LC, Moraes ME. Cleidocranial dysplasia: Importance of radiographic images in diagnosis of the condition. J Oral Sci 2006;48:161–166.
27. Hefti F. Pediatric Orthopedics in Practice, ed 2. Hinchliffe R (trans). Berlin: Springer, 2015.
28. Ornitz DM, Marie PJ. FGF signaling pathways in endochondral and intramembranous bone development and human genetic disease. Genes Dev 2002;16:1446–1465.
29. Otto F, Thornell AP, Crompton T, et al. Cbfa1, a candidate gene for cleidocranial dysplasia syndrome, is essential for osteoblast differentiation and bone development. Cell 1997;89:765–771.
30. Ten Cate AR. Oral Histology: Development, Structure, and Function, ed 4. St. Louis: Mosby, 1994.
31. Bath-Balogh M, Fehrenbach MJ, Thomas P. Illustrated Dental Embryology, Histology, and Anatomy, ed 2. St. Louis: Elsevier, 2006.
32. Basdra EK, Komposch G. Osteoblast-like properties of human periodontal ligament cells: An in vitro analysis. Eur J Orthod 1997;19:615–621.
33. Fujii S, Maeda H, Wada N, Tomokiyo A, Saito M, Akamine A. Investigating a clonal human periodontal ligament progenitor/stem cell line in vitro and in vivo. J Cell Physiol 2008;215:743–749.
34. Gay IC, Chen S, MacDougall M. Isolation and characterization of multipotent human periodontal ligament stem cells. Orthod Craniofac Res 2007;10:149–160.
35. Seo BM, Miura M, Gronthos S, et al. Investigation of multipotent postnatal stem cells from human periodontal ligament. Lancet 2004;364:149–155.
36. Seo BM, Miura M, Sonoyama W, Coppe C, Stanyon R, Shi S. Recovery of stem cells from cryopreserved periodontal ligament. J Dent Res 2005;84:907–912.
37. Tomokiyo A, Maeda H, Fujii S, Wada N, Shima K, Akamine A. Development of a multipotent clonal human periodontal ligament cell line. Differentiation 2008;76:337–347.
38. Hert J, Lisková M, Landa J. Reaction of bone to mechanical stimuli. 1. Continuous and intermittent loading of tibia in rabbit. Folia Morphol (Praha) 1971;19:290–300.
39. Lanyon LE, Baggott DG. Mechanical function as an influence on the structure and form of bone. J Bone Joint Surg Br 1976;58-B:436–443.
40. Pead MJ, Skerry TM, Lanyon LE. Direct transformation from quiescence to bone formation in the adult periosteum following a single brief period of bone loading. J Bone Miner Res 1988;3:647–656.
41. Chambers TJ, Evans M, Gardner TN, Turner-Smith A, Chow JW. Induction of bone formation in rat tail vertebrae by mechanical loading. Bone Miner 1993;20:167–178.
42. Chow JW, Wilson AJ, Chambers TJ, Fox SW. Mechanical loading stimulates bone formation by reactivation of bone lining cells in 13-week-old rats. J Bone Miner Res 1998;13:1760–1767.
43. Hasegawa S, Sato S, Saito S, Suzuki Y, Brunette DM. Mechanical stretching increases the number of cultured bone cells synthesizing DNA and alters their pattern of protein synthesis. Calcif Tissue Int 1985;37:431–436.
44. Ngan PW, Crock B, Varghese J, Lanese R, Shanfeld J, Davidovitch Z. Immunohistochemical assessment of the effect of chemical and mechanical stimuli on cAMP and prostaglandin E levels in human gingival fibroblasts in vitro. Arch Oral Biol 1988;33:163–174.
45. Saito M, Saito S, Ngan PW, Shanfeld J, Davidovitch Z. Interleukin 1 beta and prostaglandin E are involved in the response of periodontal cells to mechanical stress in vivo and in vitro. Am J Orthod Dentofacial Orthop 1991;99:226–240.
46. Neidlinger-Wilke C, Wilke HJ, Claes L. Cyclic stretching of human osteoblasts affects proliferation and metabolism: A new experimental method and its application. J Orthop Res 1994;12:70–78.
47. Harell A, Dekel S, Binderman I. Biochemical effect of mechanical stress on cultured bone cells. Calcif Tissue Res 1977;22(suppl):202–207.
48. Yeh CK, Rodan GA. Tensile forces enhance prostaglandin E synthesis in osteoblastic cells grown on collagen ribbons. Calcif Tissue Int 1984;36(suppl 1):S67–S71.
49. Sandy JR, Harris M. Prostaglandins and tooth movement. Eur J Orthod 1984;6:175–182.
50. Davidson RM, Tatakis DW, Auerbach AL. Multiple forms of mechanosensitive ion channels in osteoblast-like cells. Pflugers Arch 1990;416:646–651.
51. McDonald F, Somasundaram B, McCann TJ, Mason WT, Meikle MC. Calcium waves in fluid flow stimulated osteoblasts are G protein mediated. Arch Biochem Biophys 1996;326:31–38.
52. Sastry SK, Burridge K. Focal adhesions: A nexus for intracellular signaling and cytoskeletal dynamics. Exp Cell Res 2000;261:25–36.
53. Ingber D. Integrins as mechanochemical transducers. Curr Opin Cell Biol 1991;3:841–848.
54. Wang N, Butler JP, Ingber DE. Mechanotransduction across the cell surface and through the cytoskeleton. Science 1993;260:1124–1127.
55. Clark EA, Brugge JS. Integrins and signal transduction pathways: The road taken. Science 1995;268:233–239.
56. Shyy JY, Chien S. Role of integrins in cellular responses to mechanical stress and adhesion. Curr Opin Cell Biol 1997;9:707–713.

57. Meyer CJ, Alenghat FJ, Rim P, Fong JH, Fabry B, Ingber DE. Mechanical control of cyclic AMP signalling and gene transcription through integrins. Nat Cell Biol 2000;2:666–668.
58. Wilson E, Sudhir K, Ives HE. Mechanical strain of rat vascular smooth muscle cells is sensed by specific extracellular matrix/integrin interactions. J Clin Invest 1995;96:2364–2372.
59. Calvalho RS, Bumann A, Schwarzer C, Scott E, Yen EH. A molecular mechanism of integrin regulation from bone cells stimulated by orthodontic forces. Eur J Orthod 1996;18:227–235.
60. Kletsas D, Basdra EK, Papavassiliou AG. Mechanical stress induces DNA synthesis in PDL fibroblasts by a mechanism unrelated to autocrine growth factor action. FEBS Lett 1998;430:358–362.
61. Peverali FA, Basdra EK, Papavassiliou AG. Stretch-mediated activation of selective MAPK subtypes and potentiation of AP-1 binding in human osteoblastic cells. Mol Med 2001;7:68–78.
62. Kletsas D, Basdra EK, Papavassiliou AG. Effect of protein kinase inhibitors on the stretch-elicited c-Fos and c-Jun up-regulation in human PDL osteoblast-like cells. J Cell Physiol 2002;190:313–321.
63. Ziros PG, Gil AP, Georgakopoulos T, et al. The bone-specific transcriptional regulator Cbfa1 is a target of mechanical signals in osteoblastic cells. J Biol Chem 2002;277:23934–23941.
64. Xiao Z, Zhang S, Magenheimer BS, Luo J, Quarles LD. Polycystin-1 regulates skeletogenesis through stimulation of the osteoblast-specific transcription factor RUNX2-II. J Biol Chem 2008;283:12624–12634.
65. Xiao Z, Zhang S, Mahlios J, et al. Cilia-like structures and polycystin-1 in osteoblasts/osteocytes and associated abnormalities in skeletogenesis and Runx2 expression. J Biol Chem 2006;281:30884–30895.
66. Dalagiorgou G, Piperi C, Georgopoulou U, Adamopoulos C, Basdra EK, Papavassiliou AG. Mechanical stimulation of polycystin-1 induces human osteoblastic gene expression via potentiation of the calcineurin/NFAT signaling axis. Cell Mol Life Sci 2013;70:167–180.
67. Dalagiorgou G, Basdra EK, Papavassiliou AG. Polycystin-1: Function as a mechanosensor. Int J Biochem Cell Biol 2010;42:1610–1613.
68. Ajubi NE, Klein-Nulend J, Nijweide PJ, Vrijheid-Lammers T, Alblas MJ, Burger EH. Pulsating fluid flow increases prostaglandin production by cultured chicken osteocytes—A cytoskeleton-dependent process. Biochem Biophys Res Commun 1996;225:62–68.
69. Klein-Nulend J, Roelofsen J, Sterck JG, Semeins CM, Burger EH. Mechanical loading stimulates the release of transforming growth factor-β activity by cultured mouse calvariae and periosteal cells. J Cell Physiol 1995;163:115–119.
70. Kurata K, Heino TJ, Higaki H, Väänänen HK. Bone marrow cell differentiation induced by mechanically damaged osteocytes in 3D gel-embedded culture. J Bone Miner Res 2006;21:616–625.
71. Yoo SK, Warita H, Soma K. Duration of orthodontic force affecting initial response of nitric oxide synthase in rat periodontal ligaments. J Med Dent Sci 2004;51:83–88.
72. Birkedal-Hansen H. Role of matrix metalloproteinases in human periodontal diseases. J Periodontol 1993;64(5 suppl):474–484.
73. Birkedal-Hansen H, Moore WG, Bodden MK, et al. Matrix metalloproteinases: A review. Crit Rev Oral Biol Med 1993;4:197–250.
74. Gay CV, Weber JA. Regulation of differentiated osteoclasts. Crit Rev Eukaryot Gene Expr 2000;10:213–230.
75. Terai K, Takano-Yamamoto T, Ohba Y, et al. Role of osteopontin in bone remodeling caused by mechanical stress. J Bone Miner Res 1999;14:839–849.
76. Gowen M, Meikle MC, Reynolds JJ. Stimulation of bone resorption in vitro by a non-prostanoid factor released by human monocytes in culture. Biochim Biophys Acta 1983;762:471–474.
77. Heath JK, Saklatvala J, Meikle MC, Atkinson SJ, Reynolds JJ. Pig interleukin 1 (catabolin) is a potent stimulator of bone resorption in vitro. Calcif Tissue Int 1985;37:95–97.
78. Bertolini DR, Nedwin GE, Bringman TS, Smith DD, Mundy GR. Stimulation of bone resorption and inhibition of bone formation in vitro by human tumour necrosis factors. Nature 1986;319:516–518.
79. Lacey DL, Timms E, Tan HL, et al. Osteoprotegerin ligand is a cytokine that regulates osteoclast differentiation and activation. Cell 1998;93:165–176.
80. Yasuda H, Shima N, Nakagawa N, et al. Osteoclast differentiation factor is a ligand for osteoprotegerin/osteoclastogenesis-inhibitory factor and is identical to TRANCE/RANKL. Proc Natl Acad Sci U S A 1998;95:3597–3602.
81. Simonet WS, Lacey DL, Dunstan CR, et al. Osteoprotegerin: A novel secreted protein involved in the regulation of bone density. Cell 1997;89:309–319.
82. Jin Q, Cirelli JA, Park CH, et al. RANKL inhibition through osteoprotegerin blocks bone loss in experimental periodontitis. J Periodontol 2007;78:1300–1308.
83. Dunn MD, Park CH, Kostenuik PJ, Kapila S, Giannobile WV. Local delivery of osteoprotegerin inhibits mechanically mediated bone modeling in orthodontic tooth movement. Bone 2007;41:446–455.
84. Ogasawara T, Yoshimine Y, Kiyoshima T, et al. In situ expression of RANKL, RANK, osteoprotegerin and cytokines in osteoclasts of rat periodontal tissue. J Periodontal Res 2004;39:42–49.
85. Kanzaki H, Chiba M, Shimizu Y, Mitani H. Periodontal ligament cells under mechanical stress induce osteoclastogenesis by receptor activator of nuclear factor κB ligand up-regulation via prostaglandin E2 synthesis. J Bone Miner Res 2002;17:210–220.
86. Davidovitch Z, Nicolay OF, Ngan PW, Shanfeld JL. Neurotransmitters, cytokines, and the control of alveolar bone remodeling in orthodontics. Dent Clin North Am 1988;32:411–435.
87. Davidovitch Z. Cell biology associated with tooth movement. In: Berkovitz BKB, Moxham BJ, Newman HN (eds). The Periodontal Ligament in Health and Disease, ed 2. London: Mosby-Wolfe, 1995.
88. Dumont N, Lepage K, Côté CH, Frenette J. Mast cells can modulate leukocyte accumulation and skeletal muscle function following hindlimb unloading. J Appl Physiol (1985) 2007;103:97–104.

89. Kurokouchi K, Jacobs CR, Donahue HJ. Oscillating fluid flow inhibits TNF-α-induced NF-κB activation via an IκB kinase pathway in osteoblast-like UMR106 cells. J Biol Chem 2001;276:13499–13504.
90. Kobayashi Y, Wada H, Rossios C, et al. A novel macrolide solithromycin exerts superior anti-inflammatory effect via NF-κB inhibition. J Pharmacol Exp Ther 2013;345:76–84.
91. Ji G, Zhang Y, Yang Q, et al. Genistein suppresses LPS-induced inflammatory response through inhibiting NF-κB following AMP kinase activation in RAW 264.7 macrophages. PloS One 2012;7:e53101.
92. Szulc P, Seeman E. Thinking inside and outside the envelopes of bone: Dedicated to PDD. Osteoporos Int 2009;20:1281–1288.
93. Tommasini SM, Wearne SL, Hof PR, Jepsen KJ. Percolation theory relates corticocancellous architecture to mechanical function in vertebrae of inbred mouse strains. Bone 2008;42:743–750.
94. Kavukcuoglu NB, Denhardt DT, Guzelsu N, Mann AB. Osteopontin deficiency and aging on nanomechanics of mouse bone. J Biomed Mater Res A 2007;83:136–144.
95. Nyman JS, Roy A, Tyler JH, Acuna RL, Gayle HJ, Wang X. Age-related factors affecting the postyield energy dissipation of human cortical bone. J Orthop Res 2007; 25:646–655.
96. Jäger A. Histomorphometric study of age-related changes in remodelling activity of human desmodontal bone. J Anat 1996;189:257–264.
97. Tonna EA. [Cellular kinetics of bone and aging (report) (author's transl)] [in German]. Verh Dtsch Ges Pathol 1974;58:99–104.
98. Lee BD, White SC. Age and trabecular features of alveolar bone associated with osteoporosis. Oral Surg Oral Med Oral Pathol Oral Radiol Endod 2005;100:92–98.
99. Cao JJ, Singleton PA, Majumdar S, et al. Hyaluronan increases RANKL expression in bone marrow stromal cells through CD44. J Bone Miner Res 2005;20:30–40.
100. Chen H, Sun J, Hoemann CD, et al. Drilling and microfracture lead to different bone structure and necrosis during bone-marrow stimulation for cartilage repair. J Orthop Res 2009;27:1432–1438.
101. Boskey AL, Coleman R. Aging and bone. J Dent Res 2010;89:1333–1348.
102. Sutherland MS, Rao LG, Muzaffar SA, et al. Age-dependent expression of osteoblastic phenotypic markers in normal human osteoblasts cultured long-term in the presence of dexamethasone. Osteoporos Int 1995;5:335–343.
103. Jiang SY, Shu R, Xie YF, Zhang SY. Age-related changes in biological characteristics of human alveolar osteoblasts. Cell Prolif 2010;43:464–470.
104. Rauner M, Sipos W, Pietschmann P. Age-dependent Wnt gene expression in bone and during the course of osteoblast differentiation. Age (Dordr) 2008;30:273–282.
105. World Health Organization. Prevention and Management of Osteoporosis: Report of a WHO Scientific Group [WHO Technical Report Series 921]. Geneva, Switzerland: WHO Scientific Group on the Prevention and Management of Osteoporosis, 2000.
106. Bikle DD, Halloran BP. The response of bone to unloading. J Bone Miner Metab 1999;17:233–244.
107. Sachelarie L, Farcas DM, Dartu L, et al. Comparative study of diseases of the stomatognathic system and specific parameters of osteoporosis. Osteoporos Int 2016;27:845–848.
108. Ingber DE. Mechanobiology and diseases of mechanotransduction. Ann Med 2003;35:564–577.
109. Sapir-Koren R, Livshits G. Is interaction between age-dependent decline in mechanical stimulation and osteocyte-estrogen receptor levels the culprit for postmenopausal-impaired bone formation? Osteoporos Int 2013;24:1771–1789.
110. Lin C, Jiang X, Dai Z, et al. Sclerostin mediates bone response to mechanical unloading through antagonizing Wnt/β-catenin signaling. J Bone Miner Res 2009;24:1651–1661.
111. Joiner DM, Tayim RJ, Kadado A, Goldstein SA. Bone marrow stromal cells from aged male rats have delayed mineralization and reduced response to mechanical stimulation through nitric oxide and ERK1/2 signaling during osteogenic differentiation. Biogerontology 2012;13:467–478.
112. Zahrowski JJ. Bisphosphonate treatment: An orthodontic concern calling for a proactive approach. Am J Orthod Dentofacial Orthop 2007;131:311–320.
113. Bamias A, Kastritis E, Bamia C, et al. Osteonecrosis of the jaw in cancer after treatment with bisphosphonates: Incidence and risk factors. J Clin Oncol 2005;23:8580–8587.
114. Abu-Id MH, Acil Y, Gottschalk J, Kreusch T. [Bisphosphonate-associated osteonecrosis of the jaw]. Mund Kiefer Gesichtschir 2006;10:73–81.
115. American Dental Association Council on Scientific Affairs. Dental management of patients receiving oral bisphosphonate therapy: Expert panel recommendations. J Am Dent Assoc 2006;137:1144–1150.
116. Ruggiero SL, Dodson TB, Assael LA, Landesberg R, Marx RE, Mehrotra B; Task Force on Bisphosphonate-Related Osteonecrosis of the Jaws; American Association of Oral and Maxillofacial Surgeons. American Association of Oral and Maxillofacial Surgeons position paper on bisphosphonate-related osteonecrosis of the jaw - 2009 update. Aust Endod J 2009;35:119–130.
117. Ruggiero SL. Bisphosphonate-related osteonecrosis of the jaw (BRONJ): Initial discovery and subsequent development. J Oral Maxillofac Surg 2009;67(5 suppl):13–18.
118. Walter C, Al-Nawas B, Frickhofen N, et al. Prevalence of bisphosphonate associated osteonecrosis of the jaws in multiple myeloma patients. Head Face Med 2010;6:11.
119. Adachi H, Igarashi K, Mitani H, Shinoda H. Effects of topical administration of a bisphosphonate (risedronate) on orthodontic tooth movements in rats. J Dent Res 1994;73:1478–1486.
120. Liu L, Igarashi K, Haruyama N, Saeki S, Shinoda H, Mitani H. Effects of local administration of clodronate on orthodontic tooth movement and root resorption in rats. Eur J Orthod 2004;26:469–473.
121. Igarashi K, Adachi H, Mitani H, Shinoda H. Inhibitory effect of the topical administration of a bisphosphonate (risedronate) on root resorption incident to orthodontic tooth movement in rats. J Dent Res 1996;75:1644–1649.

122. Kim TW, Yoshida Y, Yokoya K, Sasaki T. An ultrastructural study of the effects of bisphosphonate administration on osteoclastic bone resorption during relapse of experimentally moved rat molars. Am J Orthod Dentofacial Orthop 1999;115:645–653.
123. Papachroni KK, Karatzas DN, Papavassiliou KA, Basdra EK, Papavassiliou AG. Mechanotransduction in osteoblast regulation and bone disease. Trends Mol Med 2009; 15:208–216.
124. Rubin C, Turner AS, Bain S, Mallinckrodt C, McLeod K. Anabolism. Low mechanical signals strengthen long bones. Nature 2001;412:603–604.
125. Kusumi A, Sakaki H, Kusumi T, et al. Regulation of synthesis of osteoprotegerin and soluble receptor activator of nuclear factor-κB ligand in normal human osteoblasts via the p38 mitogen-activated protein kinase pathway by the application of cyclic tensile strain. J Bone Miner Metab 2005;23:373–381.
126. Tang LL, Xian CY, Wang YL. The MGF expression of osteoblasts in response to mechanical overload. Arch Oral Biol 2006;51:1080–1085.
127. Tang L, Lin Z, Li YM. Effects of different magnitudes of mechanical strain on Osteoblasts in vitro. Biochem Biophys Res Commun 2006;344:122–128.
128. Rubin J, Murphy TC, Fan X, Goldschmidt M, Taylor WR. Activation of extracellular signal-regulated kinase is involved in mechanical strain inhibition of RANKL expression in bone stromal cells. J Bone Miner Res 2002;17:1452–1460.
129. Armstrong VJ, Muzylak M, Sunters A, et al. Wnt/β-catenin signaling is a component of osteoblastic bone cell early responses to load-bearing and requires estrogen receptor α. J Biol Chem 2007;282:20715–20727.
130. Leclerc E, David B, Griscom L, et al. Study of osteoblastic cells in a microfluidic environment. Biomaterials 2006;27:586–595.
131. Cartmell SH, Porter BD, García AJ, Guldberg RE. Effects of medium perfusion rate on cell-seeded three-dimensional bone constructs in vitro. Tissue Eng 2003;9:1197–1203.
132. Kokkinos PA, Zarkadis IK, Kletsas D, Deligianni DD. Effects of physiological mechanical strains on the release of growth factors and the expression of differentiation marker genes in human osteoblasts growing on Ti-6Al-4V. J Biomed Mater Res A 2009;90:387–395.
133. Stahl SS, Tonna EA. H3-proline study of aging periodontal ligament matrix formation: Comparison between matrices adjacent to either cemental or bone surfaces. J Periodontal Res 1977;12:318–322.
134. Oehmke MJ, Schramm CR, Knolle E, Frickey N, Bernhart T, Oehmke HJ. Age-dependent changes of the periodontal ligament in rats. Microsc Res Tech 2004;63:198–202.
135. Moxham BJ, Evans IL. The effects of aging upon the connective tissues of the periodontal ligament. Connect Tissue Res 1995;33:31–35.
136. Grant D, Bernick S. Formation of the periodontal ligament. J Periodontol 1972;43:17–25.
137. Severson JA, Moffett BC, Kokich V, Selipsky H. A histologic study of age changes in the adult human periodontal joint (ligament). J Periodontol 1978;49:189–200.
138. Kyomen S, Tanne K. Influences of aging changes in proliferative rate of PDL cells during experimental tooth movement in rats. Angle Orthod 1997;67:67–72.
139. Abiko Y, Shimizu N, Yamaguchi M, Suzuki H, Takiguchi H. Effect of aging on functional changes of periodontal tissue cells. Ann Periodontol 1998;3:350–369.
140. Mayahara K, Kobayashi Y, Takimoto K, Suzuki N, Mitsui N, Shimizu N. Aging stimulates cyclooxygenase-2 expression and prostaglandin E2 production in human periodontal ligament cells after the application of compressive force. J Periodontal Res 2007;42:8–14.
141. Ohzeki K, Yamaguchi M, Shimizu N, Abiko Y. Effect of cellular aging on the induction of cyclooxygenase-2 by mechanical stress in human periodontal ligament cells. Mech Ageing Dev 1999;108:151–163.
142. Miura S, Yamaguchi M, Shimizu N, Abiko Y. Mechanical stress enhances expression and production of plasminogen activator in aging human periodontal ligament cells. Mech Ageing Dev 2000;112:217–231.
143. Benatti BB, Silverio KG, Casati MZ, Sallum EA, Nociti FH Jr. Inflammatory and bone-related genes are modulated by aging in human periodontal ligament cells. Cytokine 2009;46:176–181.
144. Nishimura F, Terranova VP, Braithwaite M, et al. Comparison of in vitro proliferative capacity of human periodontal ligament cells in juvenile and aged donors. Oral Dis 1997;3:162–166.
145. Shiba H, Nakanishi K, Sakata M, Fujita T, Uchida Y, Kurihara H. Effects of ageing on proliferative ability, and the expressions of secreted protein, acidic and rich in cysteine (SPARC) and osteoprotegerin (osteoclastogenesis inhibitory factor) in cultures of human periodontal ligament cells. Mech Ageing Dev 2000;117:69–77.
146. Benatti BB, Silvério KG, Casati MZ, Sallum EA, Nociti FH Jr. Influence of aging on biological properties of periodontal ligament cells. Connect Tissue Res 2008;49: 401–408.
147. Goseki T, Shimizu N, Iwasawa T, Takiguchi H, Abiko Y. Effects of in vitro cellular aging on alkaline phosphatase, cathepsin activities and collagen secretion of human periodontal ligament derived cells. Mech Ageing Dev 1996;91:171–183.
148. Sawa Y, Yamaoka Y, Kuroshima S, Yoshida S. Reduction of alkaline phosphatase activity in aged human osteogenic periodontal ligament fibroblasts exhibiting short telomeres. Cell Tissue Res 2004;315:331–337.
149. Lossdorfer S, Kraus D, Jager A. Aging affects the phenotypic characteristics of human periodontal ligament cells and the cellular response to hormonal stimulation in vitro. J Periodontal Res 2010;45:764–771.
150. Stanstedt C. Einige Beiträge zur Theorie der Zahnregulierung. Nordisk Tandläkaretidskrift 1904;236–256.

CHAPTER 2

Microbial Colonization of Teeth and Orthodontic Appliances

Georgios N. Belibasakis
Anastasios Grigoriadis
Carlos Marcelo da Silva Figueredo

Principles of Microbial Colonization and Microbial Biofilm Formation

Microorganisms in nature tend to attach to and grow on surfaces. Oral bacteria are no exception to this norm, as they have the natural tendency to attach to the hard dental surfaces and grow in the form of complex polymicrobial communities known as *biofilms*. Yet teeth are not the only surfaces on which oral bacteria can attach and grow. They are also able to grow on artificial surfaces including dental restorative material,[1] osseointegrated dental implants,[2] and orthodontic appliances.[3] Clinical examples of microbial biofilm formation on natural teeth or prosthodontic restorations and dental filling materials are shown in Fig 2-1.

The adhesion of oral microorganisms to an oral surface, be it natural tissue or artificial material, is mediated by a thin layer of salivary glycoproteins termed the *acquired enamel pellicle*.[4] The calcium and phosphates of the enamel mineral form electrostatic bonds with the nitrate, phosphate, carbonate, and sulfate groups of the salivary glycoproteins, which are then adsorbed on the surface of the enamel. Microbial adhesion then follows, first with a reversible sorption stage and then with an irreversible adherence stage.[5] The sorption stage involves weak, long-range, nonspecific electrostatic forces between the glycoproteins of the salivary pellicle and the bacterial surface. The more decisive stage of adherence involves stronger, short-range, specific interactions between the involved bacteria and the glycoproteins of the pellicle. These include the molecular binding between adhesins (proteins with adhesion properties on the surface structure of the bacteria) and

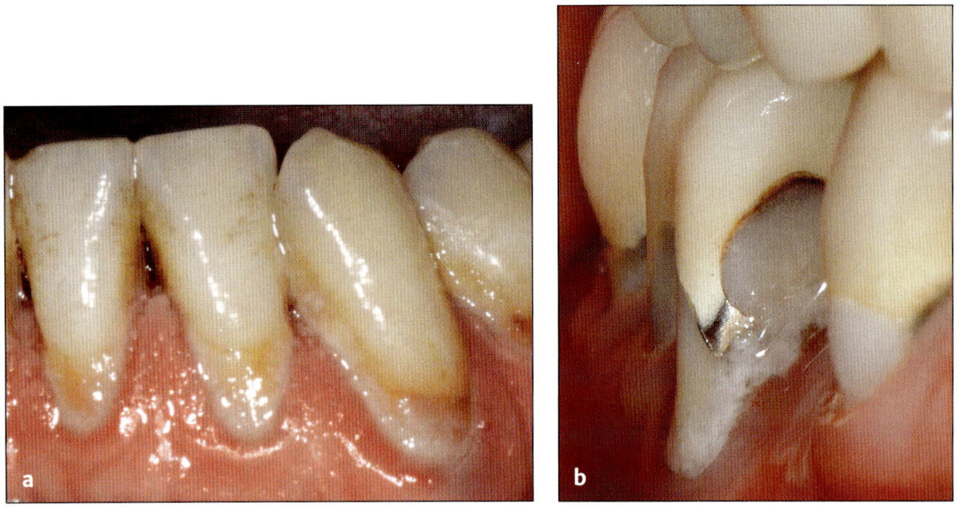

Fig 2-1 *(a)* Microbial biofilm formation on the approximal and cervical surfaces of mandibular anterior teeth. *(b)* Microbial biofilm formation on the surface of a composite and metal-ceramic restoration of a posterior tooth.

salivary glycoproteins that act as adsorbed receptors on the pellicle-coated surfaces. Typical adhesins expressed on the bacterial surface are the lectins, a family of proteins that can recognize and bind to carbohydrates. The initial colonization of the tooth surface takes place within seconds or minutes, and the earliest colonizing bacterial species include primarily streptococci and actinomycetes. The initial colonizers multiply and outgrow within hours, while more free-floating species are now able to colonize the biofilm and form its intermediate strands by co-aggregating with the initial colonizers.[6] The space between the bacterial cells becomes filled by extracellular polymeric matrix consisting of bacterial products and trapped salivary components.

There is great microbial diversity between the sequential strands of the biofilm as it gradually develops. The young biofilms consist of densely packed gram-positive nonmotile cocci and rods. Their growth rate slows down as the intermediate colonizers are incorporated into the biofilm. The intermediate strands of the microbial biofilm are less densely packed, and the constituent bacterial species continue to proliferate. The proportion of cocci and small rods now decreases, and the microbial populations of the biofilm become more diverse, enclosing more gram-negative elongated fusiform and filamentous bacteria. The outer strands of the mature biofilm are more loosely attached and can be easily detached. The diversity of the species increases further, and occasionally motile bacterial forms, such as spirochetes, can arise.

The microenvironmental conditions within the developing microbial biofilm are gradually modified. These conditions dictate the survival of specific individual species and may include temperature, redox potential, partial oxygen pressure, and nutrient availability, among others. The metabolic interactions established between the constituent species enable them to establish stronger and more coherent biofilm communities. Bacteria that are not able to survive under the newly established conditions in the biofilm are displaced by faster-growing ones and eventually become detached and removed from the loose outer layer of the biofilm.

Association of Colonizing Microbial Biofilms with Oral Disease

Under a healthy status, the microbes in the biofilm live in harmony with their human host, and in fact their interaction is beneficial to each other. Yet when the microenvironmental conditions within a niche of the oral cavity are changing in a manner that allows specific opportunistic pathogens to prevail over the rest of the community, this favors the establishment of disease.[7] This is a state of disadvantageous interaction between the host and the resident microbes that may lead to disease and is known as *dysbiosis*.[8] The most common oral diseases, including dental caries, endodontic infections, periodontal diseases, and peri-implant diseases, are the result of a dysbiotic interaction between the corresponding microbial biofilms and host tissue.[9,10] Because these are polymicrobial biofilm-associated diseases, no single bacterial species can be considered primarily responsible, but the disease results when the dysbiotic microbial community cannot be tackled efficiently by the host defenses.

Microbial Adhesion and Biofilm Formation on Orthodontic Appliances

Biofilm formation on orthodontic devices has been associated with enamel decalcification and white spot lesions as a risk of caries and opportunistic fungal infections.[11,12] Therefore, most of the recent literature has focused on the investigation of how *Candida albicans*, *Streptococcus mutans*, and lactobacilli can interact with orthodontic appliances. *C albicans* is the most prevalent fungal species of the human microbiota and colonizes healthy individuals without causing any clinical symptoms. However, it may function as an opportunistic pathogen on immunosuppressed hosts. The medical impact of *C albicans* depends on its ability to form biofilms in a range of biotic and abiotic surfaces.[13] The impact of *C albicans* in patients treated with orthodontic devices has been reviewed,[12] and it was reported that the density of *Candida* species increases and seems to be in direct association with the presence of a removable appliance and low salivary pH levels. No healthy patients appeared to develop *Candida* infection from the orthodontic appliances, yet there was a trend of conversion of non-*Candida* to *Candida* carriers following the insertion of orthodontic appliances.[12] This suggests that caution must be taken with regard to orthodontic treatment in immunocompromised children, due to increased risk of an opportunistic infection.

Regarding the adhesion and colonization of the oral cavity by *C albicans*, Gonçalves et al[14] compared the presence of *Candida* species in saliva, their adherence to oral epithelial cells, and the levels of anti–*C albicans* immunoglobulin A in children with or without orthodontic appliances. Interestingly, children with orthodontic devices exhibited more yeast cells adhering to oral epithelial cells and a higher percentage of non–*C albicans* species relative to the control group. Therefore, orthodontic appliances may favor the adherence of *Candida* to epithelial cells, though without influencing their levels in saliva. The different chemical compositions of the orthodontic device material might also influence biofilm formation and fungal virulence. Ronsani et al[15] evaluated whether metal ions can affect fungal virulence. To do so, they used culture media containing nickel (Ni^{2+}), iron (Fe^{3+}), chromium (Cr^{3+}), cobalt (Co^{2+}), or a mixture of these metal ions at concentrations similar to those released in the saliva of orthodontic patients. All ions except for Co^{2+} increased the biofilm biomass. Ni^{2+} also caused an increase in secretory aspartyl protease activity, and Fe^{3+} reduced hemolytic activity. Based on these findings, it was proposed that metal ions released during the degradation of orthodontic appliances may modulate virulence factors in *C albicans* biofilms.

Candida species may also be involved as a secondary agent in perpetuating the carious process, especially in dentinal caries.[16] Therefore, the co-existence of *C albicans*, *S mutans*, and lactobacilli in biofilms around orthodontic devices has also been a matter of concern. Several experiments have been performed to investigate how their combination could compromise dental health during the use of orthodontic devices. Beerens et al[17] studied the applicability of contemporary and conventional microbiology for caries risk assessment in orthodontic patients. The microbiologic analysis included evaluation of the total colony-forming units (CFUs) and percentages of aciduric flora for *S mutans*, *Lactobacillus* species, and *C albicans*. The authors reported that CFU counts were not predictive of white spot lesion formation in the orthodontic patients. Shukla et al[18] aimed to determine the prevalence and counts of *S mutans* and *Candida* species in patients undergoing fixed orthodontic appliance therapy and to compare the efficiency of manual and electronic toothbrushes in minimizing plaque. Orthodontic appliances were found to increase the colonization of *S mutans* and *C albicans* in the oral cavity over the period of treatment time. In fact, it has been previously shown that white spot lesion formation during multibracket appliance treatment is associated with higher counts of *Candida* and lactobacilli species, while *S mutans* was detected in all patients regardless of oral hygiene level.[19]

The use of antibiofilm products to reduce the negative effect of bacterial adhesion on orthodontic devices has been intensely studied. Taha et al[20] evaluated *(1)* the in vitro ability of esthetic, coated rectangular archwires to retain oral biofilms and *(2)* in vivo biofilm formation on these wires after 4 and 8 weeks of clinical use. Surface roughness and microbial adhesion increased after intraoral use at all time intervals. Sugii et al[21] evaluated the antibiofilm effect of iodide quaternary ammonium methacryloxy silicate (IQAMS) in light-curing adhesive resin used for braces cementation. Assays on *S mutans* demonstrated enhanced antibiofilm effect for the IQAMS-coated resin in comparison to incorporated IQAMS. Such a difference was attributed to low availability of quaternary ammonium groups at the surface of the resin when IQAMS was incorporated, hindering its antibiofilm effect.

Glass-ionomer, adhesive, and orthodontic device modifications have also been investigated for controlling microbial biofilm formation. Andrucioli et al[22] investigated the levels of *S mutans* in saliva and biofilms adjacent to orthodontic brackets retained with resin-modified glass-ionomer cement. This bonding material hindered the growth of *S mutans* in the biofilm during the study period. Similarly, differences in the levels of *S mutans* in biofilms were observed between various types of orthodontic adhesives.[23,24] Orthodontic cement containing 3% dimethylaminohexadecyl methacrylate (DMAHDM) reduced the metabolic activity, lactic acid production, and microbial load of the biofilm. Therefore, incorporation of DMAHDM provided strong antibacterial properties to a modified orthodontic cement without compromising its enamel-bonding strength.

Bracket types, conformation, and coatings have also been shown to influence the microbial adhesion and biofilm formation. Plasma-polymerized film deposition was created to modify the surface properties of metallic orthodontic brackets in order to inhibit bacterial adhesion. Tupinambá et al[25] reported that this was only effective for reducing surface roughness and bacterial adhesion in conventional brackets. Uzuner et al[26] evaluated the effect of different bracket types on the levels of *S mutans* and *Lactobacillus* species in saliva and microbial biofilms and periodontal health status. It was concluded that self-ligating brackets do not have an advantage over conventional brackets with respect to periodontal status or colonization of *S mutans* and lactobacilli. Accordingly, Fatani et al[27] reported that brackets coated with silver titanium dioxide exhibit superior antimicrobial activity and resistance to biofilm formation compared to uncoated ones.

Besides *S mutans* and *C albicans*, *Staphylococcus aureus*, a gram-positive species associated with opportunistic infections, has been investigated for its capacity to colonize orthodontic appliances. Merghni et al[28] investigated the ability of *S aureus* isolates from healthy patients with orthodontic appliances to adhere to biotic and abiotic surfaces (polystyrene and dental alloy) and demonstrated that they are indeed capable of colonizing these surfaces. They also assessed the ability of an *S aureus* biofilm to form on materials routinely used in dental practice, including stainless steel, polyethylene, and polyvinyl chloride. They demonstrated that this species exhibits higher affinity to stainless steel compared to the other tested materials and that the increased capacity for microbial biofilm formation is associated with the surface free energy.[29]

References

1. Busscher HJ, Rinastiti M, Siswomihardjo W, van der Mei HC. Biofilm formation on dental restorative and implant materials. J Dent Res 2010;89:657–665.
2. Belibasakis GN, Charalampakis G, Bostanci N, Stadlinger B. Peri-implant infections of oral biofilm etiology. Adv Exp Med Biol 2015;830:69–84.
3. Ren Y, Jongsma MA, Mei L, van der Mei HC, Busscher HJ. Orthodontic treatment with fixed appliances and biofilm formation—A potential public health threat? Clin Oral Investig 2014;18:1711–1718.
4. Marsh PD, Martin MV. The mouth as a microbial habitat. In: Oral Microbiology, ed 5. Edinburgh: Elsevier, 2009:8–23.
5. Marsh PD, Martin MV. Dental plaque. In: Oral Microbiology, ed 5. Edinburgh: Elsevier, 2009:74–102.
6. Kolenbrander PE, Palmer RJ Jr, Periasamy S, Jakubovics NS. Oral multispecies biofilm development and the key role of cell-cell distance. Nat Rev Microbiol 2010;8:471–480.
7. Marsh PD. Are dental diseases examples of ecological catastrophes? Microbiology 2003;149:279–294.
8. Hajishengallis G, Lamont RJ. Beyond the red complex and into more complexity: The polymicrobial synergy and dysbiosis (PSD) model of periodontal disease etiology. Mol Oral Microbiol 2012;27:409–419.
9. Belibasakis GN, Bostanci N. Oral biofilms and their implication in oral diseases. In: Seneviratnte CJ (ed). Oral Microbial Biofilms: Omics Biology, Antimicrobials and Clinical Implications. Boca Raton, FL: CRC, 2017:69–80.
10. Marsh PD, Zaura E. Dental biofilm: Ecological interactions in health and disease. J Clin Periodontol 2017;44(suppl 18):S12–S22.
11. Hess E, Campbell PM, Honeyman AL, Buschang PH. Determinants of enamel decalcification during simulated orthodontic treatment. Angle Orthod 2011;81:836–842.
12. Hibino K, Wong RW, Hägg U, Samaranayake LP. The effects of orthodontic appliances on *Candida* in the human mouth. Int J Paediatr Dent 2009;19:301–308.
13. Lohse MB, Gulati M, Johnson AD, Nobile CJ. Development and regulation of single- and multi-species *Candida albicans* biofilms. Nat Rev Microbiol 2018;16:19–31.
14. Gonçalves e Silva CR, Oliveira LD, Leão MV, Jorge AO. *Candida* spp. adherence to oral epithelial cells and levels of IgA in children with orthodontic appliances. Braz Oral Res 2014;28:28–32.
15. Ronsani MM, Mores Rymovicz AU, Meira TM, et al. Virulence modulation of *Candida albicans* biofilms by metal ions commonly released from orthodontic devices. Microb Pathog 2011;51:421–425.
16. Pereira D, Seneviratne CJ, Koga-Ito CY, Samaranayake LP. Is the oral fungal pathogen *Candida albicans* a cariogen? Oral Dis 2018;24:518–526.
17. Beerens MW, Ten Cate JM, van der Veen MH. Microbial profile of dental plaque associated to white spot lesions in orthodontic patients immediately after the bracket removal. Arch Oral Biol 2017;78:88–93.
18. Shukla C, Maurya R, Singh V, Tijare M. Evaluation of role of fixed orthodontics in changing oral ecological flora of opportunistic microbes in children and adolescent. J Indian Soc Pedod Prev Dent 2017;35:34–40.
19. Klaus K, Eichenauer J, Sprenger R, Ruf S. Oral microbiota carriage in patients with multibracket appliance in relation to the quality of oral hygiene. Head Face Med 2016;12:28.
20. Taha M, El-Fallal A, Degla H. In vitro and in vivo biofilm adhesion to esthetic coated arch wires and its correlation with surface roughness. Angle Orthod 2016;86:285–291.
21. Sugii MM, Ferreira FAS, Müller KC, et al. Physical, chemical and antimicrobial evaluation of a composite material containing quaternary ammonium salt for braces cementation. Mater Sci Eng C Mater Biol Appl 2017;73:340–346.
22. Andrucioli MC, Faria G, Nelson-Filho P, Romano FL, Matsumoto MA. Influence of resin-modified glass ionomer and topical fluoride on levels of *Streptococcus mutans* in saliva and biofilm adjacent to metallic brackets. J Appl Oral Sci 2017;25:196–202.
23. Ho CS, Ming Y, Foong KW, Rosa V, Thuyen T, Seneviratne CJ. *Streptococcus mutans* forms xylitol-resistant biofilm on excess adhesive flash in novel ex-vivo orthodontic bracket model. Am J Orthod Dentofacial Orthop 2017;151:669–677.
24. Feng X, Zhang N, Xu HHK, et al. Novel orthodontic cement containing dimethylaminohexadecyl methacrylate with strong antibacterial capability. Dent Mater J 2017;36:669–676.
25. Tupinambá RA, Claro CAA, Pereira CA, Nobrega CJP, Claro APRA. Bacterial adhesion on conventional and self-ligating metallic brackets after surface treatment with plasma-polymerized hexamethyldisiloxane. Dental Press J Orthod 2017;22:77–85.
26. Uzuner FD, Kaygisiz E, Cankaya ZT. Effect of the bracket types on microbial colonization and periodontal status. Angle Orthod 2014;84:1062–1067.
27. Fatani EJ, Almutairi HH, Alharbi AO, et al. In vitro assessment of stainless steel orthodontic brackets coated with titanium oxide mixed Ag for anti-adherent and antibacterial properties against *Streptococcus mutans* and *Porphyromonas gingivalis*. Microb Pathog 2017;112:190–194.
28. Merghni A, Ben Nejma M, Dallel I, et al. High potential of adhesion to biotic and abiotic surfaces by opportunistic *Staphylococcus aureus* strains isolated from orthodontic appliances. Microb Pathog 2016;91:61–67.
29. Merghni A, Bekir K, Kadmi Y, et al. Adhesiveness of opportunistic *Staphylococcus aureus* to materials used in dental office: In vitro study. Microb Pathog 2017;103:129–134.

CHAPTER 3

Changes in the Oral Microbiota During Orthodontic Treatment

William Papaioannou
Margarita Makou

Orthodontic therapy primarily aims to correct malpositioned teeth and malocclusion that can cause functional and esthetic problems for individuals. Although problems stemming from badly arranged teeth can be a source of difficulty in maintaining good daily oral health, which is vital to preserving dental and gingival health, questions do arise as to what the impact of the orthodontic appliances (brackets, bands, etc) can be on periodontal health, both in the short and long term. The close proximity of the appliances to the periodontal tissue can have an impact from both biologic and microbiologic aspects. The increased potential for the retention of dental plaque, while at the same time hindering oral hygiene, can change not only the quantity but also the quality of the resultant microbial flora. The long-term impact that these changes may have is of vital importance to address. Do the apparent changes to the periodontal tissue often seen during therapy lead to permanent damage? Are these linked to the changes in the microbiota? Are these in turn responsible for long-term or permanent effects? These are the questions that must be addressed when examining the periodontal impact of orthodontic therapy, especially considering the ever-growing number of individuals, both young and old, undergoing orthodontic treatment.

Plaque and Orthodontic Therapy

Microorganisms found in the environment exist either freely in the air or in liquids (planktonic) or are incorporated in organized bacterial communities called *biofilms*. Most microorganisms in nature are attached to surfaces, creating such biofilms. The definition most often used for these formations is a population of bacteria that is matrix enclosed and adherent to each other and/or surfaces or interfaces.[1] In this state, the behavior of bacteria can change, such as the manner of their reactions to the host or the environment. For this reason, the definition was updated to include the exhibition of an altered phenotype with respect to growth rate and gene transcription.[2]

The dental microbial plaque that forms on all oral hard surfaces comprises a central part of the human oral ecologic system. It consists of a greatly differentiated community of microorganisms united within an extracellular polymer matrix, produced by the bacterial metabolism, along with host products. This forms the dental plaque biofilm[1,3] whose composition changes over the lifetime of an individual and under certain ecologic fluctuations, or perturbations, of the oral cavity. These changes are caused by the natural transitions in the dentition—from edentulous newborn to toddler/child with a primary dentition, to adolescence and adulthood with the permanent dentition, and unfortunately sometimes a return to edentulism in old age—or occur as a result of pathologic situations, the effect of medication, or inadequate daily oral care.[4,5] Thus, the presence of a certain level of dental plaque is ubiquitous, and the oral cavity is for the most part in a state of homeostasis or balance. However, without control of the growth and accumulation of plaque, especially on the hard tooth surfaces, this state of balance is jeopardized, and a dysbiotic relationship between plaque and host is created, leading to disease.[6]

The different species of bacteria that make up a biofilm are not randomly situated microcolonies but rather exhibit a high degree of organization, both spatially and functionally.[3] The bacterial metabolisms create gradients of the parameters with an important impact on the growth and development of the bacteria (nutrients, pH, oxygen, etc). This ecologic heterogeneity allows different species of bacteria that normally would not be able to coexist to live together in a common environment. A prime example of this is the coexistence of anaerobic and aerobic bacteria in dental plaque.

Two of the most common oral diseases—caries and periodontitis—are indeed caused by the presence of the dental plaque biofilm and are especially linked to the presence of specific bacterial species. Under certain ecologic conditions, this normally symbiotic community of bacteria comprising the plaque biofilm becomes dysbiotic, and pathogenic species find the opportunity to grow and cause disease.[3,6] The start of the disease process may come many years after the establishment of pathogenic species in the oral cavity. The pathologic conditions, especially those of the periodontium, are considered chronic diseases with complex microbial composition, which contrast with acute diseases whose etiology can often be attributed to even one specific microorganism. Different hypotheses have been proposed over time for the bacterial etiology of oral disease. For many years the "nonspecific plaque hypothesis" and "specific plaque hypothesis" were at the forefront, the latter reigning up to the end of the 20th century. However, in the 1990s, P.D. Marsh proposed the "ecological plaque hypothesis,"[7] which essentially combined the previous two hypotheses. In this hypothesis, nonspecific plaque accumulations have an important role in disease initiation, creating under certain ecologic conditions a local environment conducive to the growth and dominance of specific pathogenic species. Indeed, recently the idea of keystone pathogens has been proposed, in which certain specific species act as instigators of the pathogenic potential of the bacterial plaque. This theory, which is gaining interest, is known as the "polymicrobial synergy and dysbiosis" model for disease.[8]

One of the important factors affecting the growth and maturation of dental plaque biofilm is adhesion and the protection from removal forces. The oral hard surfaces provide significant areas of attachment of bacteria, which slowly spread out and grow out of the initial adhering cells, allowing the colonization of the teeth. Different areas of the teeth have different surface morphologies and characteristics that may enhance the attachment and retention of the plaque biofilm, and natural removal forces (salivary flow, tongue movement, etc) may have an effect on the growth. Nevertheless, the nonshedding

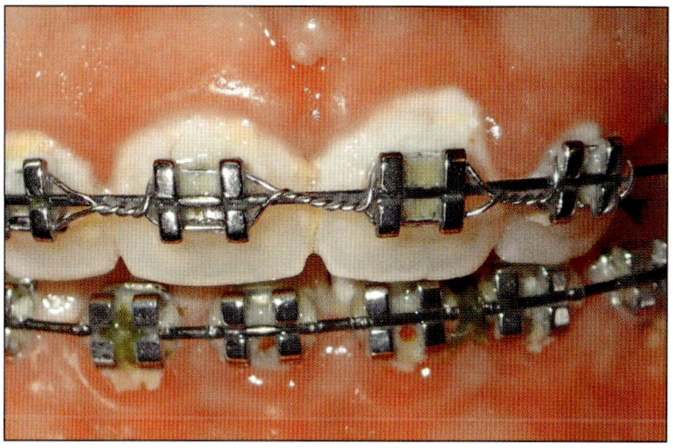

Fig 3-1 Orthodontic treatment creates conditions that facilitate and increase the tendency for higher plaque accumulation. Note the increased plaque accumulation and gingival inflammation present in this clinical case.

tooth surfaces are considered important and unique structures in the body, in turn creating unique ecologic niches for the bacteria.[9]

Apart from the supragingival tooth surface niche, there are the subgingival tooth surface niches. The soft tissues and tongue also provide separate and distinct niches for bacteria to colonize.[4,9] However, these epithelial surfaces are less than optimal for the bacteria because they continuously shed the uppermost cell layers, which usually carries away the adhering bacterial cells. Within the moist oral environment, saliva itself also provides a distinct bacterial milieu and method for the spread or translocation of bacteria within the mouth.

The nature of orthodontic therapy, requiring the placement of fixed or removable orthodontic appliances as well as other necessary materials, can have significant influence on the microbial plaque biofilm, causing significant changes in the oral environment overall. An important factor in the initial adhesion of bacteria and their ability to colonize and spread out is the lack of removal forces, primarily mechanical oral hygiene aids (eg, toothbrush, interdental brushes, etc). Orthodontic brackets, bands, ligatures, wires, and orthodontic appliances in general offer the possibility of attachment to the different oral bacteria and provide safe sites for the plaque to grow. This attachment of bacteria and their eventual colonization and growth on the various surfaces depends on many factors. These can be related to the properties of the material and its surface characteristics, design, and placement but also greatly depend on patient characteristics and oral hygiene behavior. Gingival swelling and overgrowth, which is seen in many patients, may further impede effective plaque removal.

It is generally known that orthodontic therapy leads to significant increases in the quantity[10,11] and complexity of the dental plaque.[12,13] As a result, demineralization of the tooth surfaces and caries development and/or gingival inflammation may ensue if the proper daily hygiene routines are not followed.

Orthodontic Treatment and Oral Diseases

The placement of orthodontic appliances and accessories can cause quantitative and qualitative changes in plaque bacteria in a very short time period.[10,12,13] As already mentioned, patients undergoing orthodontic treatment have a tendency for increased plaque accumulation (Fig 3-1). Without proper guidance and continual motivation, it is relatively easy for the patient to inadequately clean around the orthodontic appliances[14] and thus fail to sufficiently control the bacterial load around the teeth and the oral cavity. In this way, orthodontic therapy is considered to increase the risk of plaque-related oral disease.[15] Indeed, children with brackets have been found to

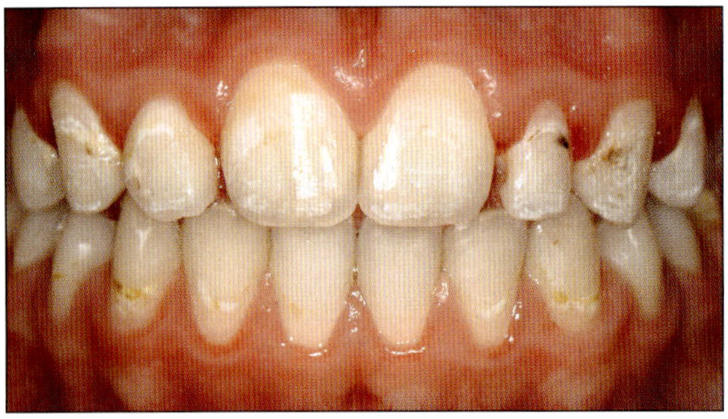

Fig 3-2 Clinical image of an orthodontic patient after therapy. Note the white spot lesions and areas of enamel demineralization in the regions around where the brackets were during orthodontic treatment.

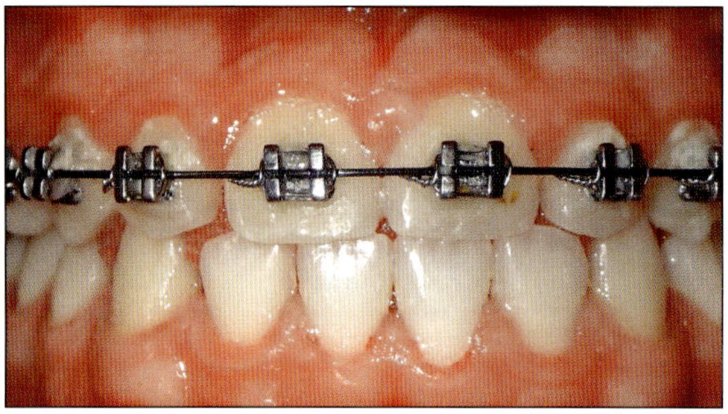

Fig 3-3 Brackets in close proximity to the gingival margin facilitate the accumulation of dental plaque that initiates changes in the health of the gingiva. Note the plaque accumulation and gingival inflammation of the maxillary lateral incisors and canines. Gingival swelling can also be noted, especially between the maxillary central incisors.

exhibit significantly higher gingival index, in tandem with an increase in plaque, when compared with a similar group without brackets.[16]

Thus, the placement of brackets on the different supragingival regions of the tooth crowns will affect the amount and balance of specific bacteria. The bacterial types adhering and forming the plaque biofilm primarily push toward a more cariogenic composition. In this way, increases in cariogenic bacteria, primarily species such as *Streptococcus mutans* and lactobacilli can be detected in patients undergoing orthodontic therapy.[13,17] These bacteria are responsible for the increase in demineralization of the enamel around the brackets and cause early caries lesions in the form of white spots (Fig 3-2). However, if the brackets are placed in close proximity to the gingival margin, then changes can also be initiated in the health of the gingiva (Fig 3-3). This is especially true when orthodontic bands are placed, which by their nature are next to the gingiva or even extend into the sulcus, especially in interdental areas. Inflammation will usually ensue as a result of the plaque-retentive properties in combination with inadequate oral hygiene and possibly the focal irritation they may cause. Corbacho de Melo et al found that adults with banded second molars presented significantly higher gingival inflammation than the control group of similar nonbanded adults.[18] These bands with the propensity for higher plaque accumulation provide the necessary conditions for the balance in the plaque composition to move toward a more complex configuration. In time, more gram-negative, anaerobic, and periodontopathic bacteria can be found within this complex biofilm bacteria, which, if allowed to overgrow, will in turn cause a further inflammatory reaction of the gingival tissues.[19,20] This has been found to be true especially in interdental regions, where the bacteria are even further protected from removal forces. In a group of adolescent orthodontic patients, Kim et al found that bands, depending on their placement in relation to the gingival margin (level with or below the margin), had a tendency for deepening the sulcus (2.9 mm when placed below the gingival margin, 2.5 mm when placed level with the gingival margin), especially compared to brackets (2.3 mm).[21] However, no important differences in the subgingival bacterial composition could be determined.

Changes toward a more periodontopathic subgingival microbiota are clearly associated with the period of orthodontic therapy that involves appliances in the oral cavity.[22–24] Very quickly after initiating the active phase of therapy (3 months after bracket placement without the use of bands), Naranjo et al,[22] using classic microbial culture techniques, found an increase in putative periodontal pathogens such as *Fusobacterium nucleatum* and *Prevotella intermedia* as well as typical periodontopathic bacteria such as *Porphyromonas gingivalis* and *Tannerella forsythia*, along with the concomitant increase in gingival inflammation (as registered by bleeding on probing), in comparison to the pretherapy situation. Superinfecting species of *Enterobacter*, *Klebsiella*, and *Serratia* were also detected.[22] In an earlier study by another group[25] using polymerase chain reaction to detect periodontal pathogens, *T forsythia*, *Treponema denticola*, and *Prevotella nigrescens* were found to be significantly more prevalent in orthodontic patients than in control patients without orthodontic treatment. However, the authors pointed out that these patients did not present with serious periodontal disease.[25]

Thornberg et al,[23] using DNA probe analysis in a large group of patients (N = 190) to detect for eight periodontopathogens, found that for six of these (*P intermedia*, *T forsythia*, *Eikenella corrodens*, *F nucleatum*, *T denticola*, and *Campylobacter rectus*) the percentages of patients with high numbers of these organisms increased significantly after 6 months of fixed orthodontic treatment, but by 12 months they returned to the levels seen before treatment. They proposed that the oral cavity found a new equilibrium for the different bacterial species, and for this reason no pathogen was found to be significantly higher after these 12 months. Moreover, they concluded that orthodontic treatment was found to be significantly protective for half of the pathogens (*E corrodens*, *F nucleatum*, *T denticola*, and *C rectus*) posttreatment, due to possible improvements in hygiene resulting from resolution of alignment problems. The improvement in both gingival condition and the levels of certain pathogens after removal of orthodontic appliances and professional prophylaxis has also been reported by Sallum et al.[26]

With completion of therapy and removal of the fixed appliances, the various studies tend to agree that the microbial composition transitions back toward one compatible to health, with reduced microbial levels, both supra- and subgingival, and improvements in periodontal parameters.[23,26–28] Clearly, although conditions during orthodontic therapy seem to become more conducive to the overgrowth of more pathogenic species, their permanent dominance is not secured, and possible future problems may answer back to the differences between individuals. These differences (genetic, environmental, etc) touch on the multifactorial nature of oral diseases and the necessity for several factors to increase disease appearance.

An interesting situation to look at is what happens to the subgingival microbiota in adults undergoing fixed orthodontic therapy who had previously been treated for chronic periodontitis. Speer et al examined seven adult patients pretreated for periodontitis without antibiotics at three distinct time points: before the start of orthodontics, 6 weeks into treatment, and 6 weeks after removal of the fixed appliances.[29] Indeed, they observed a marked reduction in the total number of bacteria in the pockets examined during orthodontic treatment, despite the clinical situation remaining unchanged. After removal of the appliances, the number of certain periodontopathogens increased slightly. They attributed this to the possible antimicrobial effect of nickel ions released through corrosion of the brackets and archwires.

Factors That May Influence the Amount and Composition of Plaque

The amount and composition of the dental plaque biofilm accumulating on fixed orthodontic appliances can be influenced by several factors: the type and design of the orthodontic devices, the material of which they are made, and of course the cements that are used for their attachment to the tooth surfaces.

TYPE OF BRACKET

Another interesting venue of research is the effect of the bracket type on the adhesion and accumulation of bacteria. Brackets are the most common component of fixed orthodontic therapy that come

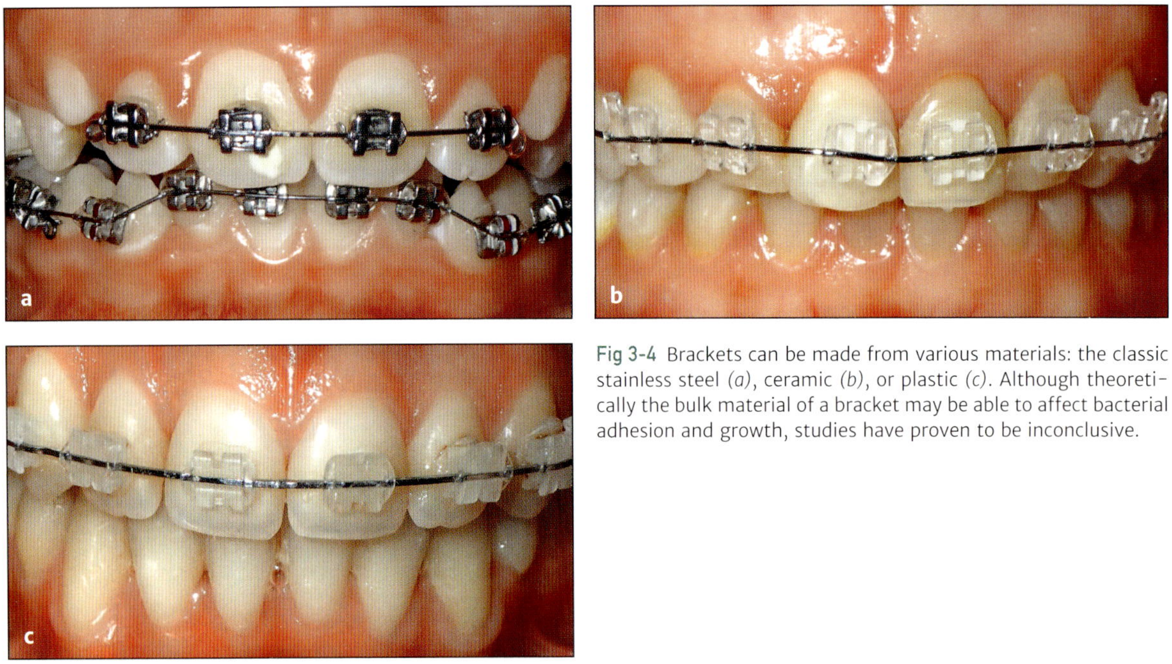

Fig 3-4 Brackets can be made from various materials: the classic stainless steel *(a)*, ceramic *(b)*, or plastic *(c)*. Although theoretically the bulk material of a bracket may be able to affect bacterial adhesion and growth, studies have proven to be inconclusive.

in intimate contact with the enamel surface of the teeth but also with the periodontal tissue. The primary factor regarding plaque accumulation concerns the bulk material of which they are made. Apart from the classic stainless steel, brackets can be made from various ceramic or plastic materials (Fig 3-4). Initial relations with bacteria in the oral cavity are through electrostatic and hydrophobic interactions, where the various characteristics of the surfaces may be a factor. However, studies in the past have shown conflicting results concerning the adherence and biofilm formation of cariogenic bacteria on plastic in comparison to stainless steel or ceramic brackets when the bacteria are allowed to interact with the clean surface.[30,31] In a more recent in vitro study concerning both cariogenic species and periodontopathogens, Papaioannou et al concluded that the bracket material alone had no significant effect on the adhesion of these bacteria.[32,33] Nonetheless, an important factor to consider is that all surfaces in the oral cavity are coated with the salivary, or acquired, pellicle, which will have a great impact on the adhesion of bacteria. This phenomenon occurs very quickly, and the resultant adsorbed film seems to further mitigate any differences in the surface characteristics while at the same time helping to promote the adhesion of bacteria, even on bracket surfaces, and the formation of *P gingivalis* biofilms.[33] This ability of periodontopathogens to form biofilms on bracket surfaces suggests that they may also act as reservoirs for pathogenic organisms.

TYPE OF LIGATION

The type of ligation used in fixed orthodontics—that is, elastomeric or stainless steel ligatures—has also been an important topic of laboratory and clinical research, as these too have been implicated in the accumulation of plaque. In an attempt to minimize the number of bacteria accumulating around brackets, researchers and clinicians have proposed the use of self-ligating brackets. These brackets were first introduced in the 1980s and are presented as having two important advantages over the classic bracket design: *(1)* They do not require the use of elastic or wire ligatures, and *(2)* they help to improve oral hygiene in that their design does not facilitate the retention of dental plaque.

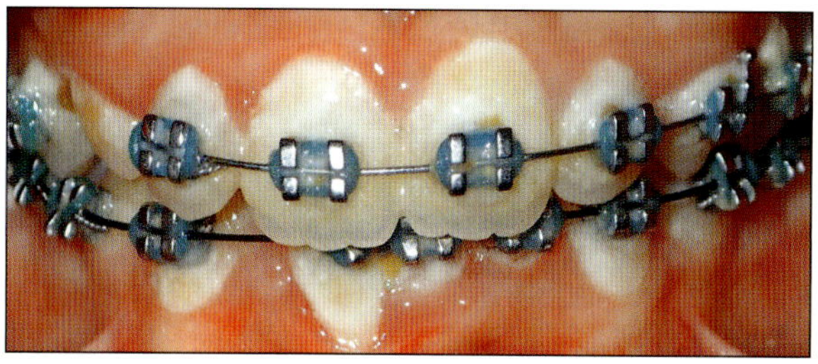

Fig 3-5 Clinical situation of a case with elastic ligatures and inadequate oral hygiene. High levels of plaque accumulation are present with a concomitant increase in gingival inflammation and enamel demineralization.

Brackets with elastic ligatures (Fig 3-5) have been found to harbor higher numbers of bacteria than similar sites with wire ligatures.[17] Another study looking at the differences between the two types of ligatures found that elastomeric rings appeared to be more conducive to gingival bleeding, a sign of gingival inflammation, due to their tendency for increased plaque accumulation.[34] These studies suggest that it would be best to avoid elastic ligatures, especially in those patients who struggle with their oral hygiene. The role that ligation in general has on plaque levels remains an open question, and for this reason many researchers suggest simply avoiding their use wherever possible.

While there are studies examining the effect of the use of self-ligating brackets on oral hygiene levels and the microbial load of the oral cavity that indeed suggest they are better than the classic brackets in this respect, overall the results tend to suggest that there is no significant difference between the two types of brackets. Pandis et al[35] found no difference in the numbers of *S mutans* in the saliva of two groups of orthodontic patients, one with self-ligating brackets and the other with conventional brackets with elastomeric ligatures. Similarly, Baka et al[36] found no differences in the plaque cariogenic buildup between the two types of brackets. In addition, there is disagreement regarding the influence of the bracket design on the periodontal condition and presence of periodontopathogens, with a previous study showing a worsening of the situation around self-ligating brackets[37] and a more recent study presenting a more positive outcome for self-ligating brackets compared to conventional brackets.[38] More recently, a systematic review concluded that only nonsignificant differences could be determined between conventional and self-ligating brackets concerning the periodontal status of adolescents undergoing orthodontic treatment.[39]

TYPE OF BONDING MATERIAL

The bonding material used to fixate the orthodontic appliances to the tooth surface can also have an impact on the adhesion and maturation of the plaque biofilm. This can be due to the characteristics of the material itself, primarily the surface roughness, as well as the junction that forms between the tooth surface and the material, factors that protect from removal forces.[40] This would allow the maturation of the biofilm that is necessary for pathogenic organisms to emerge. A promising venue of research is the investigation and modification of dental adhesives used in orthodontic bonding to retain the necessary bonding ability without facilitating the adherence and growth of bacteria.

Glass-ionomer cements can be more advantageous than composite resins in that they have an inherent antibacterial effect, especially toward cariogenic bacteria.[41] In vitro studies have shown this effect to be more potent than that exhibited by other types of bonding cements.[42] However, most cements commercially available have some degree of an antimicrobial effect.[42,43] Further increase in the antimicrobial properties of these cements is attempted by adding bioactive agents or antimicrobials to interfere with bacterial growth and/or attachment. Studies have shown that the addition of nanoparticles of silver reduced biofilm buildup and plaque accumulation around brackets in an in vitro model.[44] Similar results have been seen using antibacterial agents such as quaternary ammonium monomer dimethylaminododecyl methacrylate [45] as well as the more common antibacterial cetylpyridinium chloride (CPC).[46] CPC is a quaternary ammonium compound widely used as an adjunctive antimicrobial, mostly in oral rinses and especially for the prevention of periodontal inflammation.[47]

These studies with "enhanced" cements in orthodontics focus on the effect they may have on the cariogenic plaque bacteria, as enamel demineralization is the primary unwanted effect of plaque buildup around brackets. However, once their effect on biofilm formation is determined, there is no reason not to consider that their antibacterial effect will have a beneficial impact in those cases where the cements find themselves in more intimate contact with the periodontal tissues. Nonetheless, at this point the available clinical data is sparse. In a clinical study with orthodontic patients, Amasyali et al did not find any additional positive effect of using an antibacterial monomer in comparison with a conventional adhesive,[48] either in the clinical periodontal indices or the subgingival plaque composition, over a 6-month period.

Risk Evaluation and Oral Hygiene

In combination with the thorough clinical and radiologic examination that the orthodontic patient undergoes, an oral disease risk evaluation is necessary. This is to identify those patients who are at increased risk for developing dental and/or periodontal disease. Based on the needs and characteristics of each patient, a personalized preventive program is proposed and followed. Naturally, this is based primarily on two basic pillars: *(1)* proper and thorough oral hygiene and *(2)* proper and balanced dietary habits (primarily decreased frequency of sugar consumption).

Oral hygiene instruction and monitoring of its proper implementation is of paramount importance for the orthodontic patient and should be initiated even before the start of treatment. Patients undergoing orthodontic therapy should invest extra time and effort in performing oral hygiene because they comprise a distinct group of high-risk patients for dental disease. Therefore, time must be spent in the initial consultation to fully explain the various aspects of oral health and disease and the methods of oral hygiene that must be used. This of course must be tracked and reinforced in all subsequent consultations. Throughout the various stages of therapy, the level of oral hygiene must be evaluated and proper supplemental information given to the patient.

Conclusion

A common and undisputed observation is that orthodontic therapy does indeed have an impact on plaque accumulation and composition (both at the supragingival and subgingival levels). This can often lead to caries lesions (white spot lesions) as well as gingival inflammation, which is associated with the presence of periodontopathogens both supra- and subgingivally.

A great deal of this can be attributed to two major factors: *(1)* Orthodontic appliances provide protective surfaces for plaque bacteria to adhere to and mature on, shielded from natural removal forces, and *(2)* these same intricate surfaces make effective oral hygiene more difficult to maintain. For these reasons, proper oral hygiene instructions must be provided before and during orthodontic therapy. Moreover, electric toothbrushes may be an effective alternative to manual brushing.[49]

Besides the oral hygiene level, the periodontal condition must also be constantly monitored, especially during active treatment. Gingival inflammation that does occur, especially with increasing severity and swelling, must be treated before orthodontics can continue. Generally, after completion of therapy and removal of appliances, the periodontal and microbial situation reverts to healthy levels. Orthodontic therapy does not inherently increase the risk for severe periodontitis.

References

1. Costerton JW, Lewandowski Z, Caldwell DE, Korber DR, Lappin-Scott HM. Microbial biofilms. Annu Rev Microbiol 1995;49:711–745.
2. Donlan RM, Costerton JW. Biofilms: Survival mechanisms of clinically relevant microorganisms. Clin Microbiol Rev 2002;15:167–193.
3. Marsh PD. Dental plaque as a biofilm and a microbial community—Implications for health and disease. BMC Oral Health 2006;6(suppl 1):S14.
4. Costello EK, Stagaman K, Dethlefsen L, Bohannan BJ, Relman DA. The application of ecological theory toward an understanding of the human microbiome. Science 2012;336:1255–1262.
5. Zaura E, ten Cate JM. Towards understanding oral health. Caries Res 2015;49(suppl 1):55–61.
6. Samaranayake L, Matsubara VH. Normal oral flora and the oral ecosystem. Dent Clin North Am 2017;61:199–215.
7. Marsh PD. Microbial ecology of dental plaque and its significance in health and disease. Adv Dent Res 1994;8:263–271.
8. Hajishengalis G, Lamont RJ. Beyond the red complex and into more complexity: The polymicrobial synergy and dysbiosis (PSD) model of periodontal disease etiology. Mol Oral Microbiol 2012;27:409–419.
9. Xu X, He J, Xue J, et al. Oral cavity contains distinct niches with dynamic microbial communities. Environ Microbiol 2015;17:699–710.
10. Balenseifen JW, Madonia JV. Study of dental plaque in orthodontic patients. J Dent Res 1970;49:320–324.
11. Klukowska M, Bader A, Erbe C, et al. Plaque levels of patients with fixed orthodontic appliances measured by digital plaque image analysis. Am J Orthod Dentofacial Orthop 2011;139:e463–e470.
12. Huser MC, Baehni PC, Lang R. Effects of orthodontic bands on microbiologic and clinical parameters. Am J Orthod Dentofacial Orthop 1990;97:213–218.
13. Rosenbloom RG, Tinanoff N. Salivary *Streptococcus mutans* levels in patients before, during and after orthodontic treatment. Am J Orthod Dentofacial Orthop 1991;100:35–37.
14. Boyd RL. Longitudinal evaluation of a system for self-monitoring plaque control effectiveness in orthodontic patients. J Clin Periodontol 1983;10:380–383.
15. Sanders NL. Evidence-based care in orthodontics and periodontics: A review of the literature. J Am Dent Assoc 1999;130:521–527.
16. Cardoso-Silva C, Barbería E, Ramos Atance JA, Maroto M, Hernández A, García-Godoy F. Microbiological analysis of gingivitis in pediatric patients under orthodontic treatment. Eur J Paediatr Dent 2011;12:210–214.
17. Forsberg CM, Brattström V, Malmberg E, Nord CE. Ligature wires and elastomeric rings: Two methods of ligation, and their association with microbial colonization of *Streptococcus mutans* and lactobacilli. Eur J Orthod 1991;13:416–420.
18. Corbacho de Melo MM, Cardoso MG, Faber J, Sobral A. Risk factors for periodontal changes in adult patients with banded second molars during orthodontic treatment. Angle Orthod 2012;82:224–228.
19. Diedrich P. Periodontal relevance of anterior crowding. J Orofac Orthop 2000;61:69–79.
20. Ristic M, Vlahovic Svabic M, Sasic M, Zelic O. Effects of fixed orthodontic appliances on subgingival microflora. Int J Dent Hyg 2008;6:129–136.
21. Kim K, Heimisdottir K, Gebauer U, Persson GR. Clinical and microbiological findings at sites treated with orthodontic fixed appliances in adolescents. Am J Orthod Dentofacial Orthop 2010;137:223–228.
22. Naranjo AA, Triviño ML, Jaramillo A, Betancourth M, Botero JE. Changes in the subgingival microbiota and periodontal parameters before and 3 months after bracket placement. Am J Orthod Dentofacial Orthop 2006;130:275.e17–22.
23. Thornberg MJ, Riolo CS, Bayirli B, Riolo ML, Van Tubergen EA, Kulbersh R. Periodontal pathogen levels in adolescents before, during, and after fixed orthodontic appliance therapy. Am J Orthod Dentofacial Orthop 2009;135:95–98.
24. Kim SH, Choi DS, Jang I, Cha BK, Jost-Brinkmann PG, Song JS. Microbiologic changes in subgingival plaque before and during the early period of orthodontic treatment. Angle Orthod 2012;82:254–260.
25. Lee SM, Yoo SY, Kim HS, et al. Prevalence of putative periodontopathogens in subgingival dental plaques from gingivitis lesions in Korean orthodontic patients. J Microbiol 2005;43:260–265.
26. Sallum EJ, Nouer DF, Klein MI, et al. Clinical and microbiologic changes after removal of orthodontic appliances. Am J Orthod Dentofacial Orthop 2004;126:363–366.
27. Choi DS, Cha BK, Jost-Brinkmann PG, et al. Microbiologic changes in subgingival plaque after removal of fixed orthodontic appliances. Angle Orthod 2009;79:1149–1155.
28. van Gastel J, Quirynen M, Teughels W, Coucke W, Carels C. Longitudinal changes in microbiology and clinical periodontal parameters after removal of fixed orthodontic appliances. Eur J Orthod 2011;33:15–21.
29. Speer C, Pelz K, Hopfenmüller W, Holtgrave EA. Investigations on the influencing of the subgingival microflora in chronic periodontitis. A study in adult patients during fixed appliance therapy. J Orofac Orthop 2004;65:34–47.
30. Fournier A, Payant L, Bouclin R. Adherence of *Streptococcus mutans* to orthodontic brackets. Am J Orthod Dentofacial Orthop 1998;114:414–417.
31. Ahn SJ, Lim BS, Yang HC, Chang YI. Quantitative analysis of the adhesion of cariogenic streptococci to orthodontic metal brackets. Angle Orthod 2005;75:666–671.
32. Papaioannou W, Gizani S, Nassika M, Kontou E, Nakou M. Adhesion of *Streptococcus mutans* to different types of brackets. Angle Orthod 2007;77:1090–1095.

33. Papaioannou W, Panagopoulos A, Koletsi-Kounari H, Kontou E, Makou M. Adhesion of *Porphyromonas gingivalis* and biofilm formation on different types of orthodontic brackets. Int J Dent 2012;2012:471380.
34. Türkkahraman H, Sayin MO, Bozkurt FY, Yetkin Z, Kaya S, Onal S. Archwire ligation techniques, microbial colonization, and periodontal status in orthodontically treated patients. Angle Orthod 2005;75:231–236.
35. Pandis N, Papaioannou W, Kontou E, Nakou M, Makou M, Eliades T. Salivary *Streptococcus mutans* levels in patients with conventional and self-ligating brackets. Eur J Orthod 2010;32:94–99.
36. Baka ZM, Basciftci FA, Arslan U. Effects of 2 bracket and ligation types on plaque retention: A quantitative microbiologic analysis with real-time polymerase chain reaction. Am J Orthod Dentofacial Orthop 2013;144:260–267.
37. van Gastel J, Quirynen M, Teughels W, Coucke W, Carels C. Influence of bracket design on microbial and periodontal parameters in vivo. J Clin Periodontol 2007;34:423–431.
38. Nalçacı R, Özat Y, Çokakoğlu S, Türkkahraman H, Önal S, Kaya S. Effect of bracket type on halitosis, periodontal status, and microbial colonization. Angle Orthod 2014;84:479–485.
39. Arnold S, Koletsi D, Patcas R, Eliades T. The effect of bracket ligation on the periodontal status of adolescents undergoing orthodontic treatment. A systematic review and meta-analysis. J Dent 2016;54:13–24.
40. Quirynen M, Bollen CM. The influence of surface roughness and surface-free energy on supra- and sub-gingival plaque formation in man. A review of the literature. J Clin Periodontol 1995;22:1–14.
41. Hallgren A, Oliveby A, Twetman S. Caries associated microflora in plaque from orthodontic appliances retained with glass ionomer cement. Scand J Dent Res 1992; 100:140–143.
42. Matalon S, Slutzky H, Weiss EI. Antibacterial properties of orthodontic cements. Am J Orthod Dentofacial Orthop 2005;127:56–63.
43. Vokus RP, Cisneros GJ, Levi M. Antibacterial properties of current orthodontic cements. Pediatr Dent 1998;20:43–48.
44. Wang X, Wang B, Wang Y. Antibacterial orthodontic cement to combat biofilm and white spot lesions. Am J Orthod Dentofacial Orthop 2015;148:974–981.
45. Melo MA, Wu J, Weir MD, Xu HH. Novel antibacterial orthodontic cement containing quaternary ammonium monomer dimethylaminododecyl methacrylate. J Dent 2014;42:1193–1201.
46. Al-Musallam TA, Evans CA, Drummond JL, Matasa C, Wu CD. Antimicrobial properties of an orthodontic adhesive combined with cetylpyridinium chloride. Am J Orthod Dentofacial Orthop 2006;129:245–251.
47. Teng F, He T, Huang S, et al. Cetylpyridinium chloride mouth rinses alleviate experimental gingivitis by inhibiting dental plaque maturation. Int J Oral Sci 2016; 8:182–190.
48. Amasyali M, Enhos S, Uysal T, Saygun I, Kilic A, Bedir O. Effect of a self-etching adhesive containing an antibacterial monomer on clinical periodontal parameters and subgingival microbiologic composition in orthodontic patients. Am J Orthod Dentofacial Orthop 2011;140:e147–e153.
49. Silvestrini Biavati A, Gastaldo L, Dessì M, Silvestrini Biavati F, Migliorati M. Manual orthodontic vs. oscillating-rotating electric toothbrush in orthodontic patients: A randomised clinical trial. Eur J Paediatr Dent 2010;11:200–202.

CHAPTER 4

Pellicle Organization and Plaque Accumulation on Biomaterials

George Eliades
Theodore Eliades

Parts of this text were previously published in Dental Materials in Vivo: Aging and Related Phenomena *(Quintessence, 2005) and are reprinted with permission.*

When a biomaterial is exposed to a biologic system, organization of a noncellular acquired biofilm rapidly occurs on the biomaterial surface by spontaneous adsorption of extracellular macromolecules composed of glycoproteins and proteoglycans.[1] These films induce a conditioning effect that modifies the biomaterial surface properties and alters both the response of the subsequently attached cells and the interactions occurring at the biomaterial-host interface.[2,3] This conditioning effect is based on the differing capacities of artificial surfaces to fractionate proteins from biologic fluids, such as saliva or blood, and the ability to induce conformation and orientation changes of adsorbed proteins.[4,5]

The outcome of biofilm adsorption is dependent on the biologic fluid flow rate at the site of contact, the type of interfacial interactions involved, and the attachment strength with the substrate. Under static conditions or low flow rates, the biomaterial surface chemistry is the fundamental factor affecting the composition and organization of acquired biofilms, whereas in environments with high flow rates, substrate surface molecular motion and roughness are also important factors. In addition, when there are long exposure periods, material properties such as porosity, sorption, corrosion, and biodegradation may further modify the biomaterial-host interactions.[6] Lastly, the attachment strength of biofilms formed on biomaterial surfaces has been found capable of regulating the vitality of the contact. In cases where there is continuous adsorption/desorption of biomolecules from an artificial surface, conformational changes in the desorbed biomolecules may trigger a biochemical response from structures that are not in physical contact with the surface.[7]

The bioadhesive activity of biofilms in the biologic environment depends mainly on the composition and surface reactivity of the outer monolayers. It has been proposed that, when strong bioadhesion is required, the biomaterial surface should demonstrate a critical surface tension in the range of 30 to 40 dyn/cm, with a high proportion of polar interactive sites. In contrast, when minimal bioadhesion is sought, materials with critical surface tension of 20 to 30 dyn/cm and reduced polar sites should be chosen.[8] In the first situation, following biofilm formation, the critical surface tension may still be within the bioadhesive range, and the biofilms formed will be dense and more coherent; the conformationally changed macromolecules present will promote cell attachment. On the other hand, in surfaces of low critical surface tension, the biofilms developed are looser and more easily detached under flowing conditions; the macromolecules formed have a more native conformation and retain fewer microorganisms.[9,10]

The biofilm maturation process may induce differences in the film quality and self-organization states. However, in the absence of inhibitors, biofilm maturation may also result in calcification of the adsorbed species, either by contact activation and thrombosis on surfaces conducting blood[11] or by nonspecific ectopic calcification through nucleation of calcium phosphates on macromolecular charged groups having particular stereochemical geometry.[12,13]

Once adsorption equilibrium is established between the surfaces involved, the long-term performance of biofilms at biomaterial-host interfaces seems capable of not only influencing the cell attachment and proliferation but also in many cases modulating the phenotypic expression of attached cells and consequently the potential of interfacial tissue remodeling.

The purpose of this chapter is to review the general aspects of development and maturation of biofilms formed on biomaterial surfaces in relation to the biologic environment. This approach is intended to facilitate understanding of the complex mechanisms involved in the in vivo aging phenomena discussed in the following chapters, which eventually control the clinically functional or nonfunctional character of a biomaterial and modulate the response of tissues to orthodontic materials.

Biomaterial Surface Properties

A common definition of the term *surface* is a boundary defined by the outer atomic layer, which separates a bulk solid from an adjacent phase. However, a more realistic approach is to consider the surface as a region of variable depth and having a degree of flexibility dependent on the nature of the material.[14]

Material surfaces should be considered special states of matter with unique chemistry, organization, dynamics, and electrical properties. The major differences between surface and bulk structures arise from the direct accessibility of surface molecules for reaction with adjacent phases and the tendency for surface energy minimization to reach an equilibrium state, as mediated by the rearrangement of chemical groups, additive migration, and spontaneous adsorption of low-energy layers from the environment.[15] The effective depth of the biologically important region of biomaterials involved in interactions with protein functional groups is usually considered to be the outermost layer extending 10 nm into the material. Nevertheless, the near-surface region of 0.1 to 10 μm plays a significant role as well, as it is involved in corrosion, biodegradation, controlled release, and cell contact guidance phenomena. The biomaterial properties that influence the biologic response by selectively promoting interfacial interactions are shown in Fig 4-1 and are discussed in the following sections.

SUBSTRATE DEFINITION

The molecular and elemental composition of biomaterial surfaces is considered the determinant factor of the early response of the biologic environment. The polar or nonpolar nature, the hydrogen bonding capacity, and the electron donor or acceptor potential

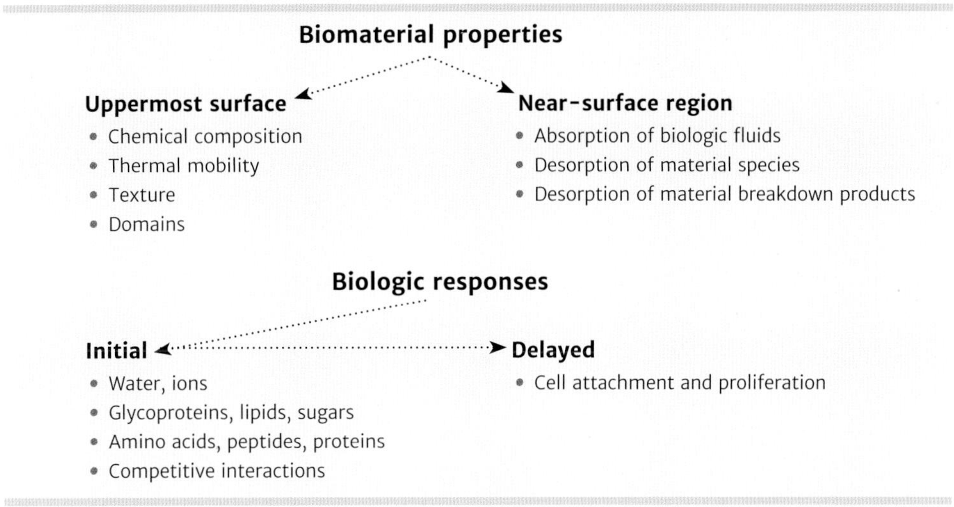

Fig 4-1 Important biomaterial surface properties and biologic responses.

seem to control the hydrophilic or hydrophobic character and the energetic state of the surfaces. In addition, surface electrical properties, such as the zeta and streaming potentials and surface charges, are also involved in interfacial interactions with biologic fluids and living cells.[16]

Surface thermal mobility is found with materials having very low elastic modulus, such as polymers in the colloidal state or soft-chain segments of hard polymers, where the majority of the material or specific regions may demonstrate active Brownian motion (ie, random particle motion in a fluid). These molecular regions are permeable to small molecules capable of modifying the conformation of biologic fluids by steric or fluctuation forces, and they demonstrate less adsorption energy. Surface mobility correlates with the degree of crystallinity; it has been well established that rigid solid crystalline phases demonstrate higher adsorption energy compared to amorphous phases, with some exceptions found for materials exposed to high flow rates.[17]

Surface texture incorporates both ultrastructural and macroscopic features, and on an ultrastructural scale, vacancies, other structural imperfections, gas entrapment, and adsorbed layers alter the surface composition. Macroscopically, surface roughness and porosity interfere with the biologic fluid flow rate by producing secondary fluid motions of enhanced or reduced shear locally, which at high flow rates may affect the shape, distribution, and aggregation of the attaching particles. At low flow rates or under static conditions, the grooves of rough surfaces may act as stagnation points, thereby promoting biofilm maturation.[18]

Because most surfaces are heterogenous at a microscopic level, the regional surface distribution of the foregoing properties may produce domains with different characteristics, inducing a variable biologic response.

SUBSTRATE MODIFICATION

The biologic responses to biomaterial surfaces (see Fig 4-1) involve a great variety of chemical species. A time sequence of the phenomena occurring on biomaterial surfaces placed in a biologic environment has been described based on experimental data and logical hypotheses[19] (Fig 4-2).

Initially, on a nanosecond scale, a water monolayer binds to a biomaterial surface by either oxygen or hydrogen bonding. Some water molecules may dissociate to hydroxyl groups, which may form

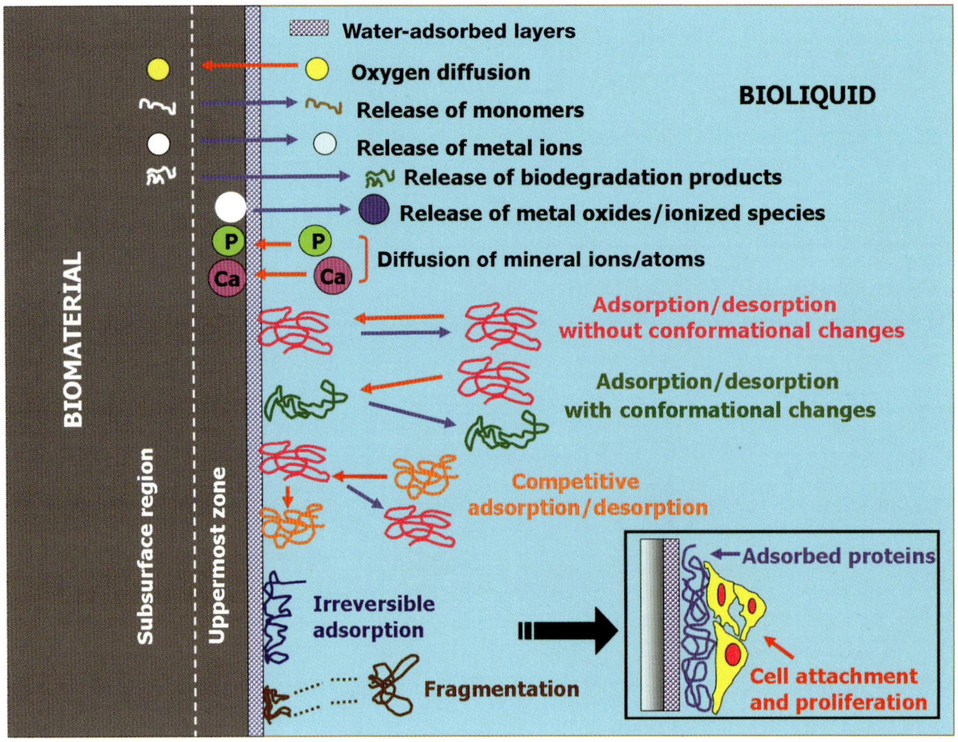

Fig 4-2 Schematic representation of the possible interactions occurring at biomaterial surfaces exposed to a biologic environment.

surface hydroxyls. Then, a second water layer binds to the first monolayer. The orientation and density of water molecules in the first adsorbed monolayer may regulate the overall hydration state of the surface, because the unique properties of water offer a wide spectrum of solvation forces in aqueous systems. On hydrophilic surfaces, for example, to which water molecules bind strongly, repulsive hydration (long-range) and steric (short-range) forces are generated when two such surfaces come in contact because of the energy required to dehydrate the surfaces; these forces are controlled by the presence of cations or pH. On hydrophobic surfaces, on the other hand, the orientation of water molecules toward the surfaces is entropically unfavorable. Thus, in the event that two such surfaces approach each other, water is ejected into the bulk solution, reducing the total free energy of the system and establishing attractive long-range hydrophobic forces between the two surfaces.[20] These phenomena are of paramount importance for biologic systems and control protein adsorption, which proceeds by nonspecific physicochemical interactions with the water- and ion-modified biomaterial surfaces.

Protein adsorption is initiated within a few milliseconds after contact with biologic fluids. The protein layers adsorbed are complex and may vary depending on the nature of the surface. In an aqueous environment, the interaction between hydrophilic surfaces with strongly attached water molecules and hydrated protein cores is weak because of the development of hydrophilic repulsive forces. Thus, on hydrated surfaces, hydrophobic and electrostatic interactions are expected to govern protein adsorption. Heavily charged macromolecules are probably the first species to be adsorbed; however, the first protein adsorbed does not determine the potential for attachment and the overall response at later stages.

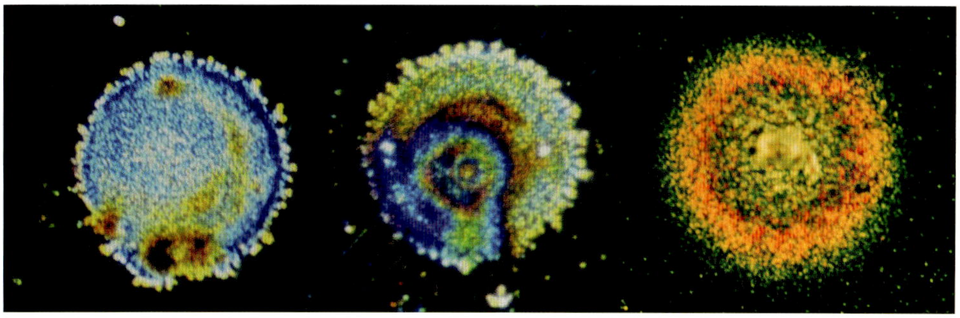

Fig 4-3 Protein adsorption on germanium minicrystals placed intraorally for 10, 30, and 60 minutes, respectively *(left to right)*. Note crystal growth at the center of the 60-minute specimen (darkfield reflected light microscopy; original magnification ×400).

In most situations, competitive adsorption occurs, with rapidly decreasing protein affinity accompanying increasing surface occupancy. The result is a sequential adsorption/desorption process and exchange of proteins on surfaces, a phenomenon known as the *Vroman effect*.[21] The adsorption/desorption sequence of proteins is not distinct because all proteins are adsorbed simultaneously at different rates and displacement occurs according to their binding affinity; the latter is associated with the spreading capacity and the energy required to denature the proteins in the solution.[22]

Proteins with high carbohydrate content and relatively uniform atomic distribution around the molecule show increased solubility, conformational stability, and minimal adsorption on hydrophobic and negatively charged surfaces, attributed to the carbohydrate shielding effect. However, when carbohydrate groups are localized, the protective effect diminishes. Lipoproteins comprise another important group having preferential adsorption on hydrophobic surfaces, especially on those possessing thermal mobility. It seems that lipid phase transition at body temperature and denaturing reactions control the adsorption process.

At protein adsorption equilibrium, biomaterial surfaces are dominated by high–molecular weight proteins. These proteins demonstrate a great number of statistical contact points in a denaturable or conformational labile state and are readily capable of interacting with the interfacial microenvironment.[22]

Adsorbed proteins may induce crystalline formation onto chemical groups of their structure that fulfill the stereochemical and surface charge requirements for crystal nucleation. If these conditions apply within a range sufficient for crystal nucleus stabilization and growth at a defined spatial orientation, then crystal growth occurs. Extracellular noncollagenous proteins are believed to be the principal components regulating crystal growth. Protein-induced mineralization in the oral environment proceeds by initial formation of potassium chloride (KCl) crystals,[23] while calcium phosphate precipitation may take place at later stages (Fig 4-3). This mode of extracellular mineralization is involved in the formation of ectopic calcified deposits on tissues and materials, including teeth, dental materials, acetabular components of hip-joint arthroplasty, and bioprosthetic valves.

CELL ATTACHMENT AND ORGANIZATION

Cell attachment onto biomaterial surfaces is a fundamental biologic process underlying numerous homeostatic functions in living organisms, as it coordinates and integrates cellular differentiation, shape, movement, and biosynthetic activity.[24] The process of cell approach to a biofilm-modified biomaterial surface requires considerably more time than that of protein adsorption and may be classified into three groups, depending on the distance between the two elements involved. The first group relates to the far-distance effects (>100 nm), the second group incorporates the intermediate-distance effects (20 to 100 nm), and the third group is controlled by the short-distance effects (<20 nm).[25]

At far distances exceeding 100 nm, cell movement is controlled by fluid dynamics and chemotaxis, which compete with repulsion forces of electrostatic origin, as both acquired protein films and cells are mostly negatively charged. At intermediate distances between 20 and 100 nm, the effect of fluid dynamic forces is reduced, and the overall response leading to the occurrence or absence of cell attachment is determined by the competitive action of van der Waals attraction, electrical repulsion, and water solvation forces. Lastly, at short distances of less than 20 nm, cell attachment occurs by nonspecific and specific bonding mechanisms.[24] The latter involve signaling transaction to cell-surface binding proteins or activation of specific transmembrane receptors, like integrins. Of particular importance is the role of heparan sulfate proteoglycans, which participate in many cellular events such as focal contacts and modification of the extracellular matrix, where they serve as reservoirs for growth factors and cytokines. Receptor mobility, cell deformability, biofluid ionic strength, and osmotic tendency of water play important roles as well. The initial cell-substrate and cell-cell contact is small. At equilibrium, a balance is set between thermodynamics and intra-aggregating factors by maximizing the number of bonds and minimizing the surface area of contact.[25] Apparently, any change in the surface-adsorbed protein composition during the lifetime of a biomaterial may lead to utilization of different cell adhesion receptors, thus altering cell behavior. This is especially important for implantable devices, where an array of reactions related to tissue inflammatory response, activation of wound-healing mechanisms, and tissue remodeling takes place. The presence of inflammatory cells at the interface initiates secondary reactions on a biomaterial surface and the surrounding cell population by secretion of proteins, enzymes, and oxidizing agents, as well as the production of oxygen radicals.[26] These agents may change the biomaterial surface reactivity by either altering the types of proteins adsorbed onto the original surface or by affecting the structure of this surface. The most common mechanisms of structural biomaterial modifications by biologic fluids involve the near-surface regions (see Fig 4-1). In general, these mechanisms may be subdivided into three groups: *(1)* the absorption of biologic species; *(2)* the desorption of ions, monomers, additives, and impurities; and *(3)* the release of breakdown products due to corrosion, wear, or enzymatic attack.

Production of wear debris at tissue-implant interfaces activates foreign-body granulomatous reactions and release of active proinflammatory substances implicated in pathologic procedures and tissue remodeling. The composition, size, and shape of the biomaterial particles released modulate the cell and tissue responses. Moreover, uptake of metals from cells and charge carrier species may affect cell differentiation and regulation of gene expression.[24] As time proceeds, the intermediate bioliquid region diminishes, and the biomaterial comes in closer contact with the tissue. At this point, cell differentiation and regulation depend on tissue vascularity and implant stability, as in skeletal tissue repair, where the distortional and hydrostatic cell strains produced at a tissue–mobile implant interface may result in fibrous growth rather than the desired osseous tissue formation.[27] The same mechanism may be responsible for the synovium-like structures developed around artificial joints.

Surface roughness may also contribute to the strength of cell and tissue attachment with the substrate. For certain types of cells, variations in substrate roughness may influence cell locomotion by contact guidance phenomena. These responses have been assigned to mechanical restrictions imposed on the formation of cell microfilament bundles at cell focal points. Contact guidance may modify the secretory and proliferative activities of cells.[28] Moreover, the surface roughness of the biomaterial may have important consequences for the tissue and biomechanical response to implants.

The basic principles of biomaterial-host interactions as reviewed above are susceptible to regional variations, which are dependent on the dynamic activity of biologic fluids and the nature of tissue response. The following discussion focuses on the interactions of dental biomaterials with saliva, soft tissues, and bone.

Saliva-Coated Biomaterials

The intraoral biofilm formed naturally on teeth and restorative materials is dental plaque, a diverse community of bacteria embedded in an organic matrix preventing colonization by exogenous microorganisms.[29] Plaque development sequentially involves formation of a conditioning film (acquired pellicle), early microbial colonization, maturation, and late colonization, leading to a dynamic equilibrium. In cases of major shifts in equilibrium, disease of hard and soft dental tissue occurs.[29,30]

The significance of surface properties on intraoral biofilm formation was realized decades ago by Glantz,[31] who for the first time introduced the analytical methodology used for traditional surface chemistry to study the surface reactivity of teeth and restorative materials. From that time, systematic efforts have been undertaken to investigate the interaction pathways of hard dental tissues and restorative materials with saliva in order to understand the interfacial phenomena involved and to achieve regulation of the complex saliva-substrate interactions.

The experimental approach used in most of these studies has been investigation of the effect of the substrate surface properties on pellicle composition, microorganism colonization, and plaque maturation.

EFFECT OF BIOMATERIAL SURFACE PROPERTIES ON PELLICLE FORMATION

Any natural or artificial surface exposed in the oral cavity will be covered within seconds by a noncellular salivary biofilm rich in acidic proteins and lipids known as *acquired pellicle*.[32,33] Pellicle has a major role in intraoral physiologic functions:

- It is a permeability barrier for ionic or macromolecular transport between surfaces and the intraoral environment.[34]
- It may act as a lubricating agent to reduce mechanical friction.[35]
- It reduces bacterial colonization by minimizing their interfacial free energy of adhesion with the substrate.[36]
- It may promote attachment of specific bacteria strains.[37]

Pellicle formation involves selective protein adsorption, employing nonspecific electrostatic and hydrophobic interactions and protein conformational changes, and it is affected by saliva flow rate and pH.[38] It has been proposed that pellicle development proceeds through three phases.[39] Initially, low-molecular weight phosphoproteins are adsorbed at a high rate, producing a tightly bound layer. Then competitive interactions take place mainly between phosphoproteins and low-molecular weight glycoproteins, creating a second, less tightly bound layer. Finally, high-molecular weight glycoproteins are adsorbed, forming a third, loosely bound layer. On enamel, the rapid pellicle adsorption period ends within 30 minutes, while the time required for adsorption equilibrium has been estimated at 90 minutes.[40,41]

Pellicle demonstrates a micellar structure, composed of negatively charged globular clusters 20 to 300 nm in diameter stabilized by calcium ions. Upon maturation, the globular structure is replaced by a homogenous layer, possibly as a result of proteolytic activity. The composition of pellicle varies on surfaces with different characteristics. Enamel

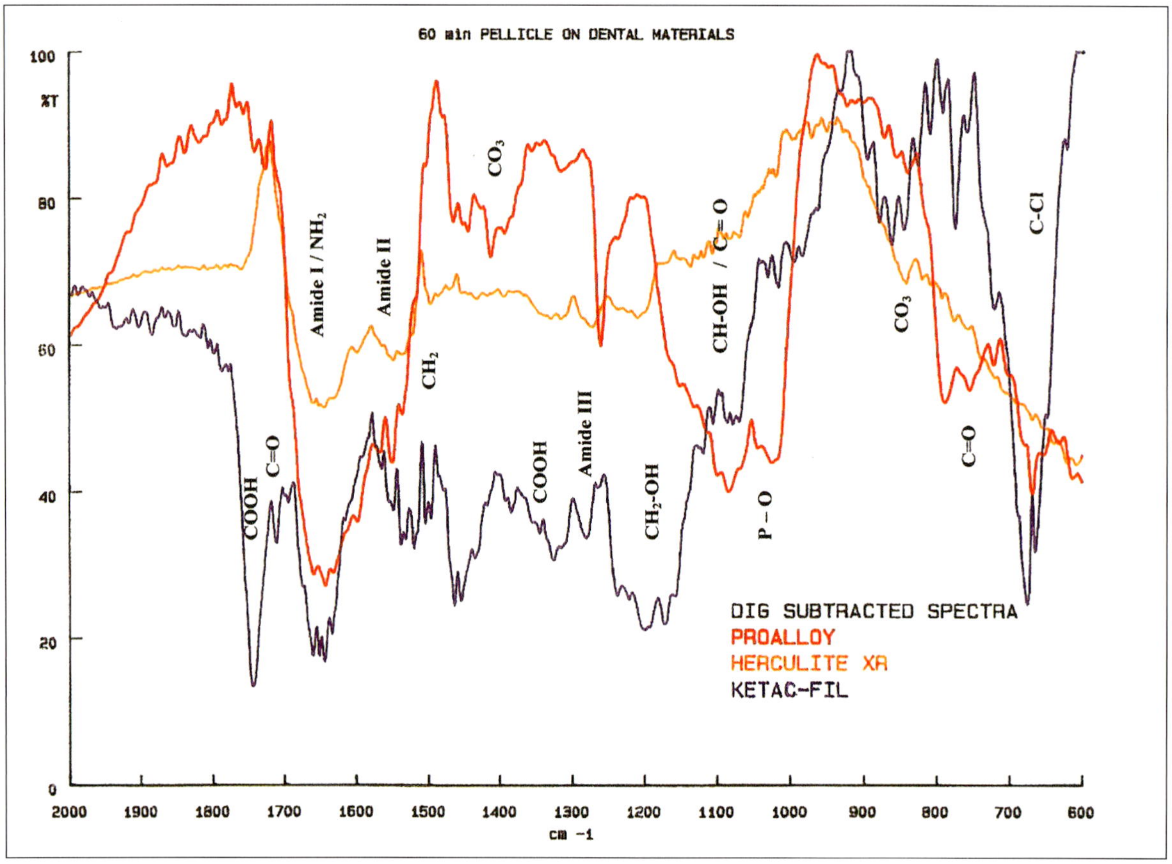

Fig 4-4 A micro multiple internal reflectance FTIR spectra showing different compositions of pellicles formed on amalgam (Proalloy, DMP Dental), resin composite (Herculite XR, Kerr), and glass-ionomer (Ketac Fil, 3M ESPE) surfaces after 60-minute simultaneous exposure of the restorative materials in the same intraoral conditions. Spectra were acquired from material surfaces and then subjected to digital subtraction interpretation to remove original material and water interferences. Note the complex profile of the adsorbed species on the hydrophilic surfaces of amalgam and glass-ionomer in comparison with the hydrophobic resin composite surface.

pellicle contains considerably higher amounts of the acidic proline proteins cysteine and lysozyme relative to cementum pellicle.[42] Extensive in vivo studies performed on pellicle formation on surfaces with well-defined characteristics, including composition, roughness, and critical surface tension, have documented that the amino acid composition[43] and packing distribution, as well as the pellicle configuration, may vary substantially.[44–46] In these studies, even though the same amount of protein was adsorbed on high- and low-energy surfaces during pellicle formation, films were found to have greater thickness and be more loosely bound on low-energy surfaces. These differences in pellicle composition and organization may reflect an inherent biologic response, where all intraorally exposed solid surfaces are transformed to the same state of bioadhesiveness.[47]

Despite the extensive study of pellicle formation on reference materials, there is a scarcity of information on pellicle composition, interaction, and organization in relation to restorative materials. Experiments employing chemical characterization techniques, which were conducted on pellicles formed in vivo on various dental materials, revealed significant differences in composition[48–52] (Fig 4-4). A transmission electron microscopy investigation of in vivo pellicle formation on a variety of restorative

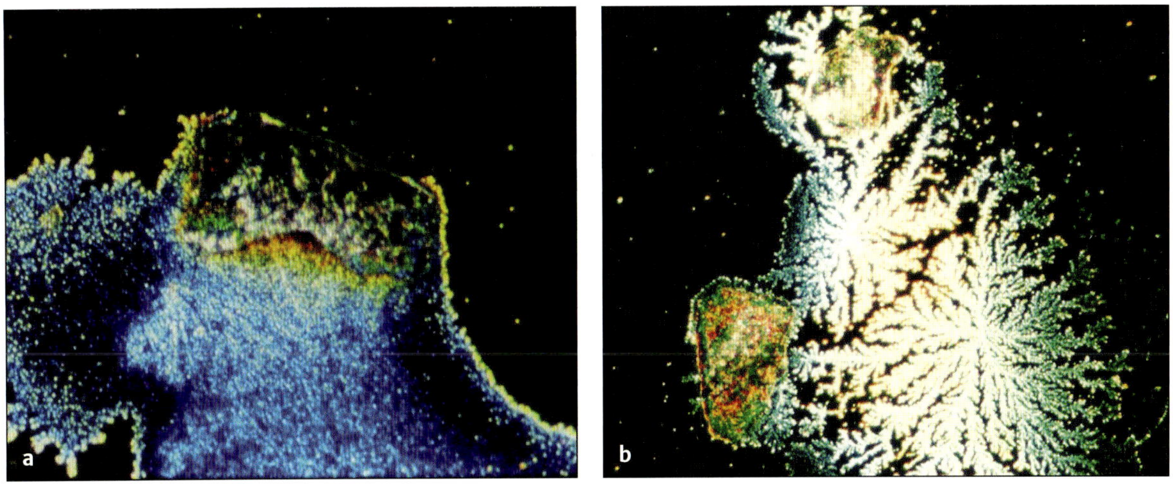

Fig 4-5 Pellicle formed on germanium microcrystals after 90-minute intraoral exposure before *(a)* and after *(b)* sucrose intake. Note the excessive bacterial colonization, dendritic aggregation, and pronounced crystal growth on surface-charged sites after sucrose intake (darkfield reflected light microscopy; original magnification ×300).

materials revealed no ultrastructural differences, implying that the initially absorbed protein layer effectively masked the substrate surface properties.[53] Nonetheless, a recent in vitro study of pellicle formation on flat and unpolished surfaces of glass-ionomer and resin composite restoratives showed that more bacteria-binding proteins (agglutinins, proline-rich proteins, and mucins) were recovered from the pellicle adjacent to the glass ionomer.[54] These findings suggest that indeed pellicle demonstrates a "memory" effect of the substrate surface properties, as mediated by the surface-protein interactions.

EFFECT OF BIOMATERIAL PROPERTIES ON PLAQUE FORMATION

Early microbial colonization of acquired pellicle (Fig 4-5) involves nonspecific forces that transfer microorganisms close to the substrate in order to establish specific bonding.[55] During this phase, the detachment shear forces (originating from salivary flow, buccal and lingual tongue movements, as well as hard food) and the surface energetic state of the substrate, as modified by pellicle, are the main factors controlling microorganism retention rate.[56] Interactions of different microbial species and strains in the bioliquid (coaggregation) or with surface-attached microorganisms (coadhesion), release of biosurfactants, production of extracellular matrix polymers, and various competitive reactions are considered important factors for formation and rapid growth of plaque.[55] After 18 to 48 hours in vivo, an equilibrium is reached, with plaque organized in cell microcolonies entrapped in a dense polysaccharide-based matrix interspersed by water channels.[57,58]

The plaque retention capacity of restorative materials has long been recognized as a major factor influencing oral health status, and efforts have been undertaken to design materials with minimal plaque growth potential. The important role of substrate surface roughness and surface free energy on in vivo plaque formation has been demonstrated in a series of studies on surfaces with well-defined characteristics. These studies showed that at supragingival regions the contribution of roughness is greater than that of the surface energy state, whereas at subgingival regions surface roughness is the determinant factor.[59] The mechanism of roughness implication on plaque formation arises from the generation of flow stagnation points on surface irregularities (ie, pores,

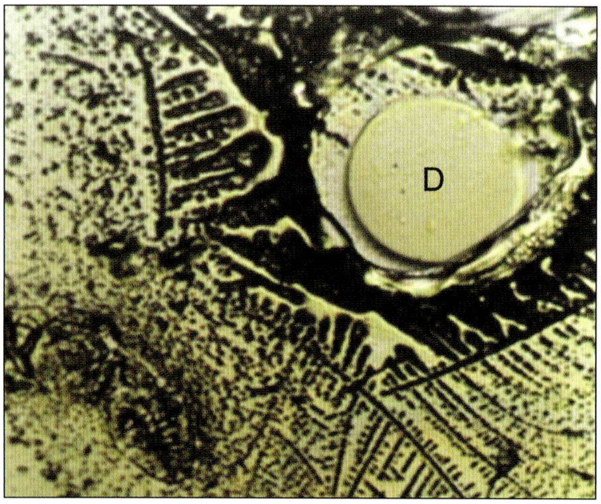

Fig 4-6 Reflected light microscopic image of the plaque developed around a defect (D) on a resin composite surface after 90 minutes of intraoral exposure. Note the thicker dendritic microbial aggregation around the protruding edges of the defect (original magnification ×250).

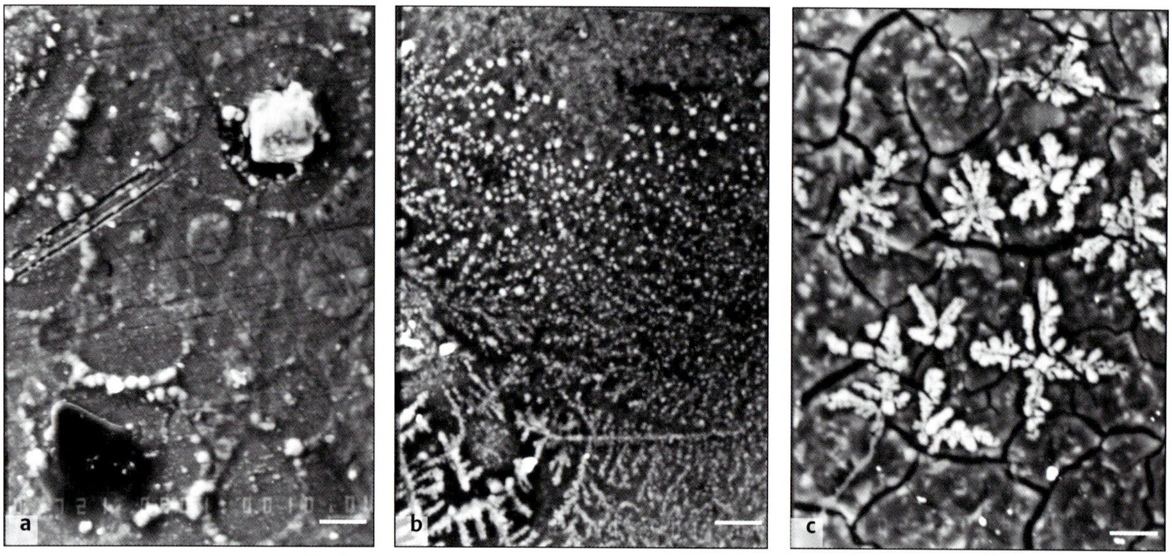

Fig 4-7 Atomic number contrast backscattered scanning electron microscopy images of the dental plaque developed on amalgam *(a)*, resin composite *(b)*, and glass-ionomer *(c)* restorative materials after 90 minutes of intraoral exposure. On the amalgam surface, crystal growth is prominent for high (white, *top*, calcium-rich) and low (gray, *bottom*, potassium-rich) mean atomic number. Bacterial colonization is apparent on the composite and glass-ionomer surfaces, with the latter being more mature (bar = 10 μm).

grooves, cracks, and scratches), which promote cell attachment, although the response of individual bacteria biofilms on rough substrates may vary[60] (Fig 4-6). Moreover, it has been documented that on low-energy (hydrophobic) surfaces, the surface area of plaque accumulation is less than that on high-energy (hydrophilic) surfaces[10] (Fig 4-7). Four possible explanations may be given for this finding:

1. The microbial binding strength is lower on low-energy surfaces.
2. High–surface energy microorganisms bind with high-energy surfaces, and vice versa. Because most of the bacteria found in human dental plaque have high surface energy,[61] colonization on low–surface energy regions is limited.

3. The surface energy regulates the cohesive strength of pellicle films against the shear detachment forces; thus, on low-energy surfaces, films with low cohesive strength are formed.
4. The increased surface area and decreased protruding height of well-spread cells may produce a geometry offering decreased flow resistance.

A limited number of in vivo studies are available where such interactions between dental materials and developing plaque have been documented.[49,50,62] However, there are in vivo studies illustrating the absence of any major structural and bacteriologic differences in the early plaque formed on various dental materials.[63–65] This finding may suggest that plaque formation is predominantly influenced by the oral environment rather than the type of substrate.[65] Nevertheless, such a mechanism fails to explain the low plaque retention clinically experienced with several materials (ie, porcelain and other ceramics).[66] Many in vitro plaque formation experiments, involving saliva incubation on dental material surfaces, have been performed as well, leading to contradictory conclusions. The results of these studies should be interpreted with caution, because shear force gradients are missing, and the pellicles formed contain more intact protein species than those developed under in vivo conditions.[67] It seems that some material surface properties are transferred through pellicle to plaque, but the detailed mechanism is not yet fully understood.[68]

At long intraoral exposure periods, the phenomena occurring at plaque-material interfaces become more complex through interactions at the near-surface region, including release of ions, monomers, and biodegradation and fretting corrosion products, which may reorganize interfacial protein adsorption and subsequently new plaque. These interactions proceed at higher rates in regions where pellicle and plaque are continuously renewed, thus establishing a more aggressive environment.[69] Of particular importance is the role of pellicle and plaque on the selective release of material species demonstrating therapeutic effect, such as fluoride. The rate of such ion-exchange interactions is strongly reduced in the presence of these natural intraoral integuments.[70]

EFFECT OF BIOMATERIAL SURFACE PROPERTIES ON CALCULUS, ORGANIC DEPOSITS, AND STAINS

Mature plaque calcification and calculus formation involve calcium and phosphate uptake from the oral environment, supersaturation, and crystal nucleation and growth. It is believed that pellicle and plaque calcification proceed only after enzymatic deactivation of certain inhibitors, such as saliva phosphoproteins and pyrophosphate, noncollagenous components including proteoglycans, and plaque lipoteichoic acid.[55,71] Plaque calcification begins at extracellular regions with deposition of the soluble calcium phosphates: octacalcium phosphate and dicalcium phosphate dihydrate. Upon maturation, carbonated hydroxyapatite and magnesium-substituted β-tricalcium phosphate are additionally formed. This structure is organized in needle-, rod-, and platelike crystals that form layers separated by organic-rich material resembling pellicle.[71]

Information on the composition of intraoral calculus on dental materials is rather limited. On denture resin polymers, the inorganic part of denture calculus is composed of carbonated hydroxyapatite and magnesium-substituted β-tricalcium phosphate.[72,73] Studies on orthodontic wires and elastomers showed that mineral deposition initially occurs by formation of KCl microcrystallites on adsorbed biofilms, followed by precipitation of calcium phosphates.[74,75] On dental alloys, the cathodic protection offered by cationic saliva corrosion inhibitors has a determinant effect on calculus formation and may explain the common clinical observation that, in patients with poor oral health, calculus is more frequently formed on gold than on amalgam.[76] For composite resins and glass ionomers, no information exists. However, the contribution of surface roughness in creating salivary flow stagnation points and biofilm calcification on composite resins has been documented in an in vivo study.[50]

On denture polymers, accumulation of amorphous dark and yellow color deposits has been observed, in addition to the presence of calculus, after prolonged intraoral exposure.[77] These deposits are strongly attached and removed only by sodium hypochlorite (NaOCl) solutions. Chemical analysis revealed that the deposit composition was different from calculus and contained much more organic material. The surface extent of these deposits did not correlate with the surface roughness of the substrate but was strongly influenced by the water absorption properties of these polymers, suggesting the role of diffusion-driven phenomena.

Extrinsic staining of dental alloys is a common observation and has been associated[76] with the surface interactions of certain elements in the alloys with thiol groups of biologic origin, resulting in the formation of nonsoluble products. With the advent of esthetic restorative materials, their surface resistance to extrinsic staining has become an important issue. Surface texture and surface free energy are considered to control the complex mechanisms for staining of tooth-colored restorative materials in the oral environment. Generally, although rough surfaces are more susceptible to staining, there are cases where the surface energetic effect overwhelms that of roughness. For example, resin composites containing acid-modified monomers (compomers), while having the same surface roughness characteristics as conventional resin composites, exhibited more staining that extended to a greater depth. This was attributed to the presence of hydrophilic carboxyl groups on the compomers and their slow neutralization rate in the oral environment.[78]

Particular importance should be given to the commonly used antiseptics and mouthrinses, because they greatly contribute to surface staining by interacting either with plaque and pellicle or with the restorative material surfaces.[79]

References

1. Baier RE. On the formation of biological films. Swed Dent J 1977;1:261–271.
2. Baier RE. Selected methods of investigation of blood-contact surfaces. Ann N Y Acad Sci 1987;516:68–77.
3. Schakenraad JM, Noordmans J, Wildevuur CRH, Arends J, Busscher JH. The effect of protein adsorption on substratum surface free energy, infrared adsorption and cell spreading. Biofuling 1986;1:193–201.
4. Schakenraad JM, Busscher HJ, Wildevuur CRH, Arends J. The influence of substrate surface free energy on growth and spreading of human fibroblasts in the presence and absence of serum proteins. J Biomed Mater Res 1989;20:773–784.
5. Chittur KR. Surface techniques to examine the biomaterial-host interface: An introduction to the papers. Biomaterials 1998;19:301–305.
6. Hoffman A. Modification of material surfaces to affect how they interact with blood. Ann N Y Acad Sci 1987;516:96–101.
7. Kasemo B, Lausmaa J. Biomaterials from a surface science perspective. In: Ratner BD (ed). Surface Characterization of Biomaterials, Progress in Biomedical Engineering, vol 6. Amsterdam: Elsevier; 1988:1–12.
8. Baier RE, Meyer AE, Natiella JR, Natiella PR, Carter JM. Surface properties determine bioadhesive outcomes: Methods and results. J Biomed Mater Res 1984;18:337–355.
9. Baier RE. Surface chemical factors presaging bioadhesive events. Ann N Y Acad Sci 1983;416:34–57.
10. Quirynen M, Marecal M, Busscher HJ, et al. The influence of surface free-energy on planimetric plaque growth in man. J Dent Res 1989;68:796–799.
11. Colman RW, Scott CF, Schmaier AH, Wachtfogel YT, Pixley RA, Edmunds LH Jr. Initiation of blood coagulation at artificial surfaces. Ann N Y Acad Sci 1987;516:253–267.
12. Addadi L, Weiner S. Interactions between acidic proteins and crystals: Stereochemical requirements for mineralization. Proc Natl Acad Sci 1985;82:4110–4114.
13. Addadi L, Borman A, Moradian O, Idak J, Weiner S. Structural and stereochemical relations between acidic macromolecules of organic matrices and crystals. Connect Tissue Res 1989;21:127–135.
14. Klauber C, Smart RSC. Solid systems. Their structure and composition. In: O'Connor DI, Sexton BA, Smart RStC (ed). Surface Analysis Methods in Materials Science, Springer Series in Surface Sciences, vol 23. Berlin: Springer, 1992:3–65.
15. Ratner BD. The surface characterization of biomaterials: How finely can we resolve surface structure. In: Surface Characterization of Biomaterials, Progress in Biomedical Engineering, vol 6. Amsterdam: Elsevier, 1988:13–36.
16. Davis JE. The importance and measurement of surface charge species in cell behaviour at the biomaterial interface. In: Ratner BD (ed). Surface Characterization of Biomaterials, Progress in Biomedical Engineering, vol 6. Amsterdam: Elsevier, 1988:219–234.
17. Merrill EW. Distinctions and correspondences among surfaces containing blood. Ann N Y Acad Sci 1987;516:196–203.

18. Karino T, Goldsmith HL, Motomiya M, Mabuchi S, Sohara Y. Flow patterns in vessels of simple and complex geometries. Ann N Y Acad Sci 1987;516:422–441.
19. Kasemo B, Lausmaa J. The biomaterial-tissue interface and its analogues in surface science and technology. In: Davies JE (ed). The Bone-Biomaterial Interface. Toronto: University of Toronto, 1991:19–32.
20. Israelachvili J. Intermolecular and Surface Forces, ed 3, San Diego: Academic, 1991:275–286.
21. Brash JL. Studies on protein adsorption to blood compatible materials. In: Missirlis YF, Lemm W (eds). Modern Aspects of Protein Adsorption on Biomaterials. Dordrecht, The Netherlands: Kluwer Academic, 1991:39–47.
22. Andrade JD, Hlady V. Plasma protein adsorption: The big twelve. Ann N Y Acad Sci 1987;516:158–172.
23. Wood SR, Kirkham J, Marsh PD, Shore RC, Nattress B, Robinson C. Architecture of intact natural human plaque biofilms studied by confocal laser scanning microscopy. J Dent Res 2000;79:21–27.
24. Leonard EF, Rahmin I, Angarska JK, Vassilief CS, Ivanov IB. The close approach of cells to surfaces. Ann N Y Acad Sci 1987;516:502–512.
25. Sauk JJ, Van Kampen CL, Somerman MJ. Role of adhesive proteins and integrins in bone and ligament cell behavior at the material surface. In: Davies JE (ed). The Bone-Biomaterial Interface. Toronto: University of Toronto, 1991:111–119.
26. Thomsen P, Ericson LE. Inflammatory cell response to bone implant surfaces. In: Davies JE (ed). The Bone-Biomaterial Interface. Toronto: University of Toronto, 1991:153–164.
27. Carter DR, Giori NJ. Effect of mechanical stress on tissue differentiation in the bony implant bed. In: Davies JE (ed). The Bone-Biomaterial Interface. Toronto: University of Toronto, 1991:367–376.
28. Brunette DM. The effect of surface topography on cell migration and adhesion. In: Ratner BD (ed). Surface Characterization of Biomaterials, Progress in Biomedical Engineering, vol 6. Amsterdam: Elsevier, 1988:203–217.
29. Marsh PD. Host defences and microbial homeostasis: Role of microbial interactions. J Dent Res 1989;68:1567–1575.
30. Gibbons RT. Bacterial adhesion to oral tissues: A model for infection diseases. J Dent Res 1989;68:750–760.
31. Glantz PO. On wettability and adhesiveness. Odontol Revy 1969;20(suppl 17):1–132.
32. Eggen KH, Rölla G. Gel filtration, ion exchange chromatography and chemical analysis of macromolecules present in acquired enamel pellicle (2 hour-pellicle). Scand J Dent Res 1982;90:182–188.
33. Slomiany BL, Murty VLN, Zdebska E, Slomiany A, Gwozdzinski K, Mandel ID. Tooth surface pellicle lipids and their role in the protection of dental enamel against lactic acid diffusion in man. Arch Oral Biol 1986;3:187–191.
34. Tabak LA, Levine MJ, Mandel ID, Ellison SA. Role of salivary mucins in the protection of the oral cavity. J Oral Pathol 1982;11:1–17.
35. Hatton MN, Levine MJ, Margarone JE, Argurre A. Lubrication and viscosity features of human saliva and commercially available saliva substitutes. J Oral Maxillofac Surg 1987;45:496–499.
36. Pratt-Terpstra IH, Weerkamp AH, Busscher HJ. Microbial factors in a thermodynamic approach of oral streptococcal adhesion to solid substrata. J Colloid Interface Sci 1989;129:568–574.
37. Pratt-Terpstra IH, Weerkamp AH, Busscher HJ. The effects of pellicle formation on streptococcal adhesion to enamel and artificial substrata with various surface free energies. J Dent Res 1989;68:463–467.
38. Vassilakos N. Some Biophysical Aspects of Salivary Film Formation [doctoral dissertation]. Malmo, Sweden: Graphic Systems AB, 1992.
39. Embery G, Hogg SD, Heaney TG, Stanbuty JB, Green RDJ. Some considerations on dental pellicle formation and early bacterial colonization: The role of high and low molecular weight proteins of the major and minor salivary glands. In: Leach SA, Arends J (eds). Bacterial Adhesion and Preventive Dentistry. Oxford: IRL, 1984:73–84.
40. Kuboki Y, Teraoka K, Okada S. X-ray photoelectron spectroscopic studies of the adsorption of salivary constituents on enamel. J Dent Res 1987;66:1016–1019.
41. Rölla G, Rykke M, Gaare D. The role of acquired enamel pellicle in calculus formation. Adv Dent Res 1995;9:403–409.
42. Ruan MS, Paola C, Mandel I. Quantitative immunochemistry of salivary proteins in vitro to enamel and cementum from caries resistant and caries susceptible human adults. Arch Oral Biol 1986;31:597–601.
43. Sönju T, Glantz PO. Chemical composition of salivary integuments formed in vivo on solids with some established surface characteristics. Arch Oral Biol 1975;20: 687–691.
44. Baier RE, Glantz PO. Characterization of oral in vivo films formed on different types of solid samples. Acta Odontol Scand 1978;76:289–301.
45. Glantz PO. Adhesion to the surfaces of teeth. In: Leach SA (ed). Dental Plaque and Surface Interactions in the Oral Cavity. Oxford: IRL, 1980:49–64.
46. Glantz PO, Baier RE, Christersson CE. Biochemical and physiological considerations for modeling biofilms in the oral cavity: A review. Dent Mater 1996:12:208–214.
47. Jendresen MD, Glantz PO. Clinical adhesiveness of selected dental materials. An in-vivo study. Acta Odontol Scand 1981:39:39–45.
48. Sönju T, Skjörland K. Pellicle composition and initial bacterial colonization on composite and amalgam in vivo. In: Stiles HM, Loesche WJ, O'Brien TC (eds). Microbial Aspects of Dental Caries. Oxford: IRL, 1976:133–141.
49. Skjörland K. Auger analysis of the integuments formed on different dental materials in vivo. Acta Odontol Scand 1982;40:129–134.
50. Palaghias G, Eliades G. Characterization of oral films adsorbed on surfaces of dental materials in vivo [abstract 668]. J Dent Res 1992;71:599.
51. Eliades T, Eliades G, Brantley W. Microbial attachment on orthodontic appliances. I. Wettability and early pellicle formation on bracket materials. Am J Orthod Dentofacial Orthop 1995;108:351–360.
52. Lee SJ, Kho HS, Lee SW, Yong WS. Experimental salivary pellicles on the surface of orthodontic materials. Am J Orthod Dentofacial Orthop 2001;119:59–66.
53. Hannig M. Transmission electron microscopic study of in vivo pellicle formation on dental restorative materials. Eur J Oral Sci 1977;105:422–433.

54. Carlen A, Nikdel K, Wennerberg A, Holmberg K, Olsson J. Surface characteristics and in vitro biofilm formation on glass ionomer and composite resin. Biomaterials 2001;22:481–487.
55. Busscher HJ, Van der Mei HC. Physico-chemical interactions on initial microbial adhesion and relevance for biofilm formation. Adv Dent Res 1977;11:24–32.
56. Christersson CE, Dunford RG, Glantz PO, Baier RE. Effect of critical surface tension on retention of oral microorganisms. Scand J Dent Res 1989;97:247–256.
57. Bowden GMW, Li YH. Nutritional influences on biofilm development. Adv Dent Res 1997;11:81–99.
58. Vasin M, Rosanova J, Sevastianov V. The role of proteins in the nucleation and formation of calcium-containing deposits on biomaterial surfaces. J Biomed Mater Res 1998:39:491–497.
59. Quirynen M, Marechal M, Busscher HJ, Weerkamp AH, Darius PL, Van Steenberghe D. The influence of surface free energy and surface roughness on early plaque formation. J Clin Periodontol 1990;17:138–144.
60. Yamauchi M, Yamamoto K, Wakabayashi M, Kawano J. In vitro adherence of microorganisms to denture base resin with different surface texture. Dent Mater J 1990;9:19–24.
61. Weerkamp AH, Quirynen M, Marechal M, Van der Mei HC, Van Steenberghe D, Busscher HJ. The role of surface energy in the early in vivo formation of dental plaque on human enamel and polymeric substrata. Microb Ecol Health Disease 1989;2:11–18.
62. Skjörland KK, Sönju T. Effect of sucrose rinses on bacterial colonization on amalgam and composite. Acta Odontol Scand 1982;40:193–196.
63. Siegrist BE, Brecx MC, Gusberti FA, Joss A, Lang NP. In vivo early human dental plaque formation on different supporting substances. A scanning electron microscopic and bacteriological study. Clin Oral Implant Res 1991;2:38–46.
64. Leonhardt Å, Olsson J, Dahlén G. Bacterial colonization on titanium, hydroxyapatite and amalgam surfaces in vivo. J Dent Res 1995;74:321–326.
65. Hannig M. Transmission electron microscopy of early plaque formation on dental materials. Eur J Oral Sci 1999;107:55–64.
66. Hahn R, Weiger R, Netuschil L, Bruch M. Microbial accumulation and vitality on different restorative materials. Dent Mater 1993;9:312–316.
67. Yao Y, Grogan J, Zehnder M, et al. Compositional analysis of human acquired enamel pellicle by mass spectrometry. Arch Oral Biol 2001;46:293–303.
68. Quirynen M, Bollen CML. The influence of surface roughness and surface-free energy on supra- and subgingival plaque formation in man. J Clin Periodontol 1995;22:1–14.
69. Jenkins GN. The Physiology and Biochemistry of the Mouth, ed 4. Oxford: Blackwell, 1978:486–487.
70. Eliades G. Chemical and biological properties of glass-ionomer cements. In: Davidson CL, Mjör IA (eds). Advances in Glass-Ionomer Cements. Chicago: Quintessence, 1999:85–101.
71. White DJ. Dental calculus: Recent insights on occurrence, formation, prevention, removal and oral health effects of supragingival and subgingival deposits. Eur J Oral Sci 1997;105:508–522.
72. Hayashi Y. High resolution electron microscopy of the interface between dental calculus and denture resin. Scanning Microsc 1995;9:419–427.
73. Gaffar A, LeGeros RJ, Gambogi RJ, Afflitto J. Inhibition of formation of calcium phosphate deposits on teeth and dental materials: Recent advances. Adv Dent Res 1995;9:419–426.
74. Eliades T, Eliades G, Watts DC. Structural conformation of in vitro and in vivo aged orthodontic elastomeric modules. Eur J Orthod 1999;21:649–658.
75. Eliades T, Eliades G, Athanasiou AE, Bradley TG. Surface characterization of retrieved NiTi orthodontic archwires. Eur J Orthod 2000;22:317–326.
76. Palaghias G. Oral corrosion and corrosion inhibition processes—an in vitro study. Swed Dent J Suppl 1985;30:1–72.
77. Zanghellini G, Dykman AG, Reinberger V, Arends J. Deposit formation on prosthetic materials in vivo after one year: A quantitative study of twelve materials. Adv Dent Res 1995;9:443–449.
78. Addy M, Moran J. Mechanisms of stain formation on teeth, in particular associated with metal ions and antiseptics. Adv Dent Res 1995;9:450–456.
79. Steflik DE, McKinney RV Jr. Epithelial attachment to ceramic dental implants. Ann N Y Acad Sci 1988;523:4–18.

SECTION II

Periodontal Considerations for the Orthodontic Patient

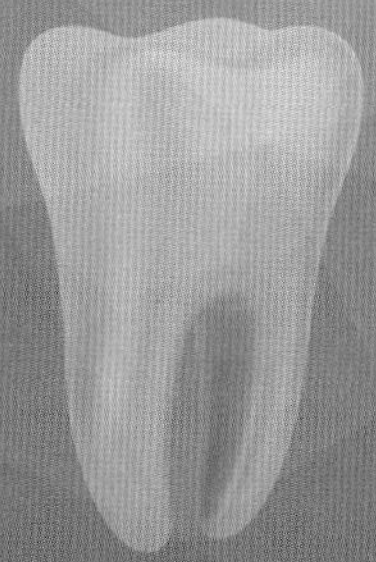

CHAPTER 5

Periodontal Examination of the Orthodontic Patient

Giovanni E. Salvi
Christoph A. Ramseier

Periodontal diseases represent inflammatory conditions initiated by oral biofilms. From a clinical point of view, redness and swelling of the gingiva as well as increased probing depths with tendency to bleeding on probing (BoP) are common characteristics of patients suffering from periodontitis. Advanced periodontitis may also be associated with gingival recessions, increased tooth mobility, and flaring of teeth. Moreover, periodontitis may be recognized in radiographs by moderate to severe loss of alveolar bone. Based on the fact that periodontitis includes gingival inflammation and progressive loss of periodontal attachment and alveolar bone, a comprehensive examination must include assessments describing such pathologic changes.

Outcomes from studies in humans have indicated that elimination of the biofilm infection and institution of plaque-control regimens result in periodontal health in most, if not all, cases. This condition forms the basis for further correction, including orthodontic therapy.

Comprehensive planning and treatment of patients with periodontal diseases and problems such as tooth malpositioning and migration should include the following:

1. A systemic phase with a smoking cessation program, if necessary
2. An initial phase of periodontal therapy
3. A corrective phase of therapy including orthodontic therapy
4. A maintenance phase including supportive periodontal care

Treatment Goals

A treatment strategy including elimination of the bacterial infection must be defined and followed. In this context, the following clinical parameters should be reached at the end of active periodontal therapy:

- Reduction of periodontal tissue inflammation as measured by BoP. A full-mouth mean BoP $\leq$ 25 % should be achieved.[1]
- Reduction in probing pocket depth (PPD) measured in millimeters. Absence of residual pockets with PPD $>$ 5 mm should be achieved.[1]
- Control of furcation involvement of multirooted teeth not exceeding grade 1.[2]
- Absence of pain and discomfort.

Following active periodontal therapy, the patient has to be enrolled in a regular supportive periodontal therapy program.[3]

Patient History and Systemic Phase

Assessment of the patient's periodontal and orthodontic problems requires an evaluation of the following aspects: chief complaint, medical history with concomitant medication(s), social and family history, dental history, oral hygiene habits, and smoking history and counseling. Prior to the initial periodontal examination, a health questionnaire should be filled out by the patient in order to immediately capture medical risk factors affecting treatment. The four major categories of medical complications encountered in patients undergoing dental treatment may be prevented by checking the medical history with respect to cardiovascular diseases, bleeding disorders, infective risks, and allergic reactions. If indicated, referral to a physician or specialist should be made to take appropriate preventive measures.

Assessment of the family history with respect to periodontal problems may also be important in order to diagnose aggressive forms of periodontitis with a hereditary component. However, based on current knowledge, it is premature to recommend a systematic genetic screening of patients with periodontal diseases and candidates for orthodontic therapy.

With respect to dental history, symptoms of periodontitis noticed by the patient such as tooth migration, increasing tooth mobility, bleeding gingiva while eating or brushing, and impaired chewing function have to be explored. Information on the patient's oral hygiene routine should also be collected, including frequency and duration of daily brushing with a manual or electric toothbrush as well as the use of interproximal cleansing devices or additional chemical agents.

Second to inadequate oral hygiene, cigarette smoking has been identified as the most important risk factor in the etiology and pathogenesis of periodontal diseases.[4,5] Therefore, in every patient, the history of tobacco use (eg, the current smoking status) must be recorded. For patients with regular tobacco use, brief interventions have to be provided in order to encourage smokers to enroll in a smoking cessation program.

Initial Phase

Following completion of a comprehensive periodontal examination, an initial phase of periodontal therapy should be conducted. This initial phase is also called *cause-related therapy*. The goal of this phase is to achieve infection-free conditions in the oral cavity through removal of all supra- and subgingival soft and hard deposits and their retentive factors (eg, root remnants, caries lesions, overhanging fillings, and reconstructions). Moreover, following individualized instructions, the patient should be motivated to perform optimal plaque control.

Repeated plaque score recordings are indicated during the initial phase of periodontal therapy (ie, infection control) and are used for the improvement of self-performed plaque control.[6]

At the end of the healing time following the initial phase (ie, 3 to 6 months), re-evaluation with a periodontal chart helps to determine the needs for additional and supportive therapies.

Corrective Phase

The need for additional therapy in the corrective phase is assessed following evaluation of the success of the initial phase. The main goal of the corrective phase is to address the sequelae of periodontal tissue destruction, and this phase includes therapies such as periodontal and implant surgery and prosthetic reconstruction.

If patient compliance is unsatisfactory, it may not be worth initiating corrective treatment procedures as they will not lead to a final improvement of periodontal health. This is supported by the outcomes of studies indicating that surgical periodontal procedures performed in patients with proper plaque control result in gain of periodontal attachment and alveolar bone, whereas periodontal surgery performed in plaque-infected dentitions may yield additional periodontal tissue destruction.[7–11]

Moreover, in patients who are candidates for dental implants, implant placement should be initiated only following the completion of successful periodontal therapy.[12]

Maintenance Phase

The aim of this phase of periodontal treatment is the prevention of reinfection and disease recurrence. During the maintenance phase, repeated assessments of clinical periodontal parameters have to be conducted. These include the assessment of residual PPD ≥ 5 mm, BoP and suppuration around teeth and implants, and the evaluation of furcation involvement. Repeated BoP recordings are recommended during the maintenance phase in order to assess periodontal stability.[13,14] It is established that self-performed plaque control combined with regular attendance of maintenance care visits following active periodontal treatment represented an effective means of controlling gingivitis and periodontitis and limiting tooth mortality over a 30-year period.[3]

It is important to emphasize that the maintenance care program must be designed to meet the individual needs of the patient. According to a periodontal risk assessment performed after completion of active therapy, some patients should be recalled every 3 months, while others may need to be checked only once a year.[15]

At the various recall visits, the following procedures should be carried out:

- Update of the medical and smoking history
- Oral examination as a cancer screening
- Recording of the full-mouth PPD ≥ 5 mm with concomitant BoP
- Reinstrumentation of bleeding sites with PPD ≥ 5 mm
- Polishing and fluoridation for caries prevention

Moreover, regular control of prosthetic reconstructions with respect to loss of retention and tooth vitality is mandatory based on the fact that loss of vitality represents a frequent complication following abutment tooth preparation.[16–18] Finally, periapical radiographs should be incorporated at regular intervals in order to detect initial interproximal caries.

Comprehensive Periodontal Examination

BASIC PERIODONTAL EXAMINATION

With every new patient, a basic periodontal examination (BPE) has to be conducted to screen for periodontal conditions and to facilitate treatment planning. The aim of the BPE is to identify patients with periodontal health, gingivitis, or periodontitis.[19] The screening of each tooth or implant is evaluated with the use of a periodontal probe. At least two sites per tooth or implant (ie, mesiobuccal and distobuccal) are probed using a light force (ie, 0.2 N) in each sextant of the dentition. The highest score in each sextant is used.

BPE scores

- Score 0: PPD ≤ 3 mm, BoP negative, absence of calculus or overhanging fillings
- Score 1: PPD ≤ 3 mm, BoP positive, absence of calculus or overhanging fillings
- Score 2: PPD ≤ 3 mm, BoP positive, presence of supra- and/or subgingival calculus and/or overhangs
- Score 3: PPD 4 to 5 mm
- Score 4: PPD ≥ 6 mm

If a single site with a PPD ≥ 6 mm is identified within a sextant, the entire sextant receives a score of 4, and no further measurement in this particular sextant is needed. The highest BPE score in any of the sextants determines the patient's overall BPE score.

Patients with BPE scores of 0, 1, or 2 belong to the periodontally healthy or gingivitis group, respectively. Patients exhibiting a sextant with BPE scores of 3 or 4 belong to the periodontitis group and should undergo a comprehensive periodontal examination.

PERIODONTAL CHARTING

The comprehensive periodontal examination is carried out by performing a full-mouth periodontal charting. This examination includes measurement of the following parameters at six sites around each tooth or implant:

- PPD
- BoP
- Clinical attachment level (CAL)
- Furcation involvement
- Tooth mobility
- Plaque index

PPD

The PPD represents the distance from the gingival margin to the bottom of the periodontal pocket and is measured by means of a graduated periodontal probe.

PPDs of 1 to 3 mm are indicated in black, while PPDs ≥ 4 mm are marked in red. This allows an immediate recognition of diseased sites in terms of both extent and severity.

BoP

If bleeding is provoked following gentle probing, the site examined is considered BoP positive and hence inflamed.

Clinical attachment level

Clinical assessment of the CAL requires measurement of the distance from the gingival margin (GM) to the cementoenamel junction (CEJ) for each tooth surface. Following the recording of these measurements, the CAL is calculated by adding the PPD to this distance. In cases with gingival recession, the distance from GM to CEJ is negative.

Furcation involvement

A detailed identification of the presence and extent of periodontal tissue destruction in the furcation area is of importance for proper diagnosis and treatment. Involvement is recorded from all furcation entrances of multirooted teeth (ie, mandibular molars, maxillary molars, and premolars). Furcation involvement is explored using a curved probe with a 3-mm graduation.

Classification of furcation involvement according to Hamp et al[20] is as follows:

- Grade 0: Furcation entrance is not detectible with the furcation probe
- Grade 1: Horizontal probing depth ≤ 3 mm
- Grade 2: Horizontal probing depth > 3 mm
- Grade 3: Open furcation (ie, "through-and-through" destruction of the supporting tissues in the furcation area)

Tooth mobility

Increased tooth mobility may be classified according to Miller[21] as the following:

- Degree 0: "Physiologic" mobility of the tooth
- Degree 1: Increased mobility of the tooth < 1 mm in horizontal direction
- Degree 2: Visually increased mobility of the tooth > 1 mm in horizontal direction
- Degree 3: Mobility of the tooth both in horizontal and vertical directions

Plaque index

In conjunction with the comprehensive periodontal examination, the patient's oral hygiene practices must be evaluated. Absence or presence of plaque on each tooth or implant surface in the dentition is recorded in a dichotomous manner.[6] The bacterial deposits are stained with a disclosing solution, facilitating their detection, and subsequently recorded.

MICROBIOLOGIC ANALYSIS

Subgingival bacterial samples for microbiologic analysis may be collected in a standardized manner from the deepest sites in each quadrant before and after the phases of periodontal therapy.

RADIOGRAPHIC ASSESSMENT

The radiographic assessment by means of periapical or panoramic radiographs provides information on both height and configuration of the interproximal bone level. Analysis of the radiographs allows the extent of horizontal and/or angular (vertical) bony defects to be estimated.

For periodontal diagnostic purposes, it is important to visualize the interdental alveolar bone height. Hence, periapical radiographs taken with a long-cone paralleling technique are recommended.[22]

PHOTOGRAPHIC STATUS AND STUDY CASTS

Following the aforementioned clinical and radiographic examinations, a photographic status and study casts of the patient may be made to complete the comprehensive periodontal examination.

PRETHERAPEUTIC SINGLE-TOOTH PROGNOSIS

Based on the results of the clinical and radiographic examination, a pretherapeutic prognosis for each tooth can be made. The following three questions may be addressed with respect to the pretherapeutic prognosis:

- Which tooth is secure?
- Which tooth is doubtful?
- Which tooth is irrational to treat?

The goal of this classification is to identify doubtful teeth before therapy and to change their prognosis to that of secure teeth. Teeth with a doubtful pretherapeutic periodontal prognosis may be identified on the basis of the following criteria:

- Furcation involvement grades 2 and 3
- Angular (ie, vertical) bony defects
- Horizontal bone loss affecting more than two-thirds of the root

Based on the comprehensive periodontal examination and pretherapeutic prognosis presented above, a diagnosis is made that will indicate how to carry out cause-related and additional periodontal treatment. Repeated examinations of the periodontal patient will have to be performed prior to and following orthodontic therapy.

In the section that follows, a case presentation illustrates the various phases of comprehensive treatment, including the periodontal re-evaluations to assess further treatment needs.

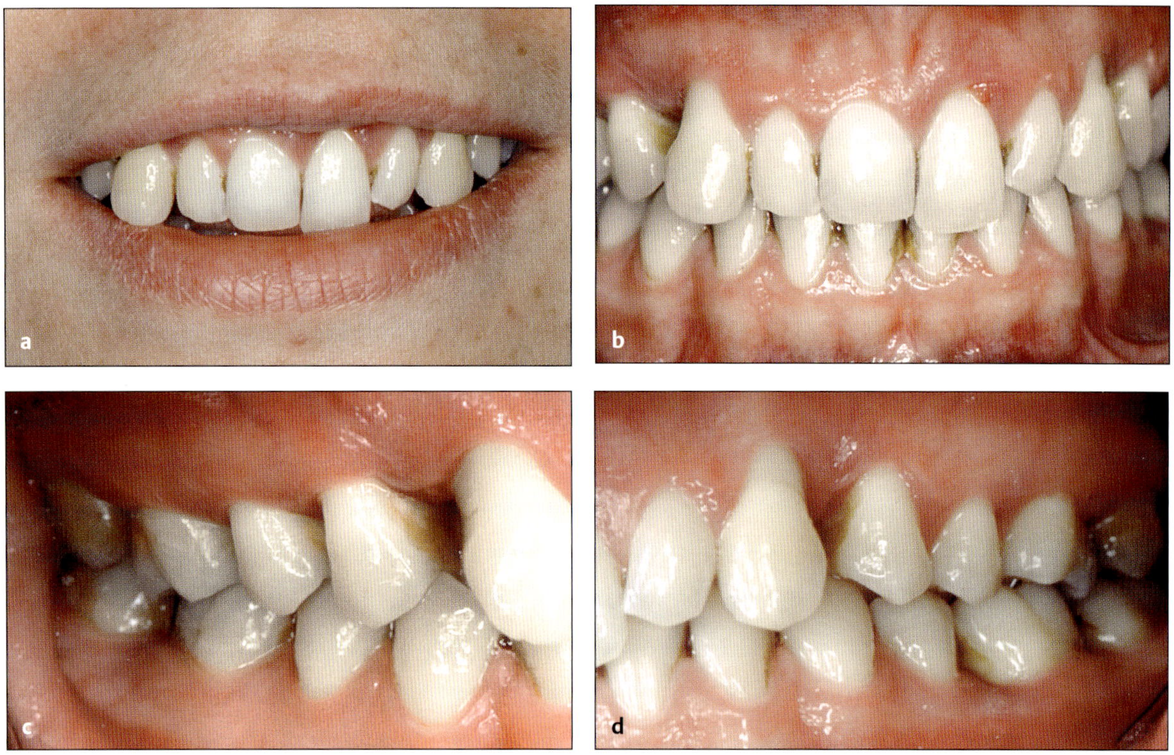

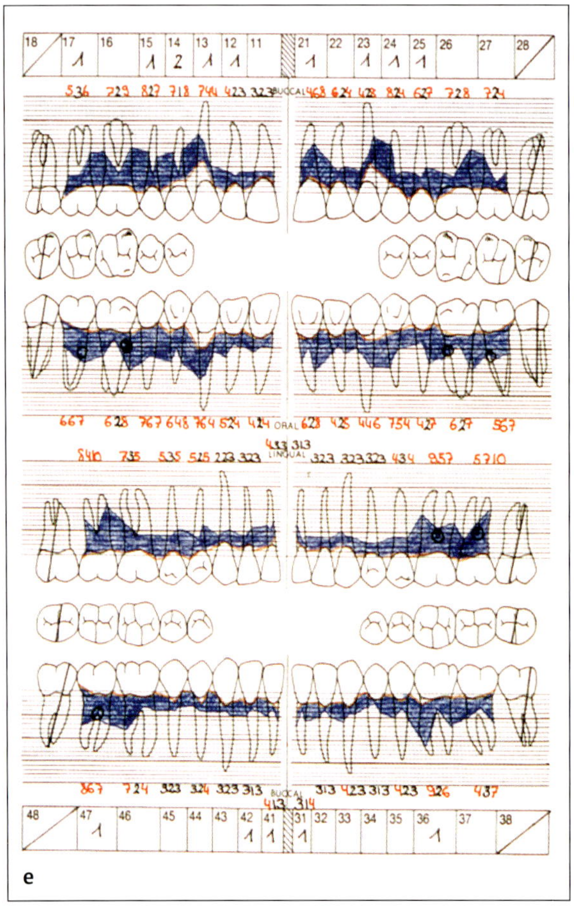

Fig 5-1 *(a to d)* Baseline smile line and clinical characteristics of the dentition. *(e)* Baseline periodontal chart. →

Case Presentation

CHIEF COMPLAINT AND BPE

A 27-year-old systemically healthy and nonsmoking woman was referred for periodontal therapy. She complained about esthetics in the maxillary anterior area, increased tooth mobility, and bleeding gingiva (Figs 5-1a to 5-1d). The baseline periodontal chart revealed generalized increased probing depths, furcation involvement, and increased tooth mobility (Fig 5-1e). The baseline periapical radiographic status revealed generalized horizontal bone loss and localized advanced bony defects at teeth 14, 15, 23, 36, and 47 (Fig 5-1f).

DIAGNOSIS

The patient was diagnosed with generalized aggressive periodontitis with furcation involvement and caries.

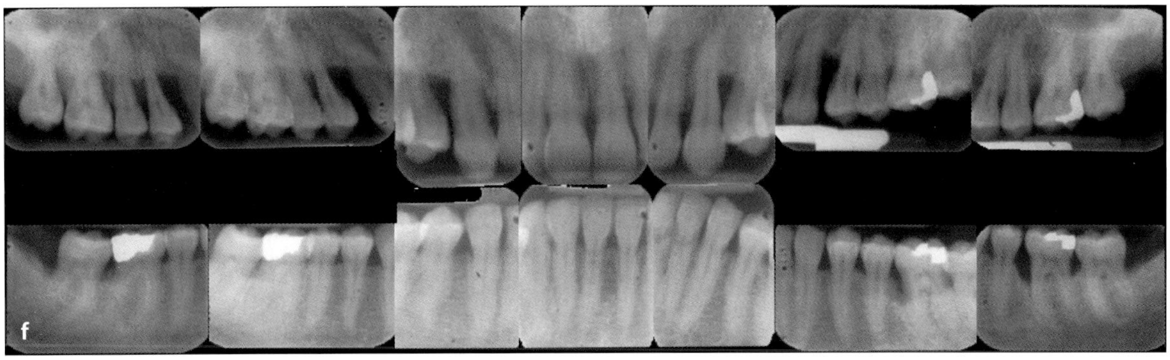

Fig 5-1f Baseline radiographs of the patient. →

TREATMENT SEQUENCE

Systemic phase

Based on the fact that the patient was systemically healthy and a nonsmoker, no medical examination or smoking cessation counseling was required.

Initial phase

The following actions were taken to treat the bacterial infection:

- Patient motivation to improve oral hygiene measures and subsequent assessments and reinstructions
- Subgingival mechanical debridement under local anesthesia
- Treatment of caries lesions at teeth 16 and 26
- Endodontic treatment of tooth 46

Re-evaluation after initial phase

Eight weeks following initial periodontal therapy, a re-evaluation of the patient's periodontal conditions was performed (Figs 5-1g to 5-1j). The results of this re-evaluation built the basis for additional corrective measures. Following completion of cause-related therapy, the patient was enrolled in a recall system aimed at preventing the recurrence of periodontitis.

Corrective phase

Based on the fact that low plaque and BoP scores (ie, 5% to 10%) were present, the corrective phase included periodontal surgery by means of open flap debridement in the maxillary left and right quadrants as well as in the mandibular molar regions (Figs 5-1k to 5-1m). Guided tissue regeneration by means of a resorbable barrier membrane was performed at the mesial aspect of tooth 36. Following completion of periodontal surgery, a re-evaluation including a periodontal chart was performed (Figs 5-1n to 5-1p).

Orthodontic therapy was performed in the maxillary anterior area to correct tooth malpositioning and improve the esthetic appearance (Figs 5-1q to 5-1s). To improve the esthetic outcome, the maxillary anterior teeth were restored with composite fillings (Figs 5-1t to 5-1v). Figures 5-1w and 5-1x show the periodontal chart and radiographic status of the patient at the final re-evaluation.

Maintenance phase

Following treatment, the patient was enrolled in a regular supportive periodontal therapy program based on an individual periodontal risk assessment.[15]

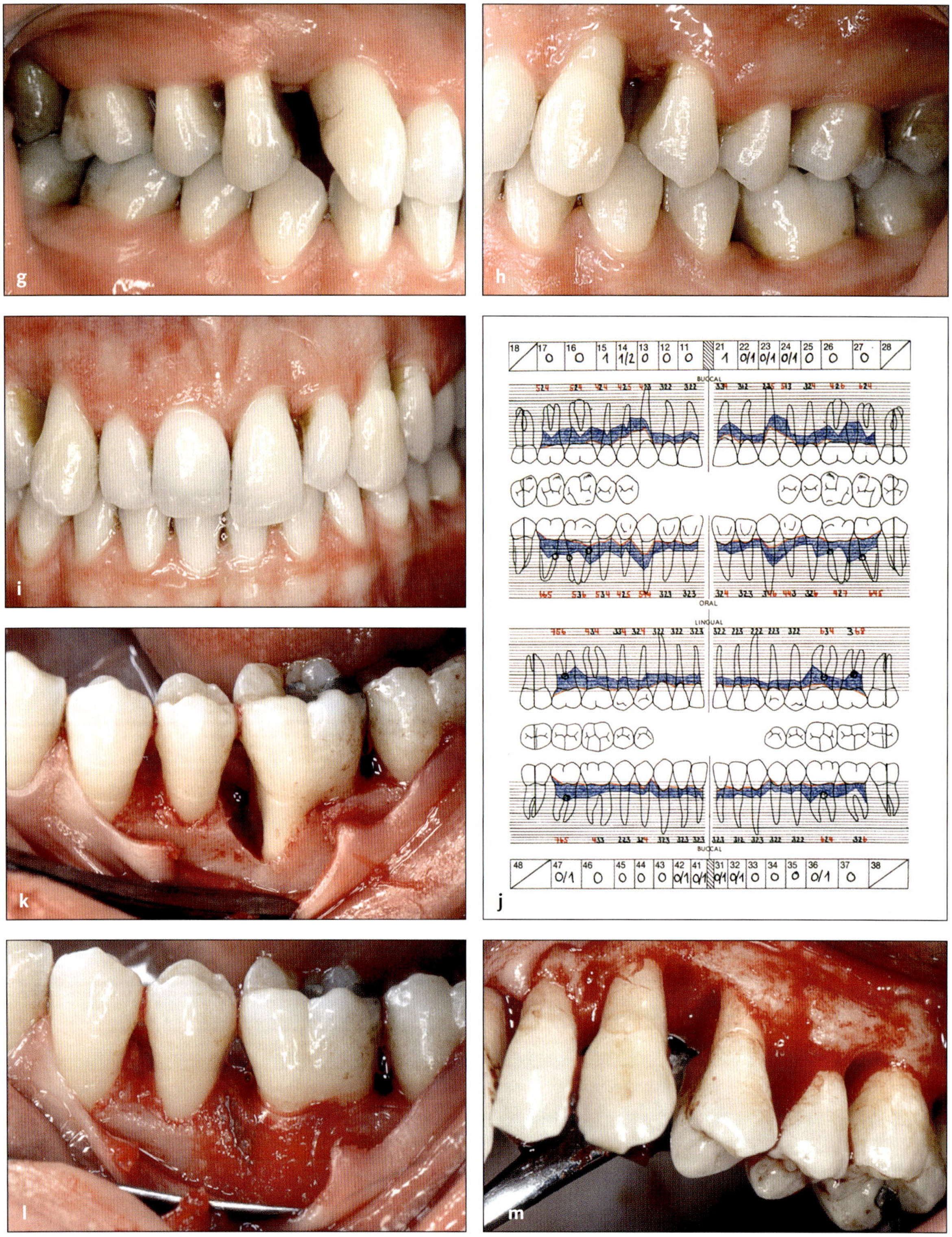

Fig 5-1 *(cont)* *(g to i)* Anterior and lateral views of the patient at re-evaluation following initial periodontal therapy. *(j)* Periodontal chart of the patient at re-evaluation after initial periodontal therapy. *(k to m)* Surgical views of the mandibular and maxillary left quadrants.

→

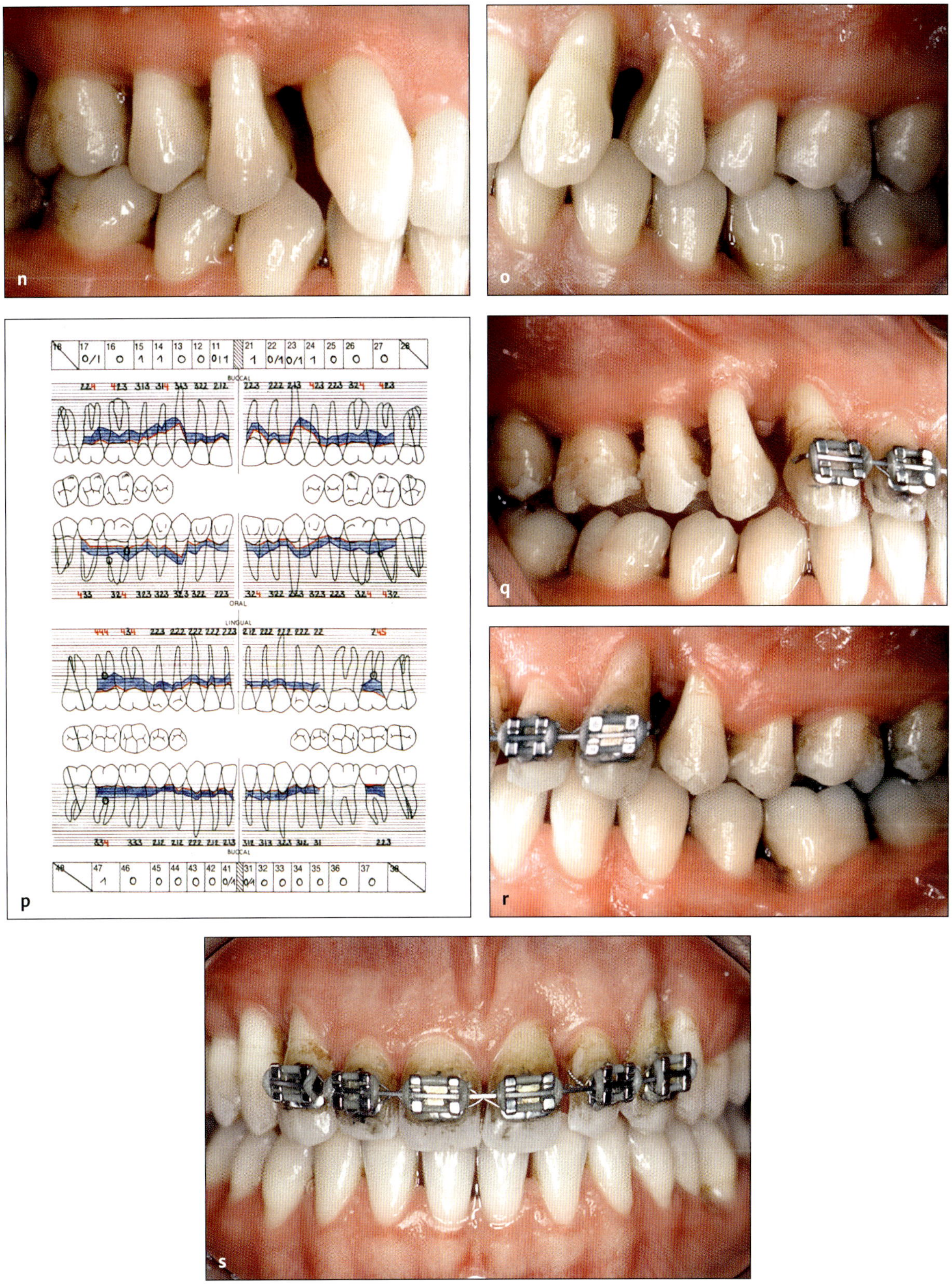

Fig 5-1 *(cont)* *(n and o)* Lateral views of the patient at re-evaluation following periodontal surgery. *(p)* Periodontal chart of the patient at re-evaluation following periodontal surgery. *(q to s)* Clinical anterior and lateral views of the patient during orthodontic therapy.

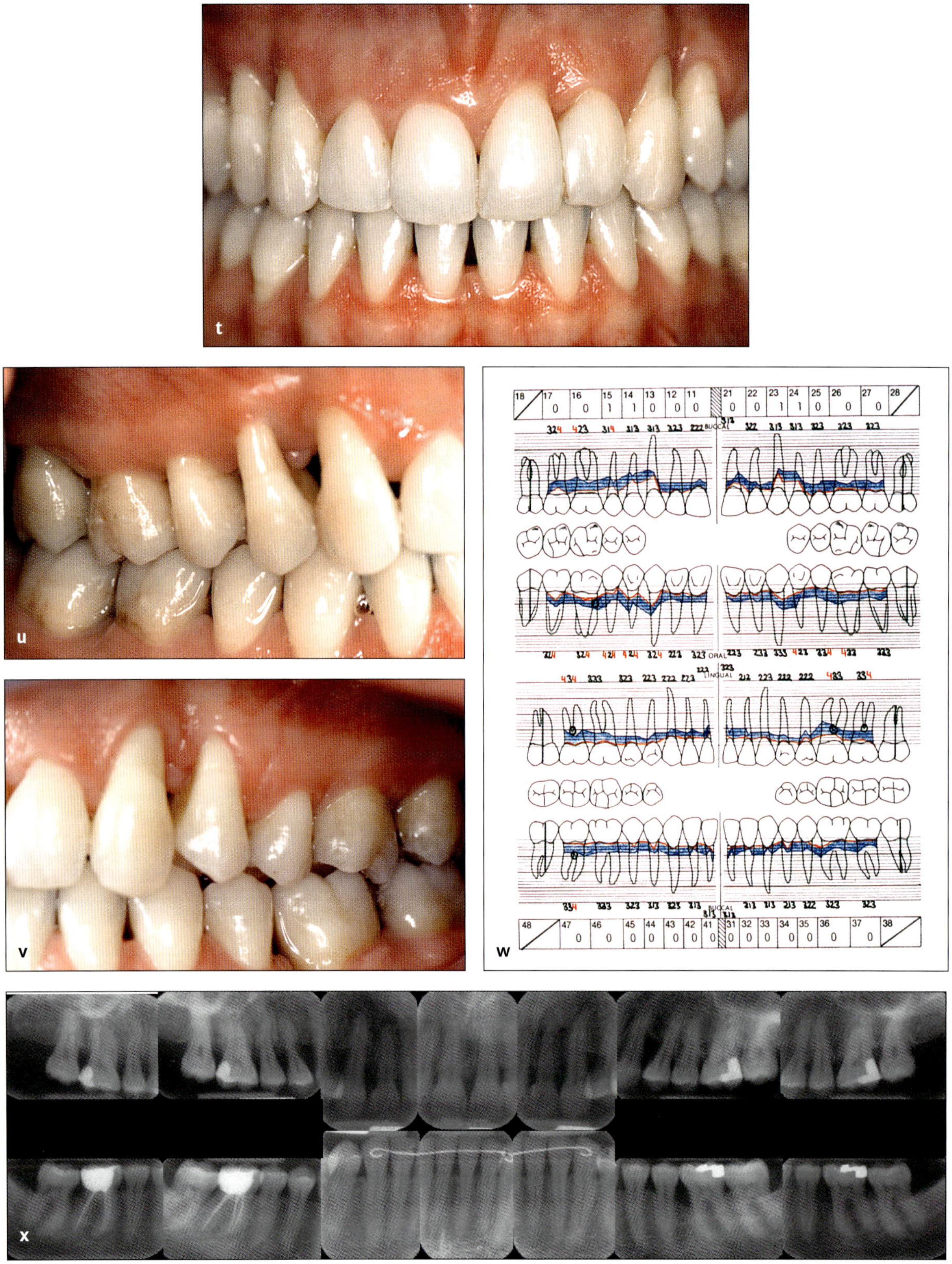

Fig 5-1 *(cont)* *(t to v)* Anterior and lateral views of the patient at the final re-evaluation. *(w)* Periodontal chart of the patient at the final re-evaluation following completion of orthodontic and restorative therapy. *(x)* Periapical radiographic status of the patient at the final re-evaluation.

Conclusion

For patients diagnosed with generalized severe periodontitis who have intact dental arches, special effort should be undertaken to maintain all teeth. Especially in the dentition of young patients, single and multiple tooth extractions may lead to a prosthetic rehabilitation involving the use of dental implants. This is particularly important when implant therapy is included in the overall treatment plan, because implant loss in patients with treated periodontal conditions is significantly higher compared with that of patients without a history of periodontitis.[23]

Provided that the fundamental principles governing the four treatment phases (ie, systemic, initial, corrective, and maintenance) are understood, deviations in the treatment plan may be accepted following discussion with the patient.

References

1. Matuliene G, Pjetursson BE, Salvi GE, et al. Influence of residual pockets on progression of periodontitis and tooth loss: Results after 11 years of maintenance. J Clin Periodontol 2008;35:685–695.
2. Salvi GE, Mischler DC, Schmidlin K, et al. Risk factors associated with the longevity of multi-rooted teeth. Long-term outcomes after active and supportive periodontal therapy. J Clin Periodontol 2014;41:701–707.
3. Axelsson P, Nyström B, Lindhe J. The long-term effect of a plaque control program on tooth mortality, caries and periodontal disease in adults. Results after 30 years of maintenance. J Clin Periodontol 2004;31:749–757.
4. Ramseier CA. Potential impact of subject-based risk factor control on periodontitis. J Clin Periodontol 2005;32(suppl 6):283–290.
5. Kinane DF, Peterson M, Stathopoulou PG. Environmental and other modifying factors of the periodontal diseases. Periodontol 2000 2006;40:107–119.
6. O'Leary TJ, Drake RB, Naylor JE. The plaque control record. J Periodontol 1972;43:38.
7. Lindhe J, Nyman S. The effect of plaque control and surgical pocket elimination on the establishment and maintenance of periodontal health. A longitudinal study of periodontal therapy in cases of advanced disease. J Clin Periodontol 1975;2:67–79.
8. Nyman S, Rosling B, Lindhe J. Effect of professional tooth cleaning on healing after periodontal surgery. J Clin Periodontol 1975;2:80–86.
9. Nyman S, Lindhe J, Rosling B. Periodontal surgery in plaque-infected dentitions. J Clin Periodontol 1977;4:240–249.
10. Rosling B, Nyman S, Lindhe J. The effect of systematic plaque control on bone regeneration in infrabony pockets. J Clin Periodontol 1976;3:38–53.
11. Rosling B, Nyman S, Lindhe J, Jern B. The healing potential of the periodontal tissues following different techniques of periodontal surgery in plaque-free dentitions. A 2-year clinical study. J Clin Periodontol 1976;3:233–250.
12. Pjetursson BE, Helbling C, Weber HP, et al. Peri-implantitis susceptibility as it relates to periodontal therapy and supportive care. Clin Oral Implants Res 2012;23:888–894.
13. Lang NP, Adler R, Joss A, Nyman S. Absence of bleeding on probing. An indicator of periodontal stability. J Clin Periodontol 1990;17:714–721.
14. Joss A, Adler R, Lang NP. Bleeding on probing. A parameter for monitoring periodontal conditions in clinical practice. J Clin Periodontol 1994;21:402–408.
15. Lang NP, Tonetti MS. Periodontal risk assessment (PRA) for patients in supportive periodontal therapy (SPT). Oral Health Prev Dent 2003;1:7–16.
16. Bergenholtz G, Nyman S. Endodontic complications following periodontal and prosthetic treatment of patients with advanced periodontal disease. J Periodontol 1984;55:63–68.
17. Lang NP, Pjetursson BE, Tan K, Brägger U, Egger M, Zwahlen M. A systematic review of the survival and complication rates of fixed partial dentures (FPDs) after an observation period of at least 5 years. II. Combined tooth-implant-supported FPDs. Clin Oral Implants Res 2004;15:643–653.
18. Lulic M, Brägger U, Lang NP, Zwahlen M, Salvi GE. Ante's (1926) law revisited: A systematic review on survival rates and complications of fixed dental prostheses (FDPs) on severely reduced periodontal tissue support. Clin Oral Implants Res 2007;18(suppl 3):63–72.
19. Mombelli A, Schmid J, Walter C, Wetzel A. Parodontologie. Qualitätsleitlinien für Zahnmedizin. Swiss Dent J 2014;124:261–267.
20. Hamp SE, Nyman S, Lindhe J. Periodontal treatment of multirooted teeth. Results after 5 years. J Clin Periodontol 1975;2:126–135.
21. Miller SC. Textbook of Periodontia; Oral Medicine, ed 3. Philadelphia: Blakiston, 1950.
22. Updegrave WJ. The paralleling extension-cone technique in intraoral dental radiography. Oral Surg Oral Med Oral Pathol 1951;4:1250–1261.
23. Sgolastra F, Petrucci A, Severino M, Gatto R, Monaco A. Periodontitis, implant loss and peri-implantitis. A meta-analysis. Clin Oral Implants Res 2015;26:e8–e16.

CHAPTER 6

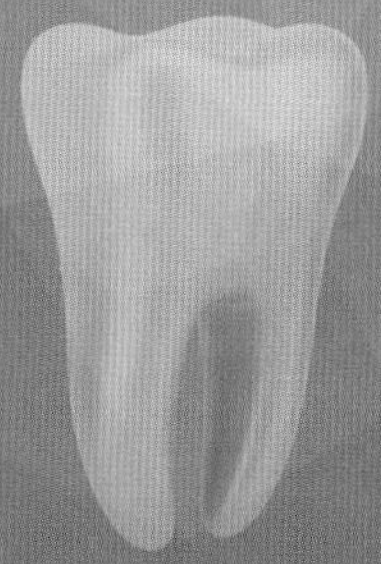

Etiology and Treatment of Gingival Recessions in Orthodontically Treated Patients

Raluca Cosgarea
Dimitrios Kloukos
Christos Katsaros
Anton Sculean

Anatomy of the Periodontium

The periodontium is a term derived from Greek (*peri* = around, *odont* = tooth) representing the structures surrounding and supporting teeth. It is composed of the periodontal ligament (PDL), the root cementum, the alveolar bone, and the tooth-facing gingiva (dentogingival junction). Each of these components has a specialized structure with different functions that interact and together ensure the proper function of the periodontium. The periodontium undergoes several age-related and/or morphologic changes as well as functionally oriented alterations.

The descriptions that follow refer to healthy periodontal tissues.

Root Cementum

The root cementum represents a hard, avascular, noninnervated, mineralized connective tissue (about 55% by weight, mainly hydroxyapatite) that covers the roots of teeth and sometimes extends over the cementoenamel junction (CEJ). Its primary function is the attachment of PDL fibers to the root. Further, root cementum contributes to repair processes of root defects, protection of the dental pulp, and adjustment of tooth positions to new conditions.[1–3]

Four types of cementum have been described according to the presence/absence of cells and the presence/absence of the collagenous matrix and its structure: acellular

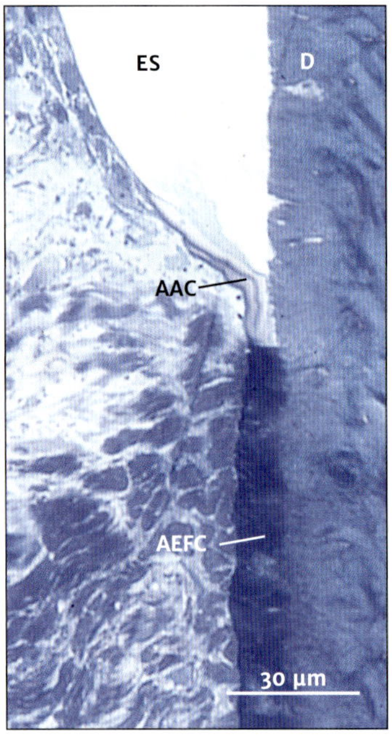

Fig 6-1 Micrograph showing AAC at the CEJ and AAC and AEFC apically. D, dentin; ES, enamel space (toluidine blue staining). (Reprinted with permission from Bosshardt.[3])

afibrillar cementum (AAC), acellular extrinsic fiber cementum (AEFC), cellular mixed stratified cementum (CMSC), and cellular intrinsic fiber cementum (CIFC)[3] (Fig 6-1). These have various functions, locations on the root surface, formation rates, biochemical compositions, and degrees of mineralization, and they are differently distributed according to the tooth type, age of the patient, and other individual variations (Table 6-1).

Cementum increases in thickness throughout the entire life of a tooth and does not undergo physiologic remodeling. The various forms of cementum have different thickening paces: AEFC, which seems to be more desirable for periodontal regenerative procedures than CIFC, grows very slowly (2 to 5 µm/year), while CIFC grows 30 times faster (in animal models) and is quickly deposited spotwise on root defects.[1,2]

Periodontal Ligament

The PDL is a soft connective tissue that is highly vascularized and innervated and rich in various types of cells; it surrounds the tooth and connects the root cementum with the adjacent alveolar bone (Fig 6-2). The PDL continues coronally to the alveolar crest with the lamina propria of the gingiva and apically with the dental pulp.[3] It has the shape of an hourglass and a width of approximately 0.25 mm (range 0.2 to 0.4 mm) that is thinnest in the middle third of the root and diminishes with age. The PDL functions as a buffer, absorbing occlusal forces during mastication or other tooth contacts and dispersing these to the alveolar bone. It plays a key role in the attachment of the tooth to the surrounding bone and is essential for tooth mobility, which is influenced mainly by the width, height, and quality of the PDL.[1-3]

Different types of cells like fibroblasts, cementoblasts, osteoblasts, osteoclasts, monocytes, macrophages, epithelial cell rests of Malassez, and undifferentiated mesenchymal progenitor and stem cells can all be found in the PDL. Thus, the PDL also functions as a cell reservoir that forms mineralized tissues and plays an essential role in wound healing/regeneration. These cells are embedded in an extracellular matrix that contains collagen fibers and noncollagenous proteins. Additionally, a multitude of blood vessels, nerve fibers, and cells are found between the fibers. The epithelial cells of Malassez (eg, remnants of the Hertwig epithelial root sheath) surround the root at a certain distance and are speculated to be implicated in periodontal homeostasis and repair. The fibroblasts are aligned along the collagen fibers and are involved in synthesizing and remodeling (ie, degrading) processes within the extracellular matrix.[1-3]

The collagen fibers are grouped in bundles that are oriented three-dimensionally between the root cementum and bone. These fibers continue within the root cementum and bone with the Sharpey fibers and differ in number according to the remodeling activity at the bone and root surface level. A small part of the fibers is represented by oxytalan fibers, which insert in the cementum and run parallel to the root.[3]

Table 6-1 Characteristics of the four root cementum types

	Location	Composition and appearance	Function
AAC	At the CEJ; may cover minor areas of the enamel	• No cells or fibrillar collagen • High noncollagenous protein content • Layered appearance	May have a sealing function
AEFC	Coronal and middle thirds of the root	• No cells • Collagenous matrix containing densely packed collagen fibers • Collagen fibers attach to the dentin on one side; on the opposite site, they continue with PDL fibers (Sharpey fibers) • At the mineralization front of AEFC, a very high number of principal PDL fibers insert (about 30,000/mm^2) • Rich in noncollagenous proteins (eg, bone sialoprotein, osteopontin) • Homogenous structure	Tooth attachment, anchorage
CMSC	Apical one- to two-thirds of the roots and furcations	• Mixture of alternating layers of AEFC and CIFC (unpredictable thickness and sequence) • Cells (cementocytes) and intrinsic fibers	Adaptive function (adjustment of the tooth to new requirements, CIFC layers), tooth anchorage (AEFC layers)
CIFC	A component of the CMSC but may also appear alone (without AEFC) anywhere on the root where resorption defects are present (mostly apical)	• Intrinsic collagen fibers (fibers produced by osteoblasts and oriented parallel to the long axis of the root) • Embedded cells (cementocytes) • Rapid matrix deposition may be responsible for the embedded cells	Repair of the resorptive and fracture defects

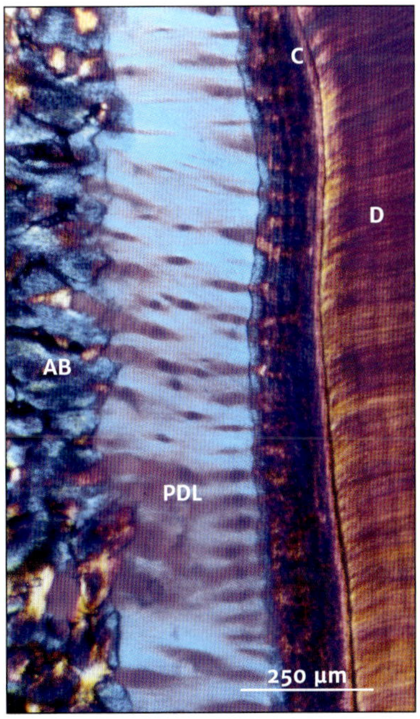

Fig 6-2 Micrograph depicting the PDL with collagen fibers, cementum (C), and alveolar bone (AB). D, dentin. (Reprinted with permission from Bosshardt.[3])

Alveolar Bone

The jawbone continues with the alveolar process in which the alveolar bone proper (alveolus) is formed in association with the tooth development. This bone has about 60% mineral weight (mainly hydroxyapatite) and can be divided into two compartments: the mineralized bone (cortical bone with outer and inner cortical plate) and the bone marrow (central spongiosa or cancellous bone).[2] The cortical bone is made up of lamellae. The inner cortical plate forms the bony alveolus (alveolar bone proper). When the alveolar process is very thin, the two cortical plates may be fused together.[3] The spongiosa contains bone trabeculae, adipocytes, vascular structures, and undifferentiated mesenchymal cells; it forms the major part of the interdental septa and a smaller part

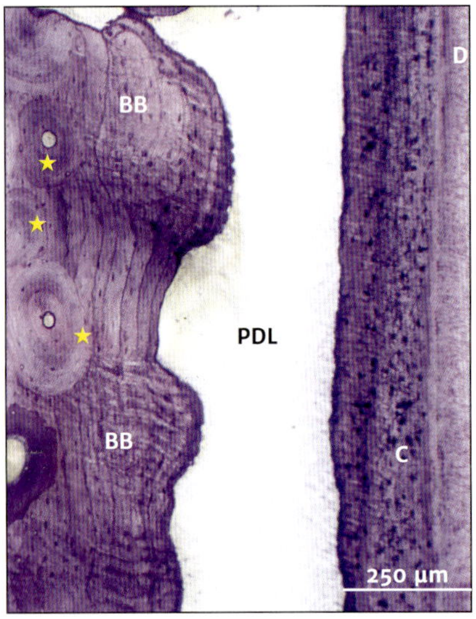

Fig 6-3 Micrograph depicting bundle bone (BB), osteons (*stars*), cementum (C), dentin (D), and the PDL. (Reprinted with permission from Bosshardt.[3])

of the buccal and palatal bone plates. The size and form of the bone trabeculae are determined genetically and change in relation to the forces applied to the teeth (ie, during mastication or orthodontic treatment).

The alveolar bone, which is formed by the inner cortical plate, is a compact bone comprised of osteons (structural unit made up of concentric layers of mineralized lamellae surrounding the Haversian canal, which houses a blood vessel; Fig 6-3) and a thin layer of bundle bone. Sometimes the bundle bone may not be found at all sites due to the constant bone-remodeling processes. The wall of the alveolar socket contains holes (Volkmann's canals) that connects the PDL with the bone marrow spaces and through which nerve fibers, blood, and lymph vessels pass. Parallel to the socket wall, thin layers of bundle bone are deposited. The bundle bone is penetrated by Sharpey fibers (see Fig 6-3).

In periodontally healthy conditions, the alveolar crest follows the CEJ about 2 mm apically.[3] The thickness of the alveolar bone varies according to the tooth region; in the molar region, the bone is thicker buccally than orally (palatal or lingual), while in the incisor and premolar areas, the buccal bone is thinner than that at the oral aspects of the teeth. The bone plate is thicker on the palatal and buccal aspects of the molars and thinner buccally in the anterior area. At the buccal aspect of the teeth, the bone may be missing, resulting in two situations: dehiscence, when the coronal portion of the roots is not covered by bone, or fenestration, when some bone is present coronally but the central part of the root is not covered by bone. In these cases, the roots are covered just by PDL and the overlying gingival tissue.[2] Such defects may also arise when teeth are displaced out of the arch.

The alveolar bone (bony alveolus) resembles the shape of the tooth within and undergoes constant modeling and remodeling according to functional demands (bone resorption and apposition). Throughout life, teeth undergo continuous eruption and mesialization in order to overcome attrition processes. In orthodontic tooth movement or when the forces are greater and/or of longer duration than physiologically acceptable, the PDL is overcompressed on one side of the tooth and the alveolar bone is resorbed; on the other side, the PDL is stretched and bone deposition is accelerated.

Gingiva

The tooth-facing part of the gingiva, also called the *marginal periodontium*, is represented by the supracrestal part of the gingiva and functions as protection for the underlying soft and hard connective tissues by preventing the microorganisms of the oral cavity and their byproducts from penetrating the periodontal tissues.

Macroscopically, the gingiva extends coronally to the gingival margin and apically to the mucogingival junction on the vestibular side (Fig 6-4a) and to the mucosa of the hard palate (Fig 6-4b), or it continues lingually with the mucosa of the floor of the mouth (Fig 6-4c). Coronally, a gingival sulcus of about 0.5 mm is generally present, while in the interdental areas the gingiva forms the gingival papillae. The gingiva can be divided into the free gingiva and the attached gingiva. Free gingiva is located coronally, can be moved mechanically with a minimal force, has a smooth surface, follows the contour of the

CEJ, and has a width of 1 to 2 mm.[1] Apically, the free gingiva sometimes has a gingival groove present and an accumulation of indentations called *stipples*. The attached gingiva resembles an orange rind, presenting stipples on its surface, and extends between the free gingiva and the alveolar mucosa/mucosa of the floor of the mouth. It has a width of 1 to 10 mm.[1] Palatally, the attached mucosa extends up to the free gingiva, and thus no mobile mucosa is present.

Histologically, the gingiva consists of three epithelia—the junctional epithelium, the oral sulcular epithelium, and the oral gingival epithelium—as well as a connective tissue component (lamina propria):

- The oral gingival epithelium is part of the masticatory mucosa and is a stratified, keratinized epithelium with four layers: stratum basale, spinosum, granulosum, and corneum. It is less permeable than the junctional epithelium.
- The oral sulcular epithelium is located between the oral gingival epithelium and the junctional epithelium. It lines the lateral wall of the sulcus and has a similar structure to the oral gingival epithelium and is often parakeratinized and less permeable than the junctional epithelium.
- The junctional epithelium lies between the bottom of the sulcus and the CEJ (about 1.5 mm away from the sulcus). It is a nonkeratinized epithelium with two layers: stratum basale and suprabasale. Its innermost cells form the epithelial attachment to the tooth consisting of basal lamina and hemidesmosomes. It has high permeability, which is important for defense mechanisms (ie, by junctional epithelial cells and leukocytes, mainly polymorphonuclear leukocytes, and tissue fluid).[4]
- The connective tissue of the gingiva contains mostly fibroblasts responsible for the formation and remodeling of collagen fibers,[4] collagen fibers arranged three-dimensionally in bundles that shape the gingiva and connect adjacent teeth, and gingival blood vessels that transport metabolites and provide macromolecules and leukocytes.

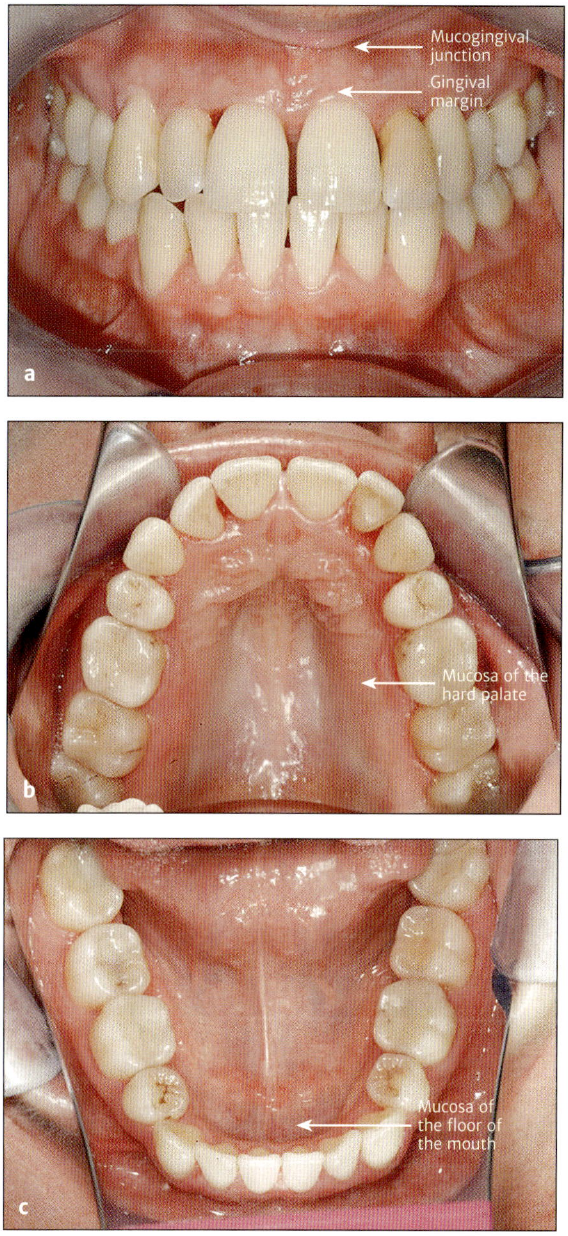

Fig 6-4 Clinical images of the gingiva. *(a)* Frontal view showing the mucogingival junction, gingival margins, and mucosa of the vestibulum. *(b)* Maxillary occlusal view showing the mucosa of the hard palate. *(c)* Mandibular occlusal view showing the mucosa of the floor of the mouth.

The structural and functional integrity of the junctional epithelium plays a major role in maintaining healthy periodontal conditions.[4] It surrounds the cervical part of the tooth, protecting the periodontal tissues against the microorganisms within the biofilm adherent to the tooth surface.

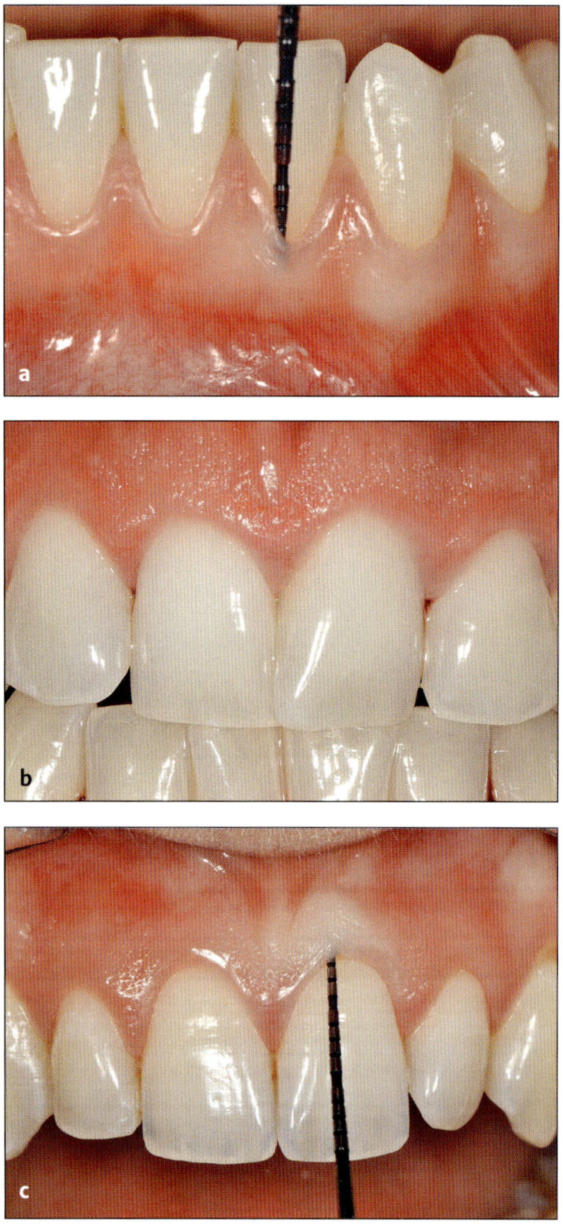

Fig 6-5 *(a)* The "thin-scalloped biotype" (cluster A1). *(b)* The thick-flat biotype (cluster B). *(c)* The thick-scalloped biotype (cluster A2).

Biotype/Phenotype of the Gingiva

Considering the morphologic characteristics of teeth and periodontium, various biotypes of gingiva have been recognized. In 1969, Ochsenbein and Ross described two main gingival phenotypes: thick-flat and thin-scalloped.[5–7] Later in 1989, Seibert and Lindhe confirmed the existence of different gingival biotypes, introducing the term *periodontal biotype*, and classified them as thick-flat and thin-scalloped.[8] According to Olsson et al,[9] the thin-scalloped periodontal biotype is characterized by the presence of long, narrow crowns with a narrow zone of attached and keratinized tissue and a pronounced scalloped gingival contour. The thick-flat periodontal biotype is rather present in individuals with short, wide crowns with a broad zone of keratinized and attached gingiva and a flat gingival contour. However, in the investigation by Olsson et al,[9] no statistically significant differences were obtained for the gingival thickness between these two biotypes.

Twenty years later in 2009, the different gingival biotypes were divided according to a cluster analysis on 100 individuals in three clusters[10]: Cluster A1 represented a thin-scalloped biotype depicting a thin gingiva with slender teeth, a narrow zone of keratinized tissue, and a highly scalloped gingival margin; this cluster was found in one-third of the investigated sample (37%) (Fig 6-5a). Cluster B described the thick-flat biotype characterized by a thick gingiva with quadratic teeth, a broad zone of keratinized tissue, and a flat gingival margin; it was found in another third of the study subjects (29%) (Fig 6-5b). The third cluster (cluster A2), found in the rest of the subjects (34%), was a mixture of the previous two clusters and was characterized by the presence of a thick gingiva around slender teeth with a high scalloped gingival margin and a narrow zone of keratinized tissue (Fig 6-5c). Moreover, confirmatory to other findings,[11,12] a statistically significant higher percentage of males showed a thick gingival biotype compared to females (84% versus 45%).[10] The existence of three gingival biotypes, namely a thin-scalloped, a thick-flat, and a thick-scalloped biotype, was confirmed in a more recent systematic review.[13] The authors found a strong positive association between gingival thickness and bone morphotype and a moderate positive association between gingival thickness and the amount of keratinized tissue; however, the dimensions of teeth, gingiva, and bone showed just a weak to moderate correlation.[13]

In the latest consensus report of the World Workshop on the Classification of Periodontal and Peri-Implant Diseases and Conditions, the term *periodontal phenotype* has been recommended to describe the appearance of the gingiva, including gingival volume and keratinized tissue width (gingival phenotype), and the thickness of the buccal bone (bone morphotype).[14,15] Moreover, in the Workshop it has been specified that the phenotype is a changeable characteristic of the gingiva attributed to environmental factors or clinical interventions.

Irrespective of the used terminology, it seems that the different architecture of the gingiva and its underlying bone influences the outcome of esthetic restorative, periodontal, and implant therapy.[16–20] Thin gingival biotypes are associated with a higher occurrence of gingival recessions,[9,16,21] less pocket formation, loss of the thin vestibular bone plate, more unpredictable healing after surgical interventions, and more extensive apical and lingual ridge resorption after extractions.[16] Gingival recessions were also described more often at the sites of immediate single-tooth implants in patients with the thin-scalloped biotype.[22,23] On the contrary, the thick-flat gingival biotype is more associated with periodontal pocket formation and bleeding on probing with edema, more predictable healing of the hard and soft tissues after surgery, and less ridge resorption after extraction.[16] This biotype has also been associated with more soft tissue rebound after crown lengthening surgeries,[24] a more predictable prognosis in recession coverage procedures, and a more successful esthetic outcome with implants.[17–20] In a recent study that evaluated the influence of periodontal biotype on the appearance of gingival recessions at the mandibular incisors during orthodontic treatment,[25] it was shown that patients with a thin periodontal biotype are more likely to undergo gingival marginal alterations, irrespective of the type of orthodontic movement. The study also showed that a thin periodontal biotype and proclination of the teeth correlate with loss of keratinized tissue.[25]

Therefore, correct assessment of the gingival biotype seems to be important for providing predictable dental treatment outcomes. Several authors investigated the various biotype features and methods of differentiation between thick and thin gingiva using direct measurement,[26] ultrasonics,[11] cone beam computed tomography (CBCT),[27] and gingival probing.[19,28] Greenberg et al[26] classified the biotypes by means of direct thickness measurement with a periodontal probe: When the gingival thickness was at least 1.5 mm, it was classified as thick; when it was less than 1.5 mm, it was classified as thin. Nonetheless, this method lacked precision, as *(1)* probe measurements are only accurate to the nearest 0.5 mm, and *(2)* probe angulation and the distortion of gingival tissue during transgingival probing may have affected probing values.

Gingival thickness can also be assessed noninvasively with an ultrasonic device; however, problems arise in determining the correct position of the device and obtaining reproducible measurements.[11,12] Gingival thickness measurements by means of CBCT are also possible and showed a good to moderate correlation with the clinical measurements.[27,29] Nonetheless, these two measurement methods imply higher costs, and the use of CBCT exposes the patient to radiation.

A widely accepted and the most commonly used method for determining the gingival biotype is visual inspection of the probe transparency through the gingiva: A visible probe relates to a thin biotype (see Fig 6-5a),[19,28] while the biotype is considered thick if the probe does not show through the gingival sulcus. This method has been shown to be highly reproducible (85% agreement between duplicate measurements), is easy to perform, and has been used in several clinical studies for biotype assessment.[22,28,30,31] This method has been also proposed by the World Workshop from 2017, indicating the presence of a thin gingiva ($\leq$ 1 mm) when the probe is visible and a thick gingiva ($\geq$ 1 mm) when the probe is not visible.[14]

Table 6-2 Miller classification for gingival recessions[34]

Miller class	*Definition*	*Clinical photograph*
Class I	The recession does not reach the mucogingival line. There is no loss of approximal periodontal tissue.	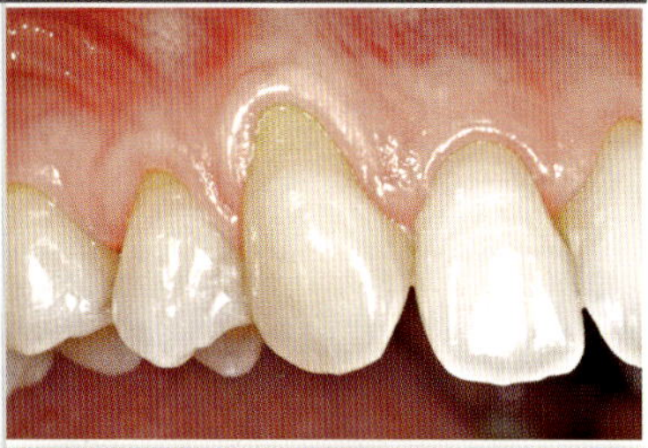
Class II	The recession extends up to/beyond the mucogingival line, but there is no loss of approximal periodontal tissue.	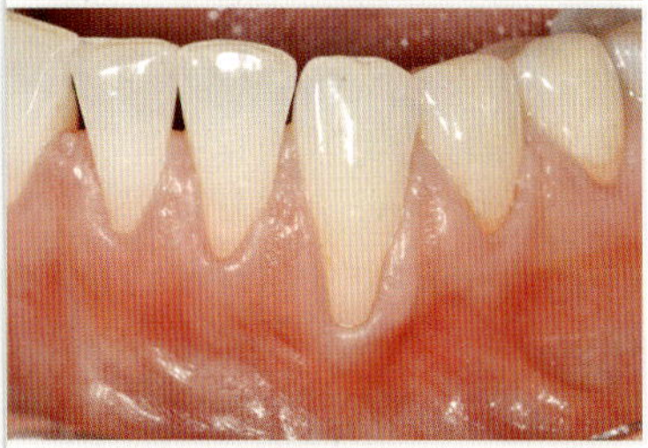
Class III	The recession extends up to/beyond the mucogingival line, and there is loss of approximal hard and soft tissue. The interdental soft tissue is displaced apically to the CEJ but situated coronally to the vestibular gingival margin.	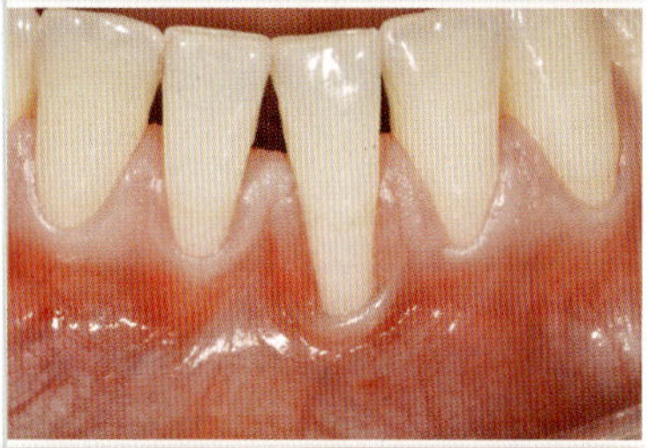
Class IV	The recession extends up to/beyond the mucogingival line, and there is advanced loss of approximal hard and soft tissue. The interdental soft tissue is displaced apically to the CEJ and to the vestibular gingival margin.	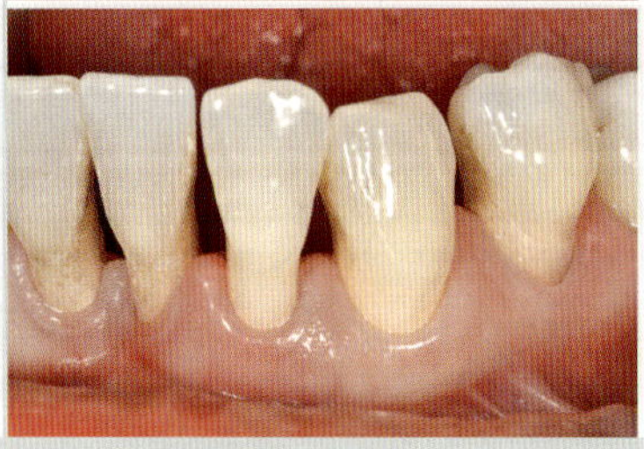

Definition and Classification of Gingival Recessions

A gingival recession represents an exposure of the root surface due to the displacement of the gingival margin[32,33] and is characterized by clinical attachment loss bucally/lingually/interproximally.[14] Several classifications for gingival recession–type defects have been proposed. The most widely used classification was developed in 1985 by Miller and is based on the amount of displaced gingiva and the loss of approximal periodontal tissue[34] (Table 6-2).

In another classification, gingival recessions have been classified into three types[35]:

- Type I: Gingival recession without interproximal attachment loss
- Type II: Gingival recession with interproximal attachment loss that is less than or equal to the buccal site
- Type III: Gingival recession with interproximal attachment loss that is more than the buccal site

This classification system was shown to be highly reproducible (intraclass correlation coefficient 0.86) and predictable for the therapeutic reduction of recession (high level of confidence, $P < .0001$).[35]

In another classification system, besides the gingival component, the presence of dental surface defects in the area of the recessions has also been considered: visible (class A) or not visible (class B) CEJ and presence (+) or absence (−) of dental surface defect. Thus, four classes exist according to this classification: A+, A−, B+ and B−.[36]

The newest classification proposed by the World Workshop on the Classification of Periodontal and Peri-Implant Diseases and Conditions is based on the interdental clinical attachment loss[14]:

- Recession type 1: A buccal/lingual gingival recession with no interproximal loss of clinical attachment, the CEJ being detectable neither at the mesial nor the distal tooth site.
- Recession type 2: A buccal/lingual gingival recession with an interproximal loss of clinical attachment not greater than the buccal clinical attachment loss.
- Recession type 3: A buccal/lingual gingival recession with an interproximal loss of clinical attachment greater than the buccal clinical attachment loss.

Prevalence and Etiologic Factors

Single or multiple gingival recessions may occur in a considerable proportion of the population, both in younger as well as in older subjects and in patients with or without adequate oral hygiene.[37–41] It seems that the occurrence of gingival recessions increases with age,[37–39,41–46] although age should not be considered an etiologic factor.[47] Surveys reveal that about 88% of persons over age 65 years and 50% of those between 18 and 64 years old have at least one site with a recession of at least 1 mm.[42–44,48] In a Norwegian periodontally well-maintained population, gingival recessions were present in over 90% of the elderly people (over 50 years of age) and in 60% of younger individuals (under 20 years of age).[37] Similar data were obtained in a French population with a prevalence of 84.6%[38] and in Brazil with 91.7% of the elderly subjects (over 60 years old) having a gingival recession at least 3 mm deep.[45] Moreover, gingival recessions seem to occur in a greater proportion of men than women,[38,42,43,45] and smoking and poor oral hygiene appear to directly influence the extent of gingival recessions.[38,42,45,49]

Several factors may lead to the appearance of gingival recessions. These can be categorized as predisposing and causative factors.[50–52]

PREDISPOSING PATHOGENETIC FACTORS

Bony vestibular dehiscences are root surface areas not covered by alveolar bone and are often overlaid by a thin, fragile gingiva. Consequently, these sites are susceptible to plaque-induced gingival inflammation and/or trauma and are at high risk of developing gingival recessions.[50–52]

Marginal lip and cheek frenula/muscle insertions may hinder a proper toothbrushing technique and thereby inhibit effective and nontraumatic self-performed oral hygiene. These areas favor plaque accumulation and consequently gingivitis and root caries. Moreover, an incorrect toothbrushing technique (ie, horizontally) may also lead to gingival trauma and thus to gingival recessions.[39,41,47,49,53–56]

The periodontal phenotype may represent another predisposing factor for gingival recessions. Studies have shown that subgingival infections in subjects with a thin phenotype result in gingival recession, whereas similar infections in subjects with a thick phenotype result in the formation of periodontal pockets.[41,48,50,52,57]

CAUSATIVE PATHOGENETIC FACTORS

Tissue trauma due to horizontal, traumatic tooth brushing with excessive pressure and hard brush bristles is one of the most common causes of gingival vestibular recessions.[39,41,49,56] Furthermore, teeth prominently positioned in the dental arch (ie, canines) where the alveolar bone is thin or absent (bony dehiscence) are prone to uneven pressure distribution during tooth brushing and consequently show gingival recessions more often. In a Swiss population of army recruits, 17% of the first molars and 8.7% of the canines showed gingival recessions.[58] Oral jewelry like in lip or tongue piercings are also traumatic triggers causing gingival recessions[59,60]: 68% of subjects with lower lip piercings presented a gingival labial recession, and 4% of these had localized periodontitis.[59]

Plaque accumulation is a further causative factor: Subgingival plaque leads to subgingival inflammation, and in cases with a thin biotype, the gingiva retracts in response to the inflammation, creating a gingival recession. In this context, subgingival incorrect marginal adaptations of dental restorations (ie, overhanging or insufficient) favor plaque retention and represent a causative factor for gingival recessions.[61,62]

Orthodontic Tooth Movement and Development of Gingival Recessions

Active orthodontic treatment can induce gingival recession when teeth are moved outside the alveolar bone.[63] Several animal experimental studies have demonstrated that when a tooth is moved through the cortical plate, a labial bone dehiscence followed by gingival recession can appear. Others, however, could not show such a relationship (for review, see Joss-Vassalli et al.[64])

At the clinical level in humans, the evidence on the association between orthodontic treatment and development of gingival recession is contradictory (for review, see Joss-Vassalli et al.[64]) Some studies found no influence of orthodontic treatment on the development of gingival recession,[65,66] whereas others reported that gingival recession was more prevalent in orthodontically treated patients than in untreated controls.[67,68] A recent retrospective study showed that the frequency values of recession in orthodontically treated patients 10 to 15 years after treatment and in matched untreated participants seeking orthodontic treatment were comparable and were in line with the report of Thomson.[66,69] The difference between the findings of these two studies[66,69] and other studies[67,68] might be due to differences in the characteristics of the control groups. Renkema et al[67] used historical controls with normal occlusion and minor tooth alignment deviations, while Gebistorf et al[69] used a control group with malocclusion left untreated for many years. Slutzkey and Levin[68] did not report the malocclusions in the control group. Also, the reported prevalence of recession sites differs substantially among the various studies,[69,70] something that could be explained by systematic differences in scoring among the raters in the various studies or differences among the assessed populations, socioeconomic status, and behavioral patterns.[69,71]

The reports in the literature are also contradictory regarding the possible association between the extent of gingival recession in orthodontic patients and the degree of therapeutic incisor proclination, the width of attached gingiva, the thickness of the mandibular symphysis, the facial type, oral hygiene, and periodontal conditions (for details, see Joss-Vassalli et al.[64])

One possible etiologic factor for the long-term development of gingival recessions is the presence of a lingual retainer. According to Pandis et al,[72] there is no clear association between the presence of fixed retainers and the development of gingival recession, but long-term fixed bonded retainers on proclined mandibular incisors could cause attachment loss. However, a recent study with a follow-up of 5 years showed that proclined mandibular incisors retained with fixed retainers have no increased risk of development of gingival recessions in comparison to nonproclined teeth.[73] Katsaros et al[74] showed that in a small fraction of orthodontic patients where fixed round flexible spiral retainers were used, the retainer became activated with time and induced unwanted tooth movements, mainly torque movements. Although retreatment in these cases is usually possible, permanent damage like bone dehiscence and gingival recession can be expected if the complications remain undetected at an early stage[75,76] (Fig 6-6).

In general, the design of the available studies does not allow us to definitively answer the question whether orthodontic tooth movement is a major risk factor for the development of gingival recession, since randomized controlled trials or prospective controlled studies are lacking in the field. The same is true regarding elucidation of the role of the individual patient-related or treatment-related contributing factors. However, despite the absence of high-quality evidence, a risk-analysis using the available evidence including age; traumatic, pathologic, anatomical, and biomechanical factors; and oral hygiene, periodontal condition, and extent of tooth movement is mandatory for every patient before any orthodontic treatment is performed.

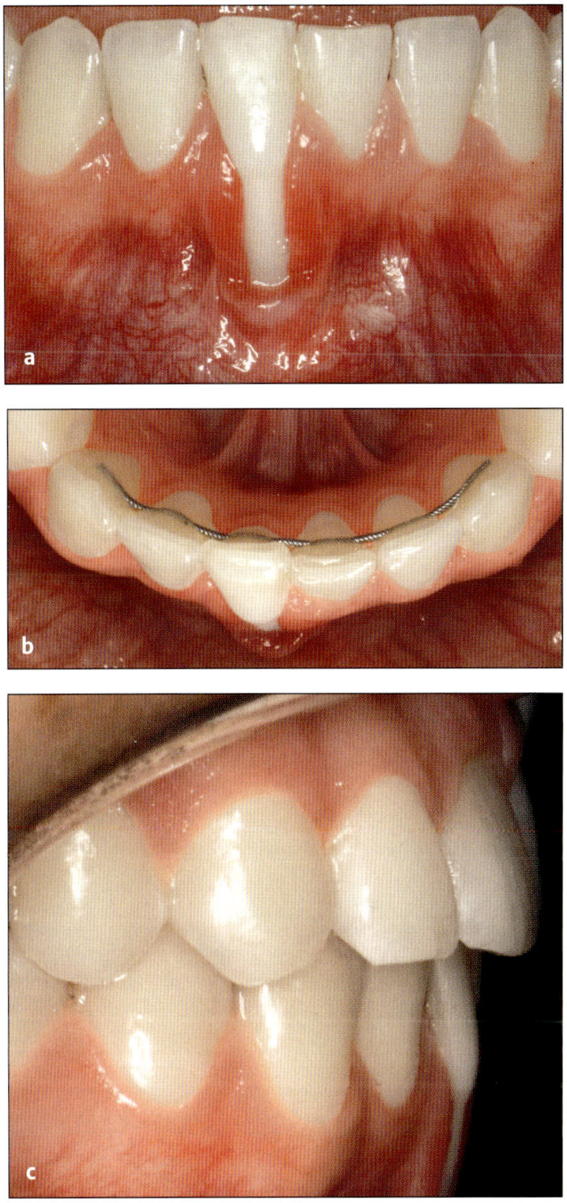

Fig 6-6 *(a to c)* Labial root torque movement of the mandibular right central incisor due to activation of the fixed flexible spiral retainer. The root movement resulted in a deep labial gingival recession. These images show the situation about 4 years after the end of orthodontic treatment.

Indications for the Treatment of Gingival Recessions

Root coverage of gingival recessions is indicated to improve the esthetic appearance, to cure/diminish tooth sensitivity, and to facilitate self-performed oral hygiene, thus preventing gingivitis, root caries, and further progression of the recession-type defects. Untreated gingival recessions are at high risk for further progression.[77–80] In a recent systematic review, 78.1% of recession-type defects showed an increase in recession depth at only 2 years posttreatment; moreover, the number of defects increased to 79.3%.[79] In another longitudinal study conducted in dental students with high standards of oral hygiene, 85% of the subjects presented with buccal gingival recessions; 10 years later, the number of sites with gingival recessions as well as the recession depth increased significantly.[80] In a study comparing surgically treated gingival recessions (gingival augmentation with free gingival graft) with untreated defects 25 years after initial examination, untreated sites showed a significant increase in the recession

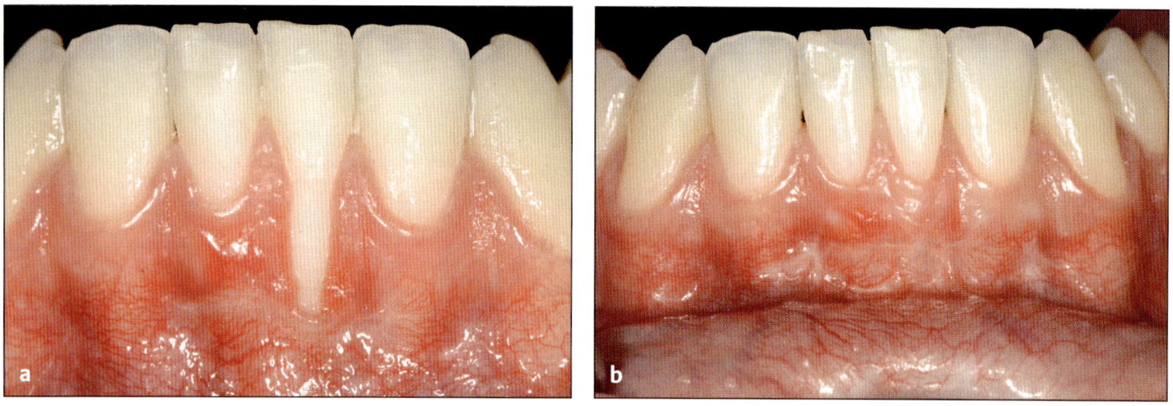

Fig 6-7 *(a)* Gingival recession at the mandibular left central incisor. *(b)* Optimal tissue blending and root coverage after treatment.

depth, whereas 83.5% of the treated sites showed a reduction.[77]

The clinical goal in recession coverage procedures is complete root coverage (100% root coverage), meaning a gingiva located at the CEJ or even slightly above it, with physiologic probing depths (1 to 3 mm) and no signs of inflammation.[81] Moreover, optimal tissue blending with no visible scars should be achieved (Fig 6-7).

Treatment Methods for Gingival Recession Coverage

The surgical therapy for root coverage involves the repositioning of different kinds of flaps onto exposed roots with or without the use of various types of grafts: autogenous grafts (ie, autogenous free gingival grafts, connective tissue grafts [CTGs]) or replacement grafts (ie, animal collagen membranes).

Flap procedures can be divided into rotational flap techniques (eg, laterally sliding flap, oblique rotated flap, double papilla flap), which include the rotation or lateral movement of a pedicle graft, or advanced flap techniques (eg, coronally repositioned flap, semilunar coronally repositioned flap, modified tunneling technique) based on the coronal displacement of a flap. These procedures may be combined with regenerative techniques like the placement of barrier membranes between the graft and the root (ie, guided tissue regeneration) or the application of enamel matrix proteins (ie, enamel matrix derivative [EMD]). According to the available width of the flap or the presence/absence of keratinized or attached mucosa at the recession site, an epithelialized or a subepithelial CTG (nonepithelialized) usually taken from the masticatory mucosa of the palate can be additionally used.

Choosing the appropriate technique depends on the number of recessions (single or multiple), the depth and width of the recession, the depth of the vestibule, the gingival phenotype, the presence or absence of keratinized/attached mucosa, and the presence of muscle attachments.

The clinical concept for the appropriate surgical technique includes the use of biologic factors (ie, EMD) to enhance periodontal healing and regeneration, the avoidance of any vertical releasing incisions if possible to minimize the formation of scar tissue, and the use of soft tissue grafts (ie, CTG) to increase gingival thickness.

For single gingival recessions, the laterally sliding flap introduced by Grupe and Warren in 1956 was considered the gold standard for many years.[82] Later, the use of soft tissue allografts was introduced also for the increase in keratinized tissue.[83] At present,

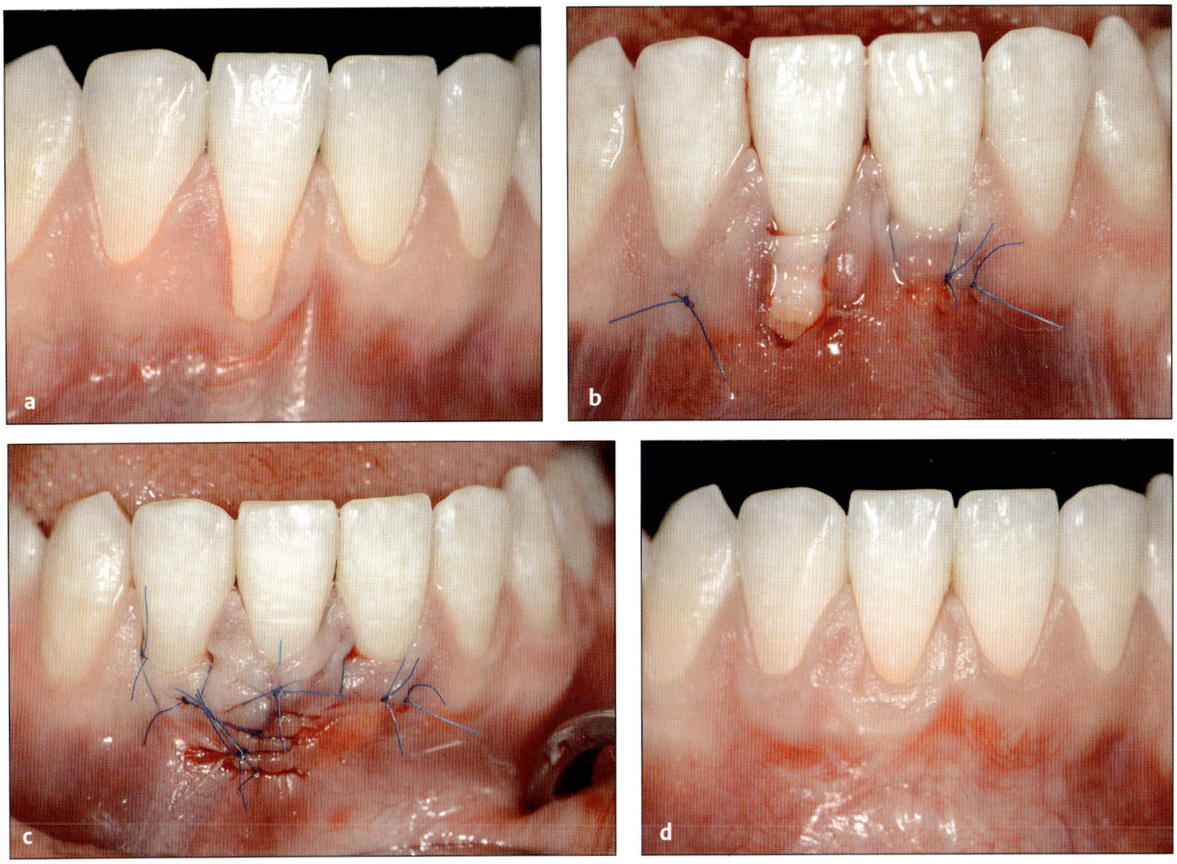

Fig 6-8 Therapy of a single Miller Class I recession in the mandible by means of a laterally closed double tunnel and a CTG. *(a)* Single Miller Class I recession at the mandibular right central incisor prior to surgical therapy. *(b)* Subepithelial CTG inserted and fixed in the tunnel. *(c)* Lateral closure of the double tunnel. *(d)* Clinical result after 12 months. (Case performed by Dr Anton Sculean.)

the coronally advanced flap (CAF) alone or combined with biologics (eg, EMD), autogenous soft tissue grafts, or soft tissue replacement materials (eg, collagen membranes) is considered the gold standard for the treatment of single and multiple gingival recessions.[84–86] More recently, the laterally closed tunnel (Fig 6-8) or the modified coronally advanced tunnel (Fig 6-9) have been shown to yield predictable outcomes in single mandibular recessions.[87]

In many clinical situations, the treatment of multiple gingival recessions is more challenging than the treatment of single defects. Anatomical variations including prominent roots, a shallow vestibule, an uneven amount of attached/keratinized tissue, and the presence of enamel-root abrasions are factors that may interfere with the preparation of the recipient site. In such situations, the surgical field is larger, thus requiring an increased amount of donor tissue, which is sometimes unavailable.

In 1970, Bernimoulin first described a treatment concept for multiple gingival recessions that included gingival augmentation with a free gingival graft and a coronally repositioned flap with two lateral vertical releasing incisions.[88] Later on, the technique was modified by Zucchelli and De Sanctis by eliminating the vertical releasing incisions, incising the papillae, and preparing a combined split-thickness, full-thickness, and again a split-thickness flap. The technique was named the *coronally advanced envelope technique*.[89] When this technique was combined

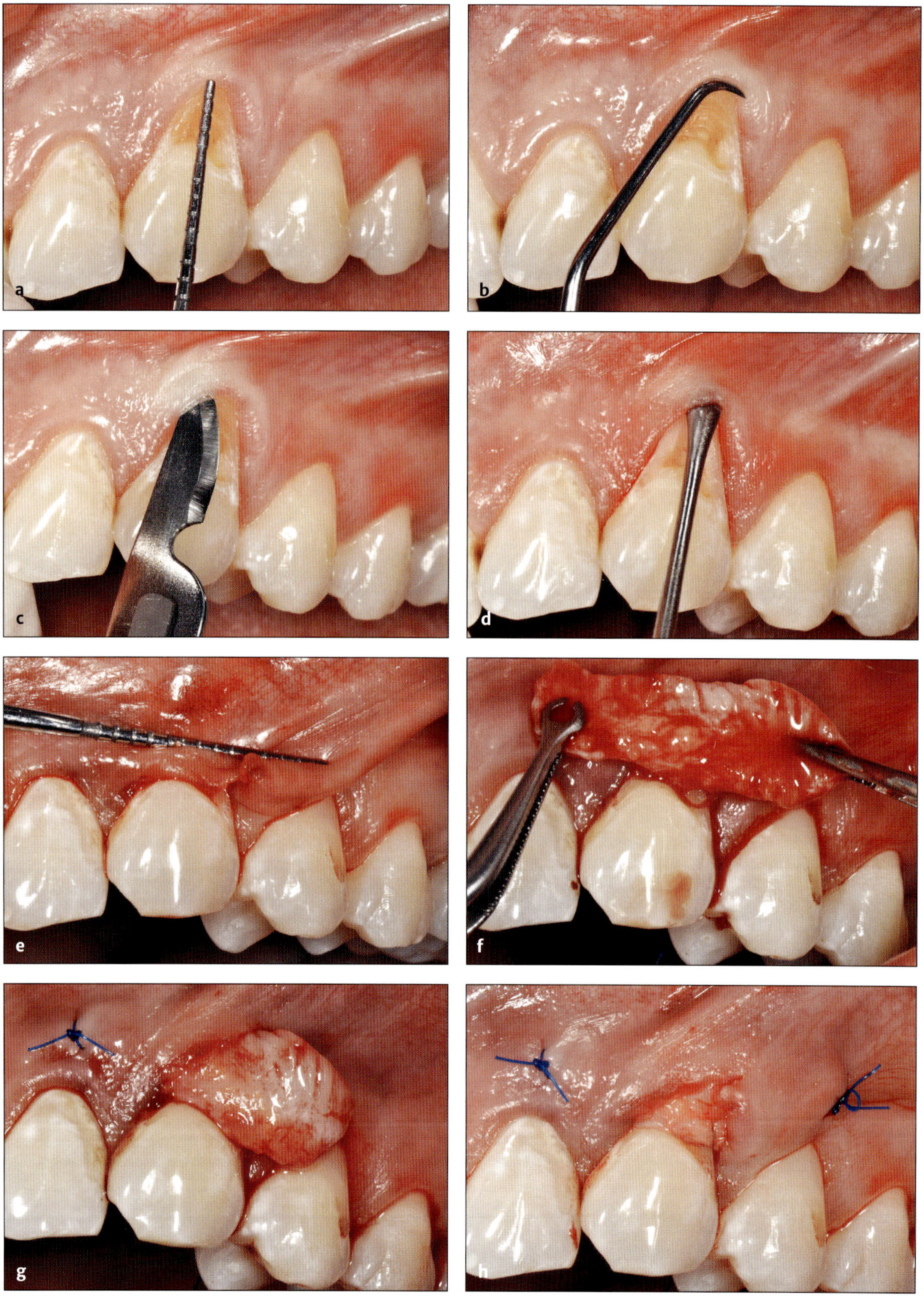

Fig 6-9 Therapy of a Miller Class I recession in the maxilla by means of the modified coronally advanced tunnel and a CTG. *(a)* Clinical situation of the maxillary left canine before surgery. *(b)* Scaling of the root surface. *(c)* Intrasulcular incision. *(d)* Preparation of the tunnel with tunnel knives. *(e)* Prepared tunnel. *(f)* CTG in place. *(g)* Fixation of the CTG in the tunnel at one end. *(h)* Fixation of the CTG in the tunnel at both ends. →

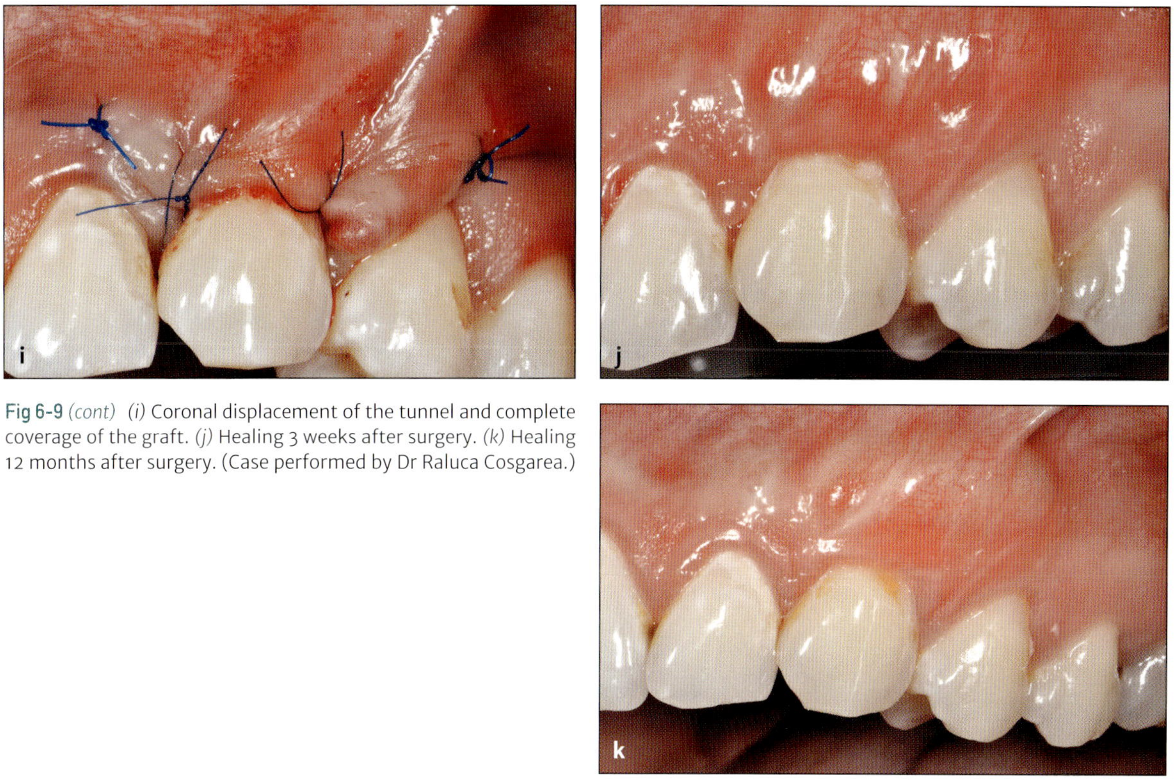

Fig 6-9 *(cont)* *(i)* Coronal displacement of the tunnel and complete coverage of the graft. *(j)* Healing 3 weeks after surgery. *(k)* Healing 12 months after surgery. (Case performed by Dr Raluca Cosgarea.)

with a CTG, 69% of the treated patients showed full coverage at 1 year as opposed to only 25% of the patients treated with the coronally advanced envelope technique alone.[90]

Another clinically efficient predictable surgical technique is the modified coronally advanced technique (MCAT), which may also be combined with soft tissue grafts or replacement membranes[84–86,91,92] (Figs 6-10 and 6-11). The advantage of the MCAT is that the preparation of the recipient bed involves a full-thickness flap, which diminishes the risk for flap perforation during preparation; moreover, no vertical releasing incisions and no incisions of the papillae are used, thus improving vascularization and wound stability.[84–86,91,92] Optimal tissue blending is ensured by the coronal displacement of the flap, thus often entirely covering the CTG. Several studies have shown predictable root coverage of multiple Miller Class I, Class II, and Class III gingival recessions when this technique was combined with a CTG.[84–86,91,92] Moreover, this technique has shown promising results when combined with a porcine collagen membrane.[84]

The use of a CTG may be associated with increased patient morbidity and risk of postoperative bleeding, reduced sensation at the donor site, limited or even lack of connective tissue, and increased surgical time. In order to overcome these aspects, various allografts and collagen-based replacement biomaterials have been used in combination with CAF or tunneling techniques.[84,92–94] The addition of an acellular dermal matrix seems to result in significant improved clinical outcomes regarding the amount of root coverage as compared to the CAF alone.[94–96] However, when compared with the additional use of a CTG, the collagen membrane alone showed statistically significantly fewer sites with complete root coverage.[92,93]

Several factors may compromise the esthetic outcome after surgical root coverage procedures. Patient- and site-related factors may or may not be controlled by the clinician, potentially hindering the treatment outcome. Patient-related factors include poor oral hygiene, traumatic tooth brushing, and smoking.[97–99] Site-specific factors include

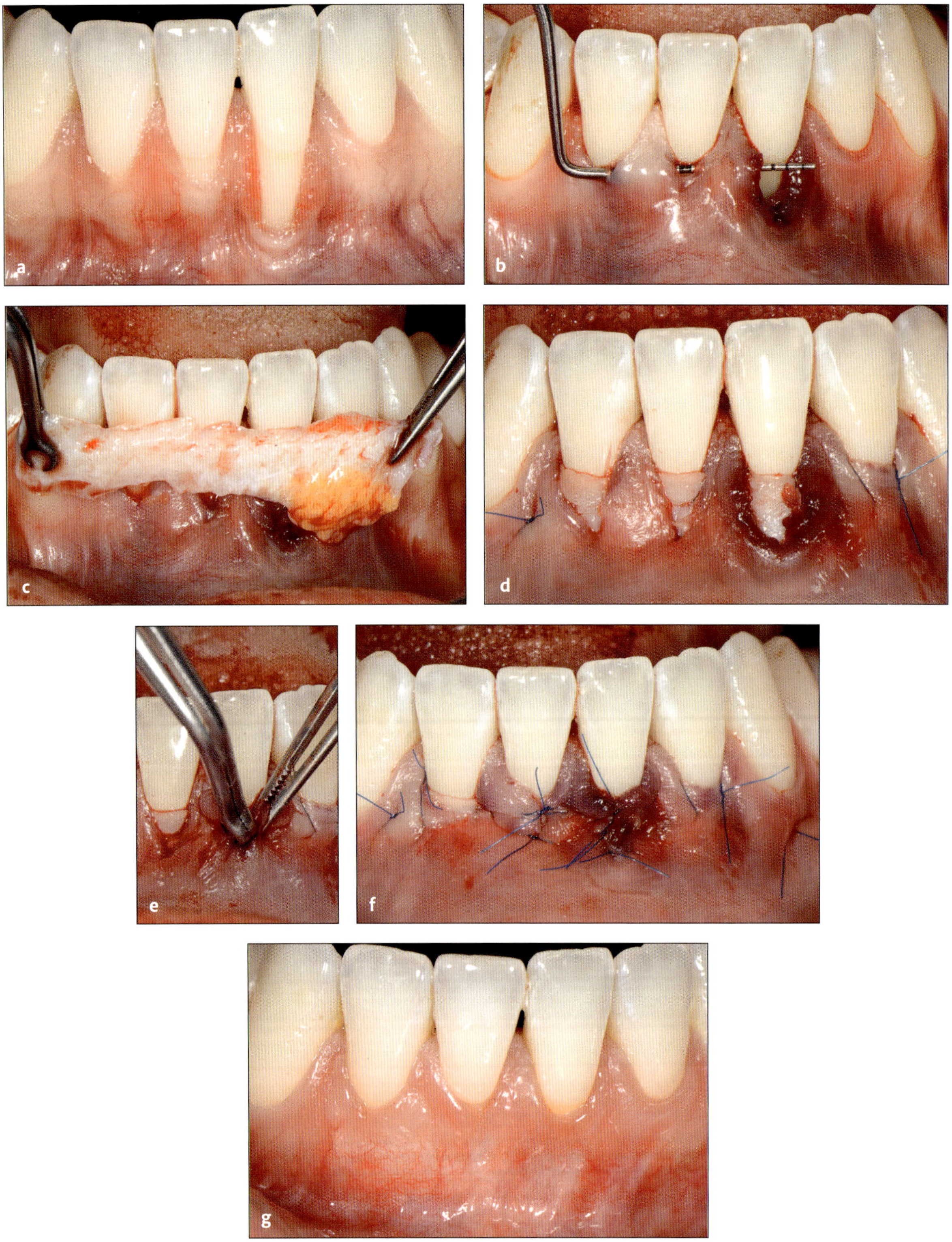

Fig 6-10 Therapy of multiple Miller Class I and Class II gingival recessions in the mandible by means of the MCAT and a CTG. *(a)* Clinical condition prior to surgery. *(b)* Prepared tunnel in the recession area. *(c)* Adaptation of the CTG at the recipient bed. *(d)* CTG inserted and fixed in the tunnel. *(e)* Tension-free adaptation of the tunnel margins. *(f)* Tension-free closure of the tunnel and coverage of the CTG and recessions. *(g)* Clinical outcome 12 months after multiple recession coverage. (Case performed by Dr Anton Sculean.)

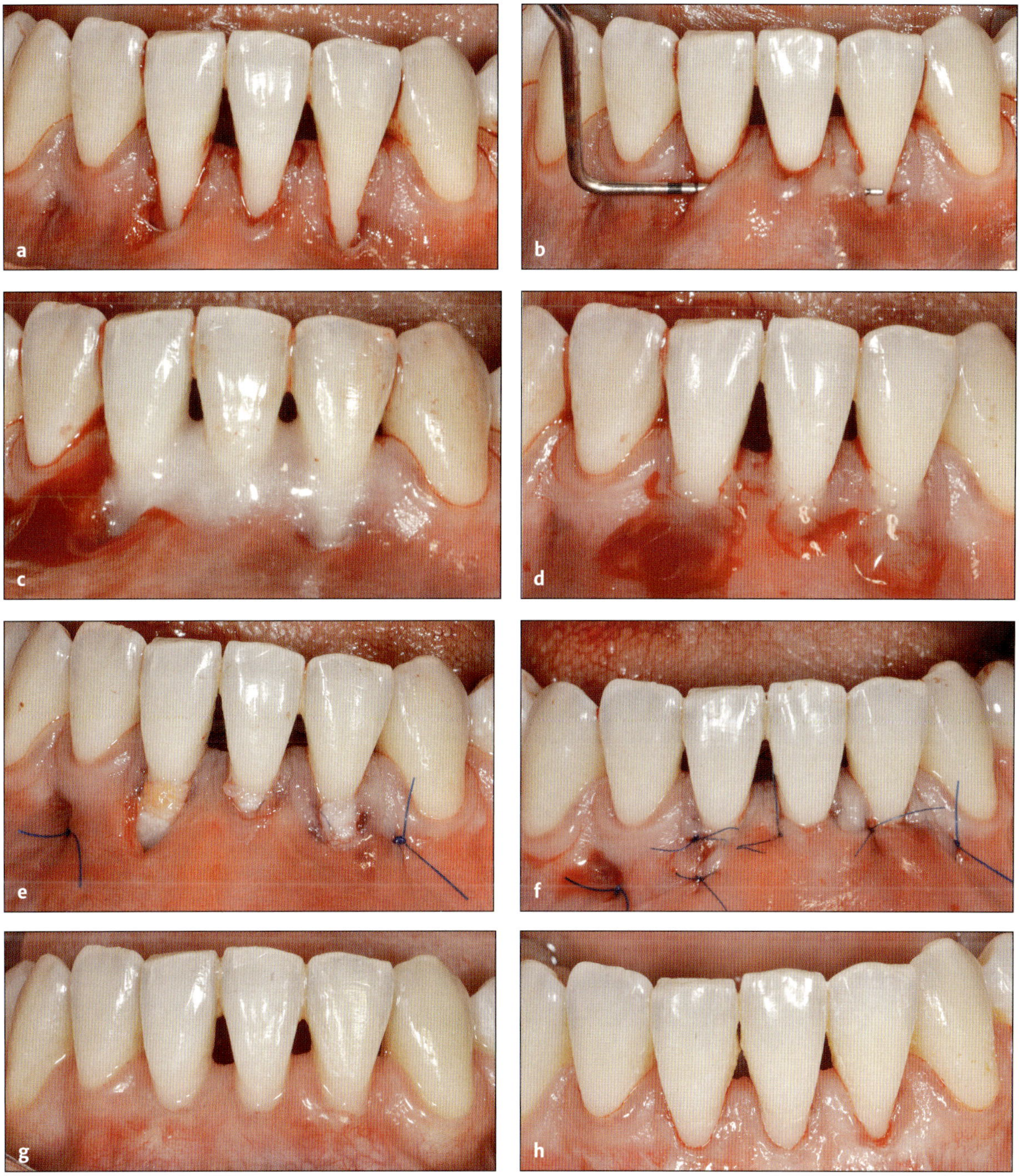

Fig 6-11 Treatment of multiple mandibular Miller Class III recessions with MCAT in combination with CTG and EMD after orthodontic treatment. *(a)* Clinical condition prior to surgery. *(b)* Preparation of the recipient bed (tunnel). *(c)* Root conditioning with PrefGel (Straumann). *(d)* Application of EMD (Emdogain, Straumann). *(e)* Inserted CTG and fixation with mattress and sling sutures. *(f)* Coronal displacement of the tunnel. *(g)* Clinical situation 3 weeks after surgery. *(h)* Clinical result 12 months after surgery. (Case performed by Dr Raluca Cosgarea.)

bulky tooth morphology, root anatomy, crowding, a high number of recessions, increased depth (at least 5 mm)[100] and width (greater than 3 mm) of the recessions, thin gingival phenotype, depth of the vestibule, and loss of interdental bone and papillae.[18,101–104] In cases with labially or lingually positioned roots, orthodontic torque movement may be indicated prior to the surgical root coverage procedure.

Technique-related factors like primary poor wound stability and blood supply (ie, vertical releasing incisions diminish the blood supply and the wound stability),[105] inappropriate flap design and tension in the flap, tension on the sutures, and the use of thick grafts[105–108] may be avoided by the clinician by choosing the appropriate surgical technique and improving the surgical skills.

References

1. Nanci A, Bosshardt DD. Structure of periodontal tissues in health and disease. Periodontol 2000 2006;40:11–28.
2. Lindhe J, Karring T, Araujo M. The anatomy of periodontal tissues. In: Lindhe JL, Niklaus P, Karring T (eds). Clinical Periodontology and Implant Dentistry, ed 5. Oxford: Blackwell, 2008:3–49.
3. Bosshardt DD. Anatomy of the periodontium in health and disease. In: Sculean A (ed). Periodontal Regenerative Therapy. London: Quintessence, 2010:5–24.
4. Bosshardt DD, Lang NP. The junctional epithelium: From health to disease. J Dent Res 2005;84:9–20.
5. Müller HP, Eger T. Gingival phenotypes in young male adults. J Clin Periodontol 1997;24:65–71.
6. Ochsenbein C, Ross S. A reevaluation of osseous surgery. Dent Clin North Am 1969;13:87–102.
7. Weisgold AS. Contours of the full crown restoration. Alpha Omegan 1977;70:77–89.
8. Seibert JS. Ridge augmentation to enhance esthetics in fixed prosthetic treatment. Compendium 1991;12: 548,550,552.
9. Olsson M, Lindhe J, Marinello CP. On the relationship between crown form and clinical features of the gingiva in adolescents. J Clin Periodontol 1993;20:570–577.
10. De Rouck T, Eghbali R, Collys K, De Bruyn H, Cosyn J. The gingival biotype revisited: Transparency of the periodontal probe through the gingival margin as a method to discriminate thin from thick gingiva. J Clin Periodontol 2009;36:428–433.
11. Müller HP, Schaller N, Eger T, Heinecke A. Thickness of masticatory mucosa. J Clin Periodontol 2000;27:431–436.
12. Vandana KL, Savitha B. Thickness of gingiva in association with age, gender and dental arch location. J Clin Periodontol 2005;32:828–830.
13. Zweers J, Thomas RZ, Slot DE, Weisgold AS, Van der Weijden FG. Characteristics of periodontal biotype, its dimensions, associations and prevalence: A systematic review. J Clin Periodontol 2014;41:958–971.
14. Jepsen S, Caton JG, Albandar JM, et al. Periodontal manifestations of systemic diseases and developmental and acquired conditions: Consensus report of workgroup 3 of the 2017 World Workshop on the Classification of Periodontal and Peri-Implant Diseases and Conditions. J Clin Periodontol 2018;45(suppl 20):S219–S229.
15. Dictionary of Biology. Oxford: Oxford University Press, 2008.
16. Kao RT, Fagan MC, Conte GJ. Thick vs. thin gingival biotypes: A key determinant in treatment planning for dental implants. J Calif Dent Assoc 2008;36:193–198.
17. Huang LH, Neiva RE, Wang HL. Factors affecting the outcomes of coronally advanced flap root coverage procedure. J Periodontol 2005;76:1729–1734.
18. Hwang D, Wang HL. Flap thickness as a predictor of root coverage: A systematic review. J Periodontol 2006;77: 1625–1634.
19. Kan JY, Rungcharassaeng K, Umezu K, Kois JC. Dimensions of peri-implant mucosa: An evaluation of maxillary anterior single implants in humans. J Periodontol 2003;74: 557–562.
20. Baldi C, Pini-Prato G, Pagliaro U, et al. Coronally advanced flap procedure for root coverage. Is flap thickness a relevant predictor to achieve root coverage? A 19-case series. J Periodontol 1999;70:1077–1084.
21. Claffey N, Shanley D. Relationship of gingival thickness and bleeding to loss of probing attachment in shallow sites following nonsurgical periodontal therapy. J Clin Periodontol 1986;13:654–657.
22. Evans CD, Chen ST. Esthetic outcomes of immediate implant placements. Clin Oral Implants Res 2008;19: 73–80.
23. Romeo E, Lops D, Rossi A, Storelli S, Rozza R, Chiapasco M. Surgical and prosthetic management of interproximal region with single-implant restorations: 1-year prospective study. J Periodontol 2008;79:1048–1055.
24. Pontoriero R, Carnevale G. Surgical crown lengthening: A 12-month clinical wound healing study. J Periodontol 2001;72:841–848.
25. Rasperini G, Acunzo R, Cannalire P, Farronato G. Influence of periodontal biotype on root surface exposure during orthodontic treatment: A preliminary study. Int J Periodontics Restorative Dent 2015;35:665–675.
26. Greenberg J, Laster L, Listgarten MA. Transgingival probing as a potential estimator of alveolar bone level. J Periodontol 1976;47:514–517.
27. Barriviera M, Duarte WR, Januário AL, Faber J, Bezerra AC. A new method to assess and measure palatal masticatory mucosa by cone-beam computerized tomography. J Clin Periodontol 2009;36:564–568.
28. Kan JY, Morimoto T, Rungcharassaeng K, Roe P, Smith DH. Gingival biotype assessment in the esthetic zone: Visual versus direct measurement. Int J Periodontics Restorative Dent 2010;30:237–243.

29. Fu JH, Yeh CY, Chan HL, Tatarakis N, Leong DJ, Wang HL. Tissue biotype and its relation to the underlying bone morphology. J Periodontol 2010;81:569–574.
30. Cook DR, Mealey BL, Verrett RG, et al. Relationship between clinical periodontal biotype and labial plate thickness: An in vivo study. Int J Periodontics Restorative Dent 2011;31:345–354.
31. Frost NA, Mealey BL, Jones AA, Huynh-Ba G. Periodontal biotype: Gingival thickness as it relates to probe visibility and buccal plate thickness. J Periodontol 2015;86: 1141–1149.
32. Armitage GC. Development of a classification system for periodontal diseases and conditions. Ann Periodontol 1999;4:1–6.
33. Wennström JL. Mucogingival therapy. Ann Periodontol 1996;1:671–701.
34. Miller PD Jr. A classification of marginal tissue recession. Int J Periodontics Restorative Dent 1985;5:8–13.
35. Cairo F, Nieri M, Cincinelli S, Mervelt J, Pagliaro U. The interproximal clinical attachment level to classify gingival recessions and predict root coverage outcomes: An explorative and reliability study. J Clin Periodontol 2011; 38:661–666.
36. Pini-Prato G, Franceschi D, Cairo F, Nieri M, Rotundo R. Classification of dental surface defects in areas of gingival recession. J Periodontol 2010;81:885–890.
37. Löe H, Anerud A, Boysen H. The natural history of periodontal disease in man: Prevalence, severity, and extent of gingival recession. J Periodontol 1992;63:489–495.
38. Sarfati A, Bourgeois D, Katsahian S, Mora F, Bouchard P. Risk assessment for buccal gingival recession defects in an adult population. J Periodontol 2010;81:1419–1425.
39. Susin C, Haas AN, Oppermann RV, Haugejorden O, Albandar JM. Gingival recession: Epidemiology and risk indicators in a representative urban Brazilian population. J Periodontol 2004;75:1377–1386.
40. Baelum V, Fejerskov O, Karring T. Oral hygiene, gingivitis and periodontal breakdown in adult Tanzanians. J Periodontal Res 1986;21:221–232.
41. Serino G, Wennström JL, Lindhe J, Eneroth L. The prevalence and distribution of gingival recession in subjects with a high standard of oral hygiene. J Clin Periodontol 1994;21:57–63.
42. Albandar JM, Kingman A. Gingival recession, gingival bleeding, and dental calculus in adults 30 years of age and older in the United States, 1988-1994. J Periodontol 1999;70:30–43.
43. Gorman WJ. Prevalence and etiology of gingival recession. J Periodontol 1967;38:316–322.
44. Murray JJ. Gingival recession in tooth types in high fluoride and low fluoride areas. J Periodontal Res 1973;8: 243–251.
45. Rios FS, Costa RS, Moura MS, Jardim JJ, Maltz M, Haas AN. Estimates and multivariable risk assessment of gingival recession in the population of adults from Porto Alegre, Brazil. J Clin Periodontol 2014;41:1098–1107.
46. Sangnes G. Traumatization of teeth and gingiva related to habitual tooth cleaning procedures. J Clin Periodontol 1976;3:94–103.
47. Khocht A, Simon G, Person P, Denepitiya JL. Gingival recession in relation to history of hard toothbrush use. J Periodontol 1993;64:900–905.
48. Kassab MM, Cohen RE. The etiology and prevalence of gingival recession. J Am Dent Assoc 2003;134:220–225.
49. Chrysanthakopoulos NA. Prevalence and associated factors of gingival recession in Greek adults. J Investig Clin Dent 2013;4:178–185.
50. Bernimoulin J, Curilović Z. Gingival recession and tooth mobility. J Clin Periodontol 1977;4:107–114.
51. Modéer T, Odenrick L. Post-treatment periodontal status of labially erupted maxillary canines. Acta Odontol Scand 1980;38:253–256.
52. Olsson M, Lindhe J. Periodontal characteristics in individuals with varying form of the upper central incisors. J Clin Periodontol 1991;18:78–82.
53. Daprile G, Gatto MR, Checchi L. The evolution of buccal gingival recessions in a student population: A 5-year follow-up. J Periodontol 2007;78:611–614.
54. Bergström J, Eliasson S. Cervical abrasion in relation to toothbrushing and periodontal health. Scand J Dent Res 1988;96:405–411.
55. Sandholm L, Niemi ML, Ainamo J. Identification of soft tissue brushing lesions. A clinical and scanning electron microscopic study. J Clin Periodontol 1982;9:397–401.
56. Heasman PA, Holliday R, Bryant A, Preshaw PM. Evidence for the occurrence of gingival recession and non-carious cervical lesions as a consequence of traumatic toothbrushing. J Clin Periodontol 2015;42(suppl 16):S237–S255.
57. Müller HP, Heinecke A, Schaller N, Eger T. Masticatory mucosa in subjects with different periodontal phenotypes. J Clin Periodontol 2000;27:621–626.
58. Rothlisberger B, Kuonen P, Salvi GE, et al. Periodontal conditions in Swiss army recruits: A comparative study between the years 1985, 1996 and 2006. J Clin Periodontol 2007;34:860–866.
59. Kapferer I, Benesch T, Gregoric N, Ulm C, Hienz SA. Lip piercing: Prevalence of associated gingival recession and contributing factors. A cross-sectional study. J Periodontal Res 2007;42:177–183.
60. Kapferer I, Beier US. Lateral lower lip piercing—Prevalence of associated oral complications: A split-mouth cross-sectional study. Quintessence Int 2012;43: 747–752.
61. Baker DL, Seymour GJ. The possible pathogenesis of gingival recession. A histological study of induced recession in the rat. J Clin Periodontol 1976;3:208–219.
62. Stetler KJ, Bissada NF. Significance of the width of keratinized gingiva on the periodontal status of teeth with submarginal restorations. J Periodontol 1987;58: 696–700.
63. Wennström JL. Mucogingival considerations in orthodontic treatment. Semin Orthod 1996;2:46–54.
64. Joss-Vassalli I, Grebenstein C, Topouzelis N, Sculean A, Katsaros C. Orthodontic therapy and gingival recession: A systematic review. Orthod Craniofac Res 2010;13: 127–141.
65. Allais D, Melsen B. Does labial movement of lower incisors influence the level of the gingival margin? A case-control study of adult orthodontic patients. Eur J Orthod 2003; 25:343–352.
66. Thomson WM. Orthodontic treatment outcomes in the long term: Findings from a longitudinal study of New Zealanders. Angle Orthod 2002;72:449–455.

67. Renkema AM, Fudalej PS, Renkema AA, Abbas F, Bronkhorst E, Katsaros C. Gingival labial recessions in orthodontically treated and untreated individuals: A case-control study. J Clin Periodontol 2013;40:631–637.
68. Slutzkey S, Levin L. Gingival recession in young adults: Occurrence, severity, and relationship to past orthodontic treatment and oral piercing. Am J Orthod Dentofacial Orthop 2008;134:652–656.
69. Gebistorf M, Mijuskovic M, Pandis N, Fudalej PS, Katsaros C. Gingival recession in orthodontic patients 10 to 15 years posttreatment: A retrospective cohort study. Am J Orthod Dentofacial Orthop 2018;153:645–655.
70. Renkema AM, Fudalej PS, Renkema A, Kiekens R, Katsaros C. Development of labial gingival recessions in orthodontically treated patients. Am J Orthod Dentofacial Orthop 2013;143:206–212.
71. Litonjua LA, Andreana S, Bush PJ, Cohen RE. Toothbrushing and gingival recession. Int Dent J 2003;53:67–72.
72. Pandis N, Vlahopoulos K, Madianos P, Eliades T. Long-term periodontal status of patients with mandibular lingual fixed retention. Eur J Orthod 2007;29:471–476.
73. Renkema AM, Navratilova Z, Mazurova K, Katsaros C, Fudalej PS. Gingival labial recessions and the post-treatment proclination of mandibular incisors. Eur J Orthod 2015;37:508–513.
74. Katsaros C, Livas C, Renkema AM. Unexpected complications of bonded mandibular lingual retainers. Am J Orthod Dentofacial Orthop 2007;132:838–841.
75. Farret MM, Farret MM, da Luz Vieira G, Assaf JH, de Lima EM. Orthodontic treatment of a mandibular incisor fenestration resulting from a broken retainer. Am J Orthod Dentofacial Orthop 2015;148:332–337.
76. Pazera P, Fudalej P, Katsaros C. Severe complication of a bonded mandibular lingual retainer. Am J Orthod Dentofacial Orthop 2012;142:406–409.
77. Agudio G, Chambrone L, Pini Prato G. Biologic remodeling of periodontal dimensions of areas treated with gingival augmentation procedure: A 25-year follow-up observation. J Periodontol 2017;88:634–642.
78. Agudio G, Cortellini P, Buti J, Pini Prato G. Periodontal conditions of sites treated with gingival augmentation surgery compared with untreated contralateral homologous sites: An 18- to 35-year long-term study. J Periodontol 2016;87:1371–1378.
79. Chambrone L, Tatakis DN. Periodontal soft tissue root coverage procedures: A systematic review from the AAP Regeneration Workshop. J Periodontol 2015;86(suppl 2):S8–S51.
80. Matas F, Sentis J, Mendieta C. Ten-year longitudinal study of gingival recession in dentists. J Clin Periodontol 2011;38:1091–1098.
81. Cairo F, Rotundo R, Miller PD, Pini Prato GP. Root coverage esthetic score: A system to evaluate the esthetic outcome of the treatment of gingival recession through evaluation of clinical cases. J Periodontol 2009;80:705–710.
82. Grupe HE, Warren RF. Repair of gingival defects by a sliding flap operation. J Periodontol 1956;27:92–95.
83. Nabers JM. Free gingival grafts. Periodontics 1966;4:243–245.
84. Cosgarea R, Juncar R, Arweiler N, Lascu L, Sculean A. Clinical evaluation of a porcine acellular dermal matrix for the treatment of multiple adjacent class I, II, and III gingival recessions using the modified coronally advanced tunnel technique. Quintessence Int 2016;47:739–747.
85. Sculean A, Cosgarea R, Stähli A, et al. The modified coronally advanced tunnel combined with an enamel matrix derivative and subepithelial connective tissue graft for the treatment of isolated mandibular Miller Class I and II gingival recessions: A report of 16 cases. Quintessence Int 2014;45:829–835.
86. Sculean A, Cosgarea R, Stähli A, et al. Treatment of multiple adjacent maxillary Miller Class I, II, and III gingival recessions with the modified coronally advanced tunnel, enamel matrix derivative, and subepithelial connective tissue graft: A report of 12 cases. Quintessence Int 2016;47:653–659.
87. Sculean A, Allen EP. The laterally closed tunnel for the treatment of deep isolated mandibular recessions: Surgical technique and a report of 24 cases. Int J Periodontics Restorative Dent 2018;38:479–487.
88. Bernimoulin JP, Lüscher B, Mühlemann HR. Coronally repositioned periodontal flap. Clinical evaluation after one year. J Clin Periodontol 1975;2:1–13.
89. Zucchelli G, De Sanctis M. Treatment of multiple recession-type defects in patients with esthetic demands. J Periodontol 2000;71:1506–1514.
90. Cairo F, Cortellini P, Pilloni A, et al. Clinical efficacy of coronally advanced flap with or without connective tissue graft for the treatment of multiple adjacent gingival recessions in the aesthetic area: A randomized controlled clinical trial. J Clin Periodontol 2016;43:849–856.
91. Aroca S, Keglevich T, Nikolidakis D, et al. Treatment of class III multiple gingival recessions: A randomized-clinical trial. J Clin Periodontol 2010;37:88–97.
92. Aroca S, Molnár B, Windisch P, et al. Treatment of multiple adjacent Miller class I and II gingival recessions with a modified coronally advanced tunnel (MCAT) technique and a collagen matrix or palatal connective tissue graft: A randomized, controlled clinical trial. J Clin Periodontol 2013;40:713–720.
93. Tonetti M, Cortellini P, Pellegrini G, et al. Multicentre multinational trial comparing coronally advanced rotated papillae flaps with connective tissue graft or collagen construct for coverage of multiple adjacent recessions [abstract]. J Clin Periodontol 2015;42:19.
94. Cardaropoli D, Tamagnone L, Roffredo A, Gaveglio L. Coronally advanced flap with and without a xenogenic collagen matrix in the treatment of multiple recessions: A randomized controlled clinical study. Int J Periodontics Restorative Dent 2014;34(suppl 3):S97–S102.
95. Ahmedbeyli C, Ipci SD, Cakar G, Kuru BE, Yilmaz S. Clinical evaluation of coronally advanced flap with or without acellular dermal matrix graft on complete defect coverage for the treatment of multiple gingival recessions with thin tissue biotype. J Clin Periodontol 2014;41:303–310.
96. Thombre V, Koudale SB, Bhongade ML. Comparative evaluation of the effectiveness of coronally positioned flap with or without acellular dermal matrix allograft in the treatment of multiple marginal gingival recession defects. Int J Periodontics Restorative Dent 2013;33:e88–e94.

97. Caffesse RG, Alspach SR, Morrison EC, Burgett FG. Lateral sliding flaps with and without citric acid. Int J Periodontics Restorative Dent 1987;7:42–57.
98. Silva CO, Sallum AW, de Lima AF, Tatakis DN. Coronally positioned flap for root coverage: Poorer outcomes in smokers. J Periodontol 2006;77:81–87.
99. Trombelli L, Scabbia A. Healing response of gingival recession defects following guided tissue regeneration procedures in smokers and non-smokers. J Clin Periodontol 1997;24:529–533.
100. Holbrook T, Ochsenbein C. Complete coverage of the denuded root surface with a one-stage gingival graft. Int J Periodontics Restorative Dent 1983;3:8–27.
101. Berlucchi I, Francetti L, Del Fabbro M, Basso M, Weinstein RL. The influence of anatomical features on the outcome of gingival recessions treated with coronally advanced flap and enamel matrix derivative: A 1-year prospective study. J Periodontol 2005;76:899–907.
102. Chambrone L, Chambrone D, Pustiglioni FE, Chambrone LA, Lima LA. The influence of tobacco smoking on the outcomes achieved by root-coverage procedures: A systematic review. J Am Dent Assoc 2009;140:294–306.
103. Clauser C, Nieri M, Franceschi D, Pagliaro U, Pini-Prato G. Evidence-based mucogingival therapy. Part 2: Ordinary and individual patient data meta-analyses of surgical treatment of recession using complete root coverage as the outcome variable. J Periodontol 2003;74:741–756.
104. Trombelli L, Schincaglia GP, Scapoli C, Calura G. Healing response of human buccal gingival recessions treated with expanded polytetrafluoroethylene membranes. A retrospective report. J Periodontol 1995;66:14–22.
105. Zucchelli G, Mele M, Mazzotti C, Marzadori M, Montebugnoli L, De Sanctis M. Coronally advanced flap with and without vertical releasing incisions for the treatment of multiple gingival recessions: A comparative controlled randomized clinical trial. J Periodontol 2009;80:1083–1094.
106. Borghetti A, Gardella JP. Thick gingival autograft for the coverage of gingival recession: A clinical evaluation. Int J Periodontics Restorative Dent 1990;10:216–229.
107. Pini Prato G, Pagliaro U, Baldi C, et al. Coronally advanced flap procedure for root coverage. Flap with tension versus flap without tension: A randomized controlled clinical study. J Periodontol 2000;71:188–201.
108. Zucchelli G, Amore C, Sforza NM, Montebugnoli L, De Sanctis M. Bilaminar techniques for the treatment of recession-type defects. A comparative clinical study. J Clin Periodontol 2003;30:862–870.

CHAPTER 7

Soft Tissue Augmentation at Maxillary and Mandibular Incisors in Orthodontic Patients

Dimitrios Kloukos
Theodore Eliades
Anton Sculean
Christos Katsaros

Gingival recession refers to the apical displacement of the gingival margin from the cementoenamel junction.[1] Gingival recessions can be localized or may involve several teeth or tooth surfaces. The resulting root surface exposure often causes esthetic concerns,[2] dentin hypersensitivity,[3] and increased susceptibility to gingivitis and/or root caries.[4] Data from epidemiologic studies have shown a prevalence of 60% in patients 20 years or younger and more than 90% in patients older than 50 years; interestingly, the individuals studied had a reasonable level of oral hygiene.[5] Gingival recessions have also been found to be more frequent in mandibular teeth than in maxillary teeth, and on facial surfaces than on lingual surfaces, especially with increasing age.[6]

As early as 1976, a justification regarding the pathogenesis of gingival recession was brought forward.[7] Localized inflammation in a "thin type" gingiva (Fig 7-1) might involve the entire volume of gingival tissue, and the consequent remodeling could lead to recession of the gingival margin. On the other hand, in a "thick type" gingiva (Fig 7-2), this inflammatory lesion could be confined to only a part of the sulcus, leaving the outer gingival tissue unaffected. This could probably predispose to pocket formation rather than recession. Although the proposal of this mechanism was based on a rat model, it may be considered as the primary concept that recognized that the thin gingival biotype (referred to as *phenotype* today) can be a risk factor for recession (see Fig 7-1). Since the late 1970s, other studies have also found a correlation between thickness of the free gingival margin and incidence of recession. For instance, gingival thickness of less than 0.5 mm has been related to more frequent and more severe recessions in mandibular anterior teeth

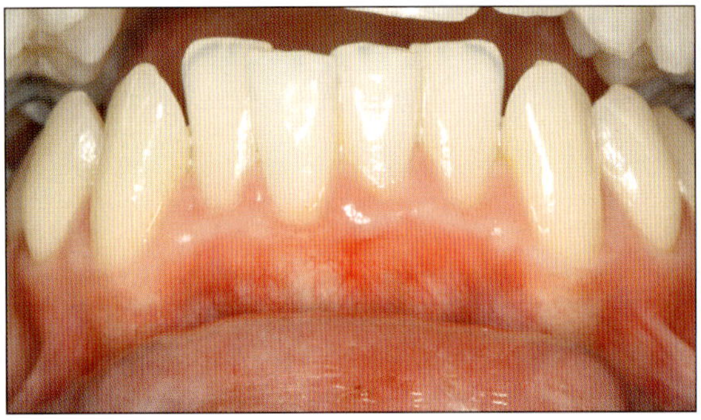

Fig 7-1 Thin gingival phenotype.

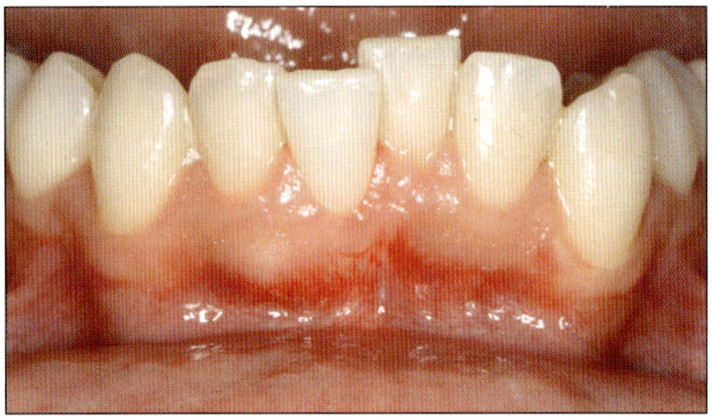

Fig 7-2 Thick gingival phenotype.

during proclination.[8] Additionally, many other factors may play a role in the development of gingival recession, not necessarily simultaneously or equally. Periodontal diseases and mechanical trauma are the two primary etiologic factors in the pathogenesis of gingival recessions.[1,2,5,9–11] Traumatic tooth brushing appears to be an important factor associated with gingival recessions.[6] Other, secondary etiologic factors might include existing bone dehiscences, smoking, and intra- and perioral piercings.[11–13]

Orthodontic Tooth Movement and Gingival Recession

A possible etiologic factor for gingival recession is the orthodontic movement of teeth, especially the movement of teeth to positions outside the labial or lingual alveolar plate, which could lead to the development of dehiscence.[14] A systematic review indicated that proclination and movement of the mandibular incisors out of the osseous envelope of the alveolar process may be associated with a higher tendency for developing gingival recessions. However, the amount of recession found in the included studies, which showed statistically significant differences between proclined and not proclined incisors, was small and the clinical consequence regarded as questionable.[15]

The precise mechanism by which orthodontic treatment influences the occurrence of recessions remains unclear. It has been assumed that the presence of bony dehiscence is a prerequisite for the development of gingival recession.[16] Because a bony dehiscence does not always lead to recession,[17] other factors, such as the ones described previously, must be present.

Among the numerous orthodontic treatment procedures and modalities, the issue of incisor proclination outside the dentoalveolar envelope as a source of gingival recession has been considered for years. Although it is broadly believed that mandibular incisor proclination leads to gingival recession, there are very few clinical studies that have actually investigated this. Some of them have shown gingival recession to be associated with proclination of the mandibular incisors,[8,18] whereas others have found no such correlation.[19–21] A series of recent retrospective studies has shown that although the change of inclination of mandibular incisors during orthodontic treatment or the degree of posttreatment inclination may not affect the development of labial recessions,[22,23] these teeth are nevertheless vulnerable to the development of recessions,[24] with their prevalence being age dependent and increasing steadily in the period before treatment and up to 15 years posttreatment.[25,26]

Gingival Augmentation

In order to prevent the development of gingival recessions in orthodontic patients, gingival augmentation to recreate the zone of attached gingiva has been proposed. The early concept for this approach was that attached gingiva is important to dissipate the force of muscle pull and unattached mucosa and could be more suitable to withstand the trauma of mastication and tooth brushing.[27–29]

Several periodontal surgical procedures have been suggested to increase the width of the attached gingiva or the volume of the facial soft tissue to prevent the development of gingival recessions. Such periodontal augmentation procedures usually include the use of free gingival grafts, a coronally advanced flap in conjunction with subepithelial connective tissue grafts (CTGs), soft tissue replacement materials, or even enamel matrix proteins. Among these, CTGs are generally considered the gold standard in gingival augmentation.[30,31] However, some clinicians consider this preventive approach to be overtreatment and prefer to wait until the potential gingival recession becomes a pathologic and clinical entity. Subsequently, the developed recession may be treated during or after orthodontic therapy.

While some guidelines exist about what constitutes an adequate width of the attached gingiva,[29] determining the sufficient width to withstand the stress and adverse effects related to the increase in mandibular incisor inclination as well as the timing of the proposed periodontal intervention remain highly subjective. Therefore, the aim of this chapter is to appraise the indication and timing of the performance of gingival augmentation in orthodontic patients, who will experience a change in the inclination of the incisors during treatment. A recently published systematic review was utilized as the basis[32] for providing the evidence discussed in this chapter, but an up-to-date literature assessment was also performed.

Available Evidence on Grafting in Conjunction with Orthodontic Treatment

Two studies provide evidence on this topic, but neither is a randomized controlled trial. One study had both prospective and retrospective data collection,[33] and the other had a retrospective design[34] (Table 7-1). Both implemented a periodontal intervention before orthodontic treatment.

Quality assessment of the studies indicated that only the retrospective study had a moderate value of evidence.[34] The other study was graded as a low level of evidence due to the poorly defined patient population (ie, no age, race, or sex specifics).[33]

An overview of the experimental setup of the included studies is given in Table 7-1. In the first study,[33] autogenous free gingival grafting was implemented as a preventive measure before orthodontic treatment in some young patients (exact number and age not given). These constituted only a part of the sample of 100 children. The mandibular central incisors were evaluated. In the second study,[34] the authors evaluated 20 patients with more than 1 mm of labial recession on one or more mandibular central incisors before treatment. These patients were divided into two groups: One group received an autogenous free gingival graft in the area of recession prior to orthodontics, and the second group (control group) received no graft before orthodontics. In both groups, the incisors were retroclined during treatment.

CLINICAL FINDINGS

Table 7-1 gives an overview of the results of these studies regarding clinical parameters. Both studies used periodontal surgery (eg, either regenerative treatment or soft tissue grafting) before orthodontic treatment. Consequently, the determination of best timing (before, during, or after orthodontic treatment) could not be assessed.

Maynard and Ochsenbein[33] stated that autogenous free gingival grafting can be recommended as an acceptable procedure prior to tooth movement in cases where orthodontic therapy is anticipated and insufficient keratinized tissue exists. According to the authors, grafts can be recommended in patients with 1 mm or less of keratinized tissue.

Ngan et al[34] found that teeth presenting true gingival recession had statistically less gingival

Table 7-1 Design, methods, and results of evaluated studies

	Maynard and Ochsenbein[33] (1975)	Ngan et al[34] (1991)
Experimental setup		
Design	Retrospective and prospective	Retrospective
Number, sex, and age of patients	100 children	20 children (12 females and 8 males) aged 11 to 16 years with labial recession
Type of orthodontic therapy	Fixed appliances	Fixed appliances
Teeth moved	Mandibular central incisors	Mandibular central incisors (retroclination)
Orthodontic treatment duration	Not reported	18–30 months (mean 24 months)
Periodontal treatment before or after orthodontic treatment	Before as preventive intervention following evaluation by clinician	Before
Procedure and type of grafting material	Autogenous gingival graft in some patients (number not reported)	Autogenous gingival graft in the area of recession (only 10 patients)
Outcome assessment	Width of keratinized gingiva and depth of gingival crevice measured via probe before and after orthodontic treatment	Gingival recessions measured on projected transparent slides of patient photographs before and after orthodontic treatment
Results		
Tooth movement achieved	Not reported	Retroclination of mandibular incisors
Change in gingival recessions	No additional recessions observed at grafted sites	Comparison of pretreatment and posttreatment recessions showed no statistically significant differences
Conclusions	Where orthodontic therapy is anticipated and there is insufficient keratinized tissue, a free gingival graft should be performed prior to tooth movement. Grafts are recommended in children with 1 mm or less of keratinized tissue.	Preorthodontic gingival grafting did not further decrease the postorthodontic gingival recession. It was postulated that eruption and maturation of the incisors during treatment contributed more to the decreased gingival recession than the graft did.

recession after being retroclined, with no difference detected between grafted and ungrafted recessions. However, because all teeth were retroclined in this study, this data cannot apply to clinical situations requiring proclination.

QUANTITATIVE SYNTHESIS

The lack of standardized protocols precluded a valid interpretation of the actual results of the studies. *Methodologic heterogeneity* refers to important differences in the interventions, participants, and outcomes of the included studies and similarly for studies other than randomized clinical trials. While both studies implemented surgical periodontal therapy before orthodontic treatment, the analysis of the indication and methodology revealed substantial differences with respect to the sample size, the type of periodontal procedure or regenerative material, and the time points of outcome assessment. Therefore, a meta-analysis was not possible.

Assessment of Grafting Timing

The inclination and the projected posttreatment position of the mandibular or maxillary incisors (obtained empirically or through a virtual treatment objective) play an important role in the diagnostic process and orthodontic treatment planning. It is frequently necessary to first establish proclination tolerance limits before treatment, especially in patients with *(1)* severe skeletal discrepancies, *(2)* arches that can accommodate only a limited number of teeth, or *(3)* an inadequate width of attached gingiva or facial soft tissue volume. These limits to estimated proclination refer to biologic factors, such as the characteristics and quality of the periodontal tissues in the area, and consequently, patients who already have thin soft tissue margins before treatment should be evaluated and treated with caution.

The development of gingival recession is not necessarily a direct consequence of incisor proclination. The findings of a systematic review failed to reveal an association between appliance-induced labial movement of mandibular incisors and gingival recession.[35] Therefore, the authors have suggested that other gingival recession–predisposing conditions of the mandibular anatomy should be considered before orthodontic planning. However, some studies have shown that excessive final incisor inclination, in addition to individual characteristics (ie, thin gingival margin) and other local or even systemic factors, can render these teeth susceptible to the development of recession defects.[8,18] On the other hand, it is reasonable to assume that in cases where the gingival margin maintains an adequate thickness after orthodontic treatment, the tissue may be more resistant and less affected by tension from excessive proclination. Consequently, the risk for developing gingival recession may be substantially reduced.

The issue of preventive periodontal intervention before orthodontic treatment, and especially before proclining or retroclining the incisors, has been long discussed in the scientific community.[33,36,37] While the evidence presented in this chapter cannot be evaluated quantitatively due to lack of consistency in methodologic approach, qualitative analysis reveals the following:

- Periodontal augmentation of labiolingual gingival dimensions before orthodontic treatment may yield satisfactory results, as far as it concerns the development or progress of gingival recessions. However, due to the lack of a high level of evidence, these results cannot yet be generalized.
- The evaluation of the attached gingiva as adequate or inadequate, and in turn the need for periodontal intervention before incisor inclination, still remains highly subjective.
- The final analysis in the included studies took place immediately after orthodontic therapy. Long-term results are clearly missing on this topic.
- In patients with a thin gingival phenotype (see Fig 7-1), soft tissue grafting might be beneficial before orthodontic tooth movement to prevent the development of gingival recession. Whether this clinical decision can be considered overtreatment still remains an open question and should be evaluated in future randomized controlled trials.

References

1. Kassab MM, Cohen RE. The etiology and prevalence of gingival recession. J Am Dent Assoc 2003;134:220–225.
2. Smith RG. Gingival recession: Reappraisal of an enigmatic condition and a new index for monitoring. J Clin Periodontol 1997;24:201–205.
3. Al-Wahadni A, Linden GJ. Dentine hypersensitivity in Jordanian dental attenders. A case control study. J Clin Periodontol 2002;29:688–693.
4. Lawrence HP, Hunt RJ, Beck JD. Three-year root caries incidence and risk modelling in older adults in North Carolina. J Public Health Dent 1995;55:69–78.
5. Löe H, Anerud A, Boysen H. The natural history of periodontal disease in man: Prevalence, severity, and extent of gingival recession. J Periodontol 1992;63:489–495.
6. Khocht A, Simon G, Person P, Denepitiya JL. Gingival recession in relation to history of hard toothbrush use. J Periodontol 1993;64:900–905.
7. Baker DL, Seymour GJ. The possible pathogenesis of gingival recession. A histological study of induced recession in the rat. J Clin Periodontol 1976;3:208–219.
8. Yared KF, Zenobio E G, Pacheco W. Periodontal status of mandibular central incisors after orthodontic proclination in adults. Am J Orthod Dentofacial Orthop 2006;130:e1–e8.
9. Litonjua LA, Andreana S, Bush PJ, Cohen RE. Toothbrushing and gingival recession. Int Dent J 2003;53:67–72.
10. Rawal SY, Claman LJ, Kalmar JR, Tatakis DN. Traumatic lesions of the gingiva: A case series. J Periodontol 2004;75:762–769.
11. Levin L, Zadik Y, Becker T. Oral and dental complications of intra-oral piercing. Dent Traumatol 2005;21:341–343.
12. Albandar JM, Streckfus CF, Adesanya MR, Winn DM. Cigar, pipe, and cigarette smoking as risk factors for periodontal disease and tooth loss. J Periodontol 2000;71:1874–1881.
13. Susin C, Haas AN, Oppermann RV, Haugejorden O, Albandar JM. Gingival recession: Epidemiology and risk indicators in a representative urban Brazilian population. J Periodontol 2004;75:1377–1386.
14. Wennström JL, Lindhe J, Sinclair F, Thilander B. Some periodontal tissue reactions to orthodontic tooth movement in monkeys. J Clin Periodontol 1987;14:121–129.
15. Joss-Vassalli I, Grebenstein C, Topouzelis N, Sculean A, Katsaros C. Orthodontic therapy and gingival recession: A systematic review. Orthod Craniofac Res 2010;13:127–141.
16. Wennström JL. Mucogingival considerations in orthodontic treatment. Semin Orthod 1996;2:46–54.
17. Thilander B, Nyman S, Karring T, Magnusson I. Bone regeneration in alveolar bone dehiscences related to orthodontic tooth movements. Eur J Orthod 1983;5:105–114.
18. Årtun J, Krogstad O. Periodontal status of mandibular incisors following excessive proclination. A study in adults with surgically treated mandibular prognathism. Am J Orthod Dentofacial Orthop 1987;91:225–232.
19. Ruf S, Hansen K, Pancherz H. Does orthodontic proclination of lower incisors in children and adolescents cause gingival recession? Am J Orthod Dentofacial Orthop 1998;114:100–106.
20. Djeu G, Hayes C, Zawaideh S. Correlation between mandibular central incisor proclination and gingival recession during fixed appliance therapy. Angle Orthod 2002;72:238–245.
21. Allais D, Melsen B. Does labial movement of lower incisors influence the level of the gingival margin? A case-control study of adult orthodontic patients. Eur J Orthod 2003;25:343–352.
22. Renkema AM, Fudalej PS, Renkema A, Bronkhorst E, Katsaros C. Gingival recessions and the change of inclination of mandibular incisors during orthodontic treatment. Eur J Orthod 2013;35:249–255.
23. Renkema AM, Navratilova Z, Mazurova K, Katsaros C, Fudalej PS. Gingival labial recessions and the post-treatment proclination of mandibular incisors. Eur J Orthod 2015;37:508–513.
24. Renkema AM, Fudalej PS, Renkema AA, Abbas F, Bronkhorst E, Katsaros C. Gingival labial recessions in orthodontically treated and untreated individuals: A case-control study. J Clin Periodontol 2013;40:631–637.
25. Renkema AM, Fudalej PS, Renkema A, Kiekens R, Katsaros C. Development of labial gingival recessions in orthodontically treated patients. Am J Orthod Dentofacial Orthop 2013;143:206–212.
26. Gebistorf M, Mijuskovic M, Pandis N, Fudalej PS, Katsaros C. Gingival recession in orthodontic patients 10 to 15 years posttreatment: A retrospective cohort study. Am J Orthod Dentofacial Orthop 2018;153:645–655.
27. Corn H. Periosteal separation: Its clinical significance. J Periodontol 1962;33:140–153.
28. Carranza FA, Carraro JJ. Mucogingival techniques in periodontal surgery. J Periodontol 1970;41:294–299.
29. Lang NP, Löe H. The relationship between the width of keratinized gingiva and gingival health. J Periodontol 1972;43:623–627.
30. Chambrone L, Tatakis DN. Periodontal soft tissue root coverage procedures: A systematic review from the AAP Regeneration Workshop. J Periodontol 2015;86(2 suppl):S8–S51.
31. Chambrone L, Chambrone D, Pustiglioni FE, Chambrone LA, Lima LA. Can subepithelial connective tissue grafts be considered the gold standard procedure in the treatment of Miller Class I and II recession defects? J Dent 2008;36:659–671.
32. Kloukos D, Eliades T, Sculean A, Katsaros C. Indication and timing of soft tissue augmentation at maxillary and mandibular incisors in orthodontic patients. A systematic review. Eur J Orthod 2014;36:442–449.
33. Maynard JG Jr, Ochsenbein C. Mucogingival problems, prevalence and therapy in children. J Periodontol 1975;46:543–552.
34. Ngan PW, Burch JG, Wei SH. Grafted and ungrafted labial gingival recession in pediatric orthodontic patients: Effects of retraction and inflammation. Quintessence Int 1991;22:103–111.
35. Aziz T, Flores-Mir C. A systematic review of the association between appliance-induced labial movement of mandibular incisors and gingival recession. Aust Orthod J 2011;27:33–39.
36. Mehta P, Lim LP. The width of the attached gingiva—Much ado about nothing? J Dent 2010;38:517–525.
37. Johal A, Katsaros C, Kiliardis S, et al. State of the science on controversial topics: Orthodontic therapy and gingival recession (a report of the Angle Society of Europe 2013 meeting). Prog Orthod 2013;14:16.

CHAPTER 8

Periodontal Considerations in Orthodontic and Orthopedic Expansion

Andrew Dentino
T. Gerard Bradley

The use of orthopedic forces to expand the maxilla as a way to treat transverse maxillary skeletal deficiency was first reported by Angell over 150 years ago.[1] Since that time, there have been concerns about the potential deleterious effects of such movement on the periodontal tissues. These effects appear to be dependent on technique, age, and probably biologic phenotype. Among these effects, the best documented are root resorption, loss of buccal crestal alveolar bone height and thickness, apical migration of the buccal gingival margin, dental tipping, and an increase in thickness of palatal bone. This chapter reviews the periodontal effects of the different techniques used in different age groups and summarizes the current understanding of the periodontal effects of rapid palatal expansion (RPE). It also suggests future directions for research that could help clarify current controversies.

Devices Employed for Palatal Expansion

The Hyrax expander (Fig 8-1) is a completely tooth-borne expander, whereas the Haas appliance shown in Fig 8-2 provides both a tooth- and tissue-borne force. The Haas expander was developed as a way to try to gain more skeletal change than simple dental tipping in the preadolescent or early adolescent patient. Both appliances employ a jack screw to cause steady separation at a rapid or semirapid rate depending on the frequency of activation of the jack screw. Once the maxillary midline suture ossifies in the late teenage years, expansion can only be accomplished with surgery. Surgically assisted rapid palatal expansion (SARPE) requires

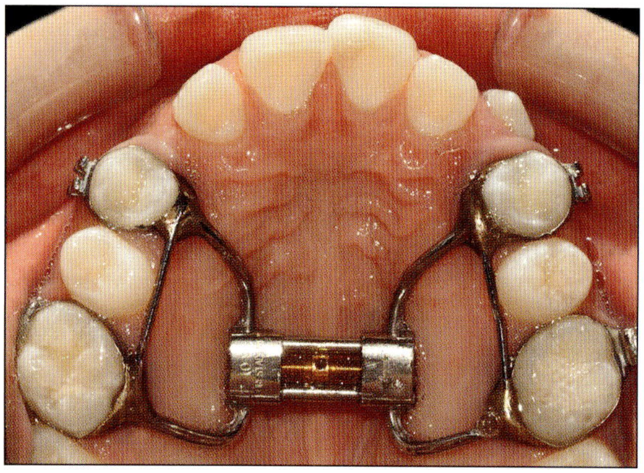

Fig 8-1 Hyrax expander.

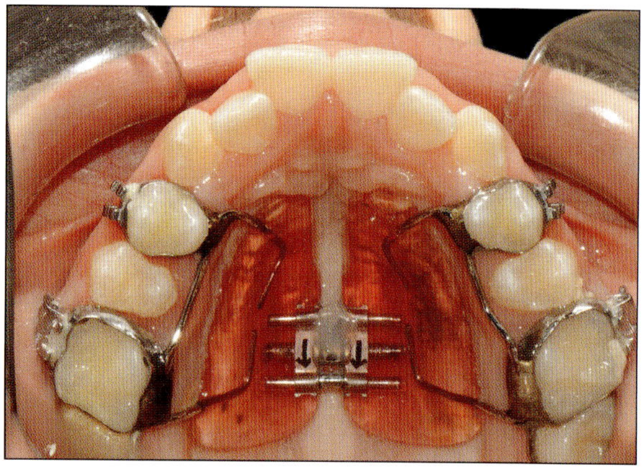

Fig 8-2 Haas expander.

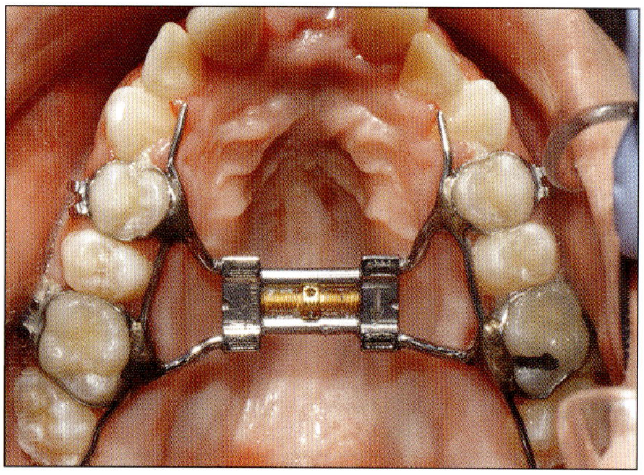

Fig 8-3 Surgically assisted rapid palatal expansion device.

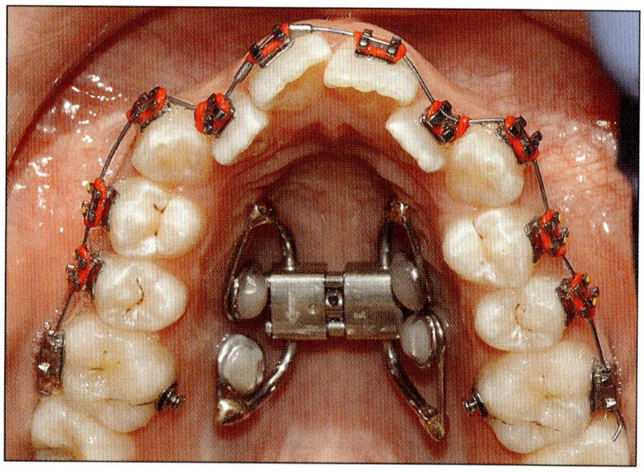

Fig 8-4 Expander using temporary anchorage devices.

surgical intervention followed by activation of an expansion device. Figure 8-3 shows such a device that can be used in adults after appropriate surgical intervention to create mobile bony segments through corticotomy. An appliance using temporary anchorage devices to try to achieve skeletal change is shown in Fig 8-4.

Clinical Indications for Palatal Expansion

In 1970, Haas suggested five clinical situations where palatal expansion was clinically useful.[2] These included surgical and nonsurgical Class III cases, cases of real and relative maxillary deficiency, inadequate nasal capacity, mature cleft palate patients, and selected arch length cases where tooth removal would lead to profile discrepancies, which remains a controversial topic.

Since that time, a range of different techniques for accomplishing palatal expansion have been used in the practice of orthodontics. Semirapid or slow palatal expansion (SPE, about 1.0 mm/week, light continuous forces of 450 to 900 g) and RPE (0.5 mm/day, orthopedic forces ranging from 10 to 20 lbs) using either tooth-borne or tissue/tooth-borne appliances have been commonly used. Both approaches appear to yield the same results in terms of skeletal and dental changes to achieve the desired expansion. These techniques have been employed primarily in preadolescent and adolescent patients, whereas SARPE has been used in adult populations where the maxillary suture has closed.[3] More recently, there have been attempts at skeletal expansion in adults using temporary anchorage devices, with little to no evidence on their efficacy at this time.

General considerations regarding the use of the different techniques have been recently laid out.[4,5] These include avoidance of RPE in the primary dentition in favor of SPE, because RPE can lead to facial esthetic problems if employed in young children. Beyond the early and late mixed dentition stage, RPE can be used with excellent results up until closure of the maxillary suture, usually around the middle teen years. In preadolescents, expansion techniques, whether SPE or RPE, yield significant arch expansion with approximately one-half to one-third of the change coming from true skeletal expansion and the other half to two-thirds of the change actually coming from dental changes such as tipping. Palatal expansion can be done up to the end of the adolescent growth spurt. The use of RPE had been seen as a way to increase skeletal change via separation of the maxillary suture while limiting dental changes such as tipping of the teeth. However, the slow deposition of bone at the suture borders after RPE leads to more dental tipping than originally thought during the stabilization period.[6]

Two landmark papers illustrating the age-appropriate use of palatal expansion include Geran et al,[7] who used an acrylic tooth-borne splint for semirapid expansion (0.25 mm/day) in a group of young patients (mean age, 8 years 10 months), and McNamara et al,[8] who employed a Haas appliance with RPE (0.5 mm/day) in subjects with a mean age of 12 years 2 months. The long-term follow-up in these studies showed very good orthodontic outcomes for post-teen subjects compared with models taken from untreated age-matched controls. Unfortunately, there was no evaluation of periodontal effects of the treatment compared with the controls.

RPE is contraindicated in mature patients as well as in open bite cases and in subjects who already present with recession of bone on the buccal aspects of the maxillary posterior teeth. In mature patients where the maxillary suture has ossified, surgically assisted forms of palatal expansion have generally been employed. These techniques involve various Le Fort procedures with maxillary midline corticotomies and in some cases pterygomaxillary dysjunction.

Potential Periodontal Problems with RPE

There have been two relatively recent systematic reviews that have noted a slight tendency toward recession in post-orthodontic patients.[9,10] The Bollen et al review[9] looked at orthodontic treatment of all kinds, whereas the Joss-Vassalli et al review[10] looked more specifically at incisor proclination. While both reviews did find evidence for post-orthodontic recession, they cautioned about the clinical significance of such findings or the strength of the evidence. Neither review looked specifically at palatal expansion cases. One retrospective study used bone-sounding measurements to assess crestal bone height levels in RPE patients compared with SPE patients and untreated controls and noted some loss of crestal height, but the authors felt this was not of major significance.[11]

RECESSION AND BONE THINNING OR BONE LOSS

One of the most common periodontal sequelae of palatal expansion is recession and dehiscence formation. The movement of teeth in the alveolar housing has limits, as demonstrated in animal models in dogs[12] and monkeys.[13–15] These groups published some rather striking observations. They showed that teeth orthodontically moved outside the normal bony housing would consistently show loss of alveolar bone with tipping or bodily labial movement, and often, but not always, gingival recession developed as well. Bone dehiscences could often be improved, at least to some degree, with movement back into the alveolar housing. This was most often observed if the animals were on a strict hygiene regimen. Soft tissue recession, however, was not so readily reversed. In a more recent study in rats, Danz et al pecifically evaluated the effects of force on the phenomenon of recession and bone thinning/dehiscence formation.[16] In this animal model, they showed that the dehiscence formation was similar whether conventional or low force was applied during the tooth movement.

Human Studies on Palatal Expansion Using CBCT

With the advent of advanced radiologic techniques such as cone beam computed tomography (CBCT), it has become possible to do more stringent analysis of orthodontic treatment on the alveolar housing. Timock et al have demonstrated the accuracy and reliability of CBCT in assessing crestal bone height and thickness.[17] It has been suggested that in humans, age-appropriate use of palatal expansion can achieve a good orthodontic result,[4] and yet there is a growing body of evidence that palatal expansion can result in thinning of the alveolar buccal bone and reduction of crestal bone height, which puts teeth at risk for future gingival recession.[18–21] These studies included a range of appliances and techniques from RPE to SPE in preadolescent to adolescent children. The findings are boringly consistent.

Moreover, recession has been clearly documented in all forms of palatal expansion from SPE to RPE and even different forms of SARPE.[22–25] The widespread use of CBCT has been a major source of confirmation regarding loss of bone height even in the absence of obvious clinical recession.[26–29] Unfortunately, there are no truly long-term follow-up studies that specifically look at the periodontal effects of palatal expansion therapies. While Fields and Proffit state that loss of bone with subsequent recession may be avoided or at least minimized if the proper technique is used in the proper patient,[4] it appears that the boundaries of proper and improper use of these techniques have not been precisely defined at present.

It is clear, however, that as patients age and the maxillary suture closes, the prospect of skeletal expansion via orthopedic appliances decreases, and the inevitability of dental tipping and alveolar bending increases. According to Vanarsdall,[30] these types of orthodontic movement not only result in thinning of the buccal alveolus but also lead to elongation of the clinical crown and likely reduction of the buccal alveolar crest. These observations warrant caution on the part of clinicians who want to expand the maxillary arch.

In an attempt to help define more precisely the limits of palatal expansion, Vanarsdall and Secchi have suggested that transverse skeletal discrepancy is the most critical risk factor for identifying subjects susceptible to recession and clinical attachment loss when considering palatal expansion.[31] They report that individuals with a maxillomandibular discrepancy greater than 5 mm will show recession over time and that palatal expansion will accentuate this problem. They also note that because maxillary transverse skeletal growth is essentially finished by 15 years of age, expansion appliances in preadolescents yield increased arch width stemming from 50% skeletal change and 50% dental tipping, whereas in adolescents the skeletal component of the change is reduced to 35%, and the dental component increases to 65%.[31] What has yet to be evaluated in any significant way is the role that periodontal phenotype/gingival biotype[32] may play in long-term periodontal effects in palatal expansion cases. This would be a fruitful area for research because tissue thickness seems to play a critical role in susceptibility to recession.[33]

ROOT RESORPTION

Root resorption has been clearly demonstrated in humans on the buccal aspect of maxillary premolars after RPE.[34,35] Both groups of researchers demonstrated that the resorption was at least to some degree reversible toward the coronal aspect of the teeth depending on how long they were in retention prior to extraction; the apical aspect of the roots did not show as clear a pattern of reversal. Others have shown similar resorption complications in an animal model.[36]

INTERPROXIMAL PERIODONTAL BONE LOSS

This finding has been demonstrated in animals as well as in humans and is widely accepted as a problem in any type of orthodontic tooth movement in the presence of uncontrolled periodontal inflammation.[30] Though a concern in all forms of palatal expansion, there has been clear and repeated documentation of bone loss in various cases of SARPE.[25,37,38] Cureton and Cuenin further suggested careful consideration of root proximity in the central incisor area and called for orthodontic separation of the roots prior to surgical intervention to avoid an asymmetric corticotomy, which would lead to very significant defects in the esthetic zone that can be impossible to correct.[37]

Future Considerations

The scarcity of long-term follow-up on prospective clinical trials for the many different palatal expansion techniques is still problematic. In addition, the absence of any studies looking at palatal expansion techniques while accounting for the thickness of gingival tissue, commonly known as *periodontal phenotype* or *gingival biotype*, further limit our knowledge.[39,40] Techniques such as ultrasound as used by Müller and Eger,[39] the convergence of CBCT DICOM (Digital Imaging and Communications in Medicine) files with intraoral scanning of barium-coated stents,[41] as well as the more exotic optical coherence tomography[42] provide noninvasive ways to quantify soft tissue thickness with precision. These techniques could help shed light on the limits of palatal expansion in different gingival biotypes. In addition, the more widespread use of CBCT data to identify the buccolingual tooth position within the arch along with assessments of soft tissue thickness might be used to optimize when a tooth is centrally located within the alveolar bone.

Perhaps even more intriguing is the possible application of preorthodontic guided bone regeneration as a way to alter the periodontal biotype or to carry out the augmentation as part of periodontally accelerated osteogenic orthodontics.[43] Such an approach has the potential to counteract the thinning of the alveolar bone and loss of buccal bone height, especially in more mature patients whose expansion will lead to more dental tipping and alveolar bending rather than any significant skeletal expansion.[44–46] More work needs to be done in this area to determine the feasibility of such an approach, because very limited human histology exists to show that true bone generation has been accomplished, and more long-term follow-up is needed as well as randomized controlled trials.

References

1. Angell E. Treatment of irregularity of permanent or adult teeth. Dent Cosmos 1860;1:540–544.
2. Haas AJ. Palatal expansion: Just the beginning of dentofacial orthopedics. Am J Orthod 1970;57:219–255.
3. Lee SC, Park JH, Bayome M, Kim KB, Araujo EA, Kook YA. Effect of bone-borne rapid maxillary expanders with and without surgical assistance on the craniofacial structures using finite element analysis. Am J Orthod Dentofacial Orthop 2014;145:638–648.
4. Fields HW Jr, Proffit WR. Treatment of skeletal problems in children and preadolescents. In: Fields HW Jr, Proffit WR, Sarver, DM (eds). Contemporary Orthodontics. St Louis: Elsevier, 2013:476–480.
5. Kokich VG, Kokich VO. Interrelationship of orthodontics with periodontics and restorative dentistry. In: Nanda R (ed). Esthetics and Biomechanics in Orthodontics. St Louis: Elsevier, 2015:560–581.
6. Cobourne MT, DiBiase AT. Orthodontics and orthognathic surgery. In: Handbook of Orthodontics, ed 2. Edinburgh: Elsevier, 2016:475–476.
7. Geran RG, McNamara JA Jr, Baccetti T, Franchi L, Shapiro LM. A prospective long-term study on the effects of rapid maxillary expansion in the early mixed dentition. Am J Orthod Dentofacial Orthop 2006;129:631–640.
8. McNamara JA Jr, Baccetti T, Franchi L, Herberger TA. Rapid maxillary expansion followed by fixed appliances: A long-term evaluation of changes in arch dimensions. Angle Orthod 2003;73:344–353.

9. Bollen AM, Cunha-Cruz J, Bakko DW, Huang GJ, Hujoel PP. The effects of orthodontic therapy on periodontal health: A systematic review of controlled evidence. J Am Dent Assoc 2008;139:413–422.
10. Joss-Vassalli I, Grebenstein C, Topouzelis N, Sculean A, Katsaros C. Orthodontic therapy and gingival recession: A systematic review. Orthod Craniofac Res 2010;13:127–141.
11. Greenbaum KR, Zachrisson BU. The effect of palatal expansion therapy on the periodontal supporting tissues. Am J Orthod 1982;81:12–21.
12. Karring T, Nyman S, Thilander B, Magnusson I. Bone regeneration in orthodontically produced alveolar bone dehiscences. J Periodontal Res 1982;17:309–315.
13. Batenhorst KF, Bowers GM, Williams JE Jr. Tissue changes resulting from facial tipping and extrusion of incisors in monkeys. J Periodontol 1974;45:660–668.
14. Engelking G, Zachrisson BU. Effects of incisor repositioning on monkey periodontium after expansion through the cortical plate. Am J Orthod 1982;82:23–32.
15. Wennström JL, Lindhe J, Sinclair F, Thilander B. Some periodontal tissue reactions to orthodontic tooth movement in monkeys. J Clin Periodontol 1987;14:121–129.
16. Danz JC, Bibby BM, Katsaros C, Stavropoulos A. Effects of facial tooth movement on the periodontium in rats: A comparison of conventional and low force. J Clin Periodontol 2016;43:229–237.
17. Timock AM, Cook V, McDonald T, et al. Accuracy and reliability of buccal bone height and thickness measurements from cone-beam computed tomography imaging. Am J Orthod Dentofacial Orthop 2011;140:734–744.
18. Garib DG, Henriques JF, Jandon G, de Freitas MR, Fernandes AY. Periodontal effects of rapid maxillary expansion with tooth-tissue-borne and tooth-borne expanders: A computed tomography evaluation. Am J Orthod Dentofacial Orthop 2006;129:749–758.
19. English JD, Akyalcin S, Peltomaki T, Litschel K. Oral hygiene: Possible problems and complications. In: Mosby's Orthodontic Review, ed 2. St Louis: Mosby, 2015:265–270.
20. Corbridge JK, Campbell PM, Taylor R, Ceen RF, Buschang PH. Transverse dentoalveolar changes after slow maxillary expansion. Am J Orthod Dentofaial Orthop 2011;140:317–325.
21. Domann CE, Kau CH, English JD, Xia JJ, Souccar NM, Lee RP. Cone beam computed tomography analysis of dentoalveolar changes immediately after maxillary expansion. Orthodontics (Chic) 2011;12:202–209.
22. Northway WM, Meade JB Jr. Surgically assisted rapid maxillary expansion: A comparison of technique, response, and stability. Angle Orthod 1997;67:309–320.
23. Carmen M, Marcella P, Giuseppe C, Roberto A. Periodontal evaluation in patients undergoing maxillary expansion. J Craniofac Surg 2000;11:491–494.
24. Handelman CS, Wang L, BeGole EA, Haas AJ. Nonsurgical rapid maxillary expansion in adults: Report on 47 cases using the Haas expander. Angle Orthod 2000;70:129–144.
25. Williams BJ, Currimbhoy S, Silva A, O'Ryan FS. Complications following surgically assisted rapid palatal expansion: A retrospective cohort study. J Oral Maxillofac Surg 2012;70:2394–2402.
26. Rungcharassaeng K, Caruso JM, Kan JY, Kim J, Taylor G. Factors affecting buccal bone changes of maxillary posterior teeth after rapid maxillary expansion. Am J Orthod Dentofacial Orthop 2007;132:428.e1–428.e8.
27. Landes CA, Laudemann K, Schübel, et al. Comparison of tooth- and bone-borne devices in surgically assisted rapid maxillary expansion by three-dimensional computed tomography monitoring: Transverse dental and skeletal maxillary expansion, segmental inclination, dental tipping, and vestibular bone resorption. J Craniofac Surg 2009;20:1132–1141.
28. Sygouros A, Motro M, Ugurly F, Acar A. Surgically assisted rapid maxillary expansion: Cone-beam computed tomography evaluation of different surgical techniqes and their effects in the maxillary dentoskeletal complex. Am J Orthod Dentofacial Orthop 2014;146:748–757.
29. Baka ZM, Akin M, Ucar FI, Ileri Z. Cone-beam computed tomography evaluation of dentoskeletal changes after asymmetric rapid maxillary expansion. Am J Orthod Dentofacial Orthop 2015;147:61–71.
30. Vanarsdall RL. Orthodontics and periodontal therapy. Periodontol 2000 1995;9:132–149.
31. Vanarsdall RL, Secchi AG. Periodontal-orthodontic interrelationships. In: Graber LW, Vanarsdall RL, Vig KWL (eds). Orthodontics: Current Principles and Techniques. Philadelphia: Mosby, 2012:807–841.
32. Cook DR, Mealey BL, Verrett RG. Relationship between clinical periodontal biotype and labial plate thickness: An in vivo study. Int J Periodontics Restorative Dent 2011;31:345–354.
33. Webbström JL. Mucogingival considerations in orthodontic treatment. Semin Orthod 1996;2:46–54.
34. Barber AF, Sims MR. Rapid maxillary expansion and external root resorption in man: A scanning electron microscope study. Am J Orthod 1981;79:630–652.
35. Odenrick L, Karlander EL, Pierce A, Kretschemar U. Surface resorption following two forms of rapid maxillary expansion. Eur J Orthod 1991;13:264–270.
36. Vardimon AD, Graber TM, Pitaru S. Repair process of external root resorption subsequent to palatal expansion treatment. Am J Orthod Dentofacial Orthop 1993;103:120–130.
37. Cureton SL, Cuenin M. Surgically assisted rapid palatal expansion: Orthodontic preparation for clinical success. Am J Orthod Dentofacial Orthop 1999;116:46–59.
38. Laudemann K, Petruchin O, Nafzger M, et al. Long-term 3D cast model study: Bone-borne vs. tooth-borne surgically assisted rapid maxillary expansion due to secondary variables. Oral Maxillofac Surg 2010;14:105–114.
39. Müller HP, Eger T. Gingival phenotypes in young male adults. J Clin Periodontol 1997;24:65–71.
40. Müller HP, Eger T. Masticatory mucosa and periodontal phenotype: A review. Int J Periodontics Restorative Dent 2002;22:172–183.
41. Gallucci GO, Finelle G, Papadimitriou DE, Lee SJ. Innovative approach to computer-guided surgery and fixed provisionalization assisted by screw-retained transitional implants. Int J Oral Maxillofac Implants 2015;30:403–410.
42. Ajdaharian J, Dadkhan M, Sabokpey S, et al. Multimodal imaging of the effects of a novel dentifrice on oral biofilm. Lasers Surg Med 2014;46:546–552.

43. Brugnami F, Caiazzo A. Orthodontically driven corticotomy: Tissue engineering to expand basal bone, modify the periodontal biotype and lower the risks of orthodontic damage to the periodontium. In: Orthodontically Driven Corticotomy: Tissue Engineering To Enhance Orthodontic and Multidisciplinary Treatment. Ames, IA: Wiley, 2015:189–218.
44. Einy S, Horwitz J, Aizenbud D. Wilckodontics—An alternative adult orthodontic treatment method: Rationale and application. Alpha Omegan 2011;104:102–111.
45. Wilcko MT, Wilcko WM, Pulver JJ, Bissada NF, Bouquot JE. Accelerated osteogenic orthodontics technique: A 1-stage surgically facilitated rapid orthodontic technique with alveolar augmentation. J Oral Maxillofac Surg 2009; 67:2149–2159.
46. Wilcko WM, Wilcko T, Bouquot JE, Ferguson DJ. Rapid orthodontics with alveolar reshaping: Two case reports of decrowding. Int J Periodontics Restorative Dent 2001;21:9–19.

CHAPTER 9

Surgical Lengthening of the Clinical Crown

Spyridon I. Vassilopoulos
Phoebus N. Madianos
Ioannis Vrotsos

The restorability of a tooth or a root is not determined solely by its orientation within the dental arch or its periodontal-endodontic prognosis. The inadequate amount of remaining supracrestal tooth substance is a common cause of failure of full-coverage restorations. An insufficient amount of sound tooth structure may reduce optimal retention and resistance to dislodging forces encountered during function. Although this may be improved by modifying tooth preparations with slots, grooves, or pinholes, another option is to increase the dimensions of the clinical crown by surgical or orthodontic procedures.[1] This chapter addresses only the surgical approach.

Crown lengthening procedures are indicated for several clinical situations, including pathologic or iatrogenic conditions, prosthetic needs, esthetic demands, and orthodontic needs (Box 9-1 and Fig 9-1).

BOX 9-1 Indications for crown lengthening procedures

Pathologic or iatrogenic condition
- Caries lesions at or below the gingival margin
- Subgingival or subcrestal extension of tooth fractures
- Previously placed restoration margins in close proximity to bone crest
- Teeth with excessive occlusal or incisal wear
- Gingival overgrowth (see Fig 9-1)
- Root perforation or resorption (coronal part of the root)

Prosthetic needs
- Inadequate amount of supracrestal tooth structure for optimal retention
- Teeth with inadequate interocclusal space for proper restorative procedures

Esthetic demands
- Short clinical or anatomical crown (see Fig 9-1)
- Asymmetric gingival margin contour

Orthodontic needs
- Short clinical crown may impede easy placement of orthodontic attachments and eventually hinder proper oral hygiene procedures (see Fig 9-1)

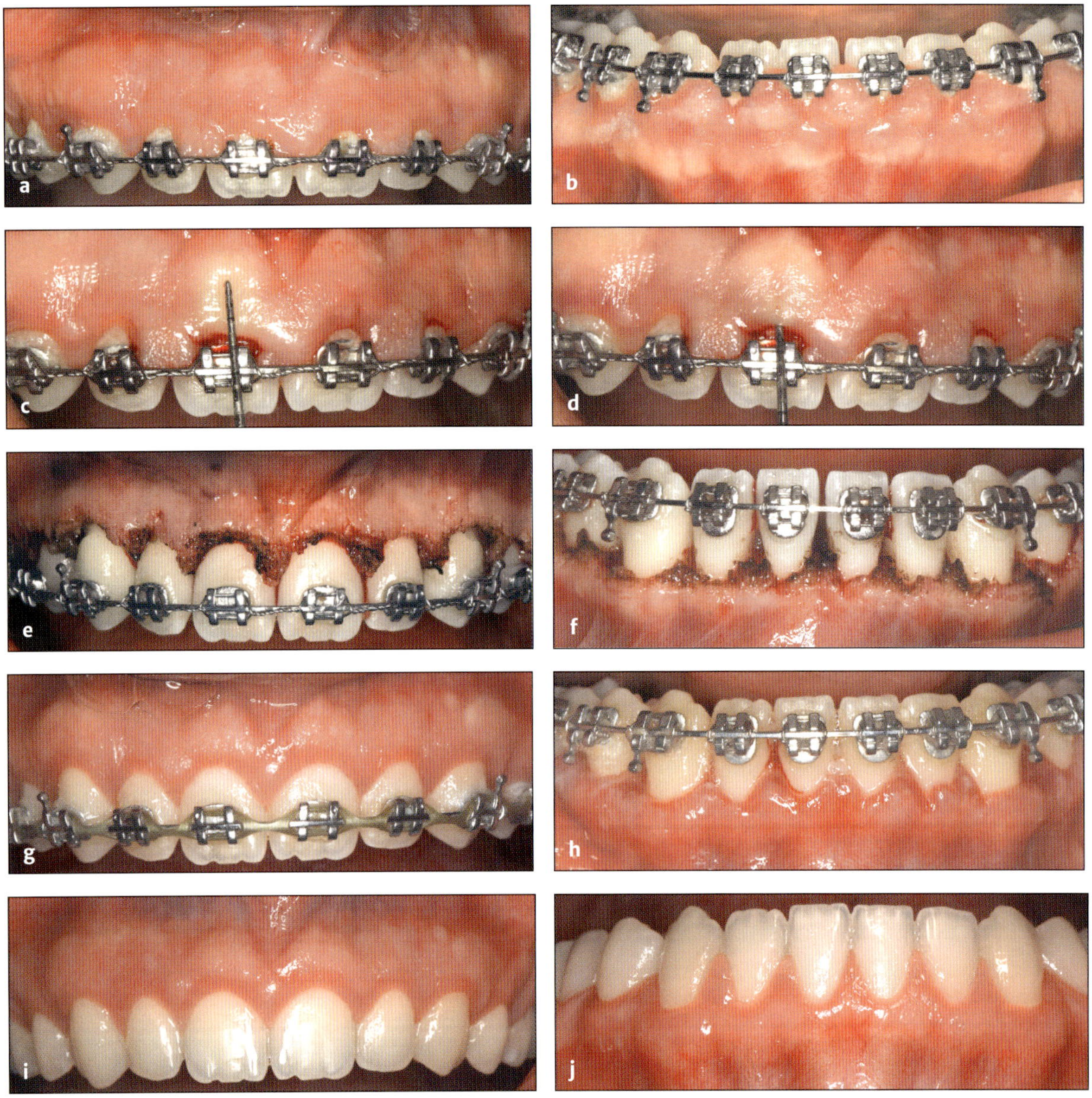

Fig 9-1 Case of gingival overgrowth treated with crown lengthening. *(a and b)* Pretreatment condition. *(c)* Much of the clinical crown is hidden beneath the overgrown gingival tissue. This will hinder proper oral hygiene around the orthodontic appliances. *(d)* Bone sounding. *(e and f)* Surgical crown lengthening has been performed to expose more of the clinical crowns utilizing a scalpel and an Nd:YAG (neodymium-doped yttrium aluminum garnet) laser. *(g and h)* After healing. *(i and j)* After removal of the orthodontic appliances.

Pretreatment Planning

Prior to crown lengthening procedures, a periodontal-endodontic and restorative prognosis must be established. Clinical examination and radiographic analysis employing intraoral periapical radiography should be consulted to determine the amount of remaining tooth structure, the periodontal condition, the endodontic status, and the root length and form[2] (see Fig 9-2). Diagnostic casts may also be included in the pretreatment evaluation in order to facilitate provisional preparation and surgical guide fabrication, especially when crown lengthening is scheduled in the esthetically demanding anterior maxillary region.

The following factors must be considered during this diagnostic phase.

MINIMUM DIMENSIONAL REQUIREMENTS

In cases where bone is to be resected to provide adequate sound tooth structure for restorative requirements, the maintenance of space for re-establishment of a normal dentogingival junction is a necessity of primary importance. This dimension has been referred to as the *biologic width* and comprises the summation of the supracrestal connective tissue attachment and the junctional epithelium.[3]

Gargiulo et al originally reported the average distance between the alveolar crest and the gingival margin as 2.73 mm, with a range of 2.17 to 3.05 mm.[4] They recorded connective tissue attachment lengths of 0.44 to 1.56 mm (mean value, 1.07 mm), epithelial attachment lengths of 0.71 to 1.35 mm (mean value, 0.97 mm), and sulcular depths of 0 to 2.79 mm (mean value, 0.69 mm). Vacek et al examined human cadaver specimens and reported mean values of 0.77 mm for the connective tissue attachment and 1.14 mm for the epithelial attachment.[5]

A recent systematic review concluded that a universal dimension of the biologic width does not exist and that the use of mean values as a treatment objective could mask the actual clinical situation.[6] Considerable inter- and intrasubject variations have been demonstrated, and each case should be individualized after periodontal and transgingival probing regarding the length of the biologic width. The biologic width also seems to be reduced in patients with gingival inflammation as well as in patients with attachment loss or untreated chronic periodontitis.[4,6–8] Nonetheless, any violation of this critical minimal dimension will produce a persistent inflammatory response similar to that of ligature-induced experimental gingivitis in animals. Placing restorative margins in close proximity to the bone crest will impinge on the supracrestal connective tissue attachment, thereby resulting in this inflammatory response. This iatrogenic chronic inflammation may lead to bone resorption.[9]

Several investigators suggested that 1 to 2 mm should be added coronal to the average biologic width of 2.04 mm as an optimal distance between the bone crest and a restorative margin.[3,10,11] This dimension is applied to each surface of each tooth and establishes a minimum distance of 3 to 4 mm coronal to the alveolar crest that is necessary to reduce the risk of periodontal attachment loss induced by subgingival restorative margins and to permit proper restoration of the tooth.[12] In cases of sustained tooth damage where little supragingival tooth structure remains or the integrity of the pulp is compromised, endodontic treatment and concomitant placement of a post and core is often necessary for a full-crown tooth restoration (Fig 9-2). Care should be taken to provide adequate sound tooth structure for the formation of a ferrule, which is thought to increase the resistance of a pulpless tooth to fracture by counteracting functional lever forces as well as the wedging effects and lateral cementation forces of dowels.[13,14] The best ferrule design according to Sorensen and Egelman is a 360-degree metal collar of the crown that surrounds the parallel walls of the dentin and extends at least 1 mm coronal to the shoulder of the preparation.[15] This additional surgical exposure of 1 mm of tooth structure is provided in addition to the minimum 3 to 4 mm coronal to the alveolar crest. Wagenberg et al determined that 5.0 to 5.5 mm of clinical crown should be exposed (measured from

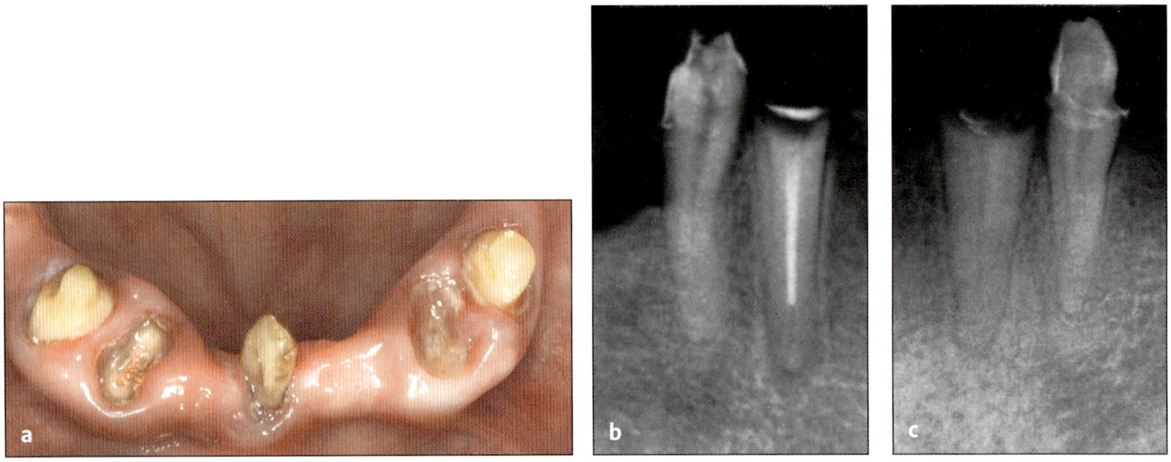

Fig 9-2 Fractured and subgingivally decayed mandibular teeth. The right central incisor is extracted due to its hopeless prognosis. *(a)* Pretreatment condition. *(b and c)* Periapical radiographs of the remaining teeth.

the alveolar crest) to achieve an adequate dimension of clinical crown after healing in cases of post and core–restored teeth.[16] When extensive bone removal is required to expose 5 mm of tooth structure, alternative treatments should be considered because the bone removal could compromise the biomechanical tooth leverage (see Fig 9-3).

POSTSURGICAL CROWN-TO-ROOT RATIO

While the crown-to-root ratio is no longer considered a determining factor for tooth prognosis, in cases where the remaining periodontal support is severely compromised and the crown-to-root ratio is 1, the tooth should be considered hopeless and should be replaced by a fixed or removable partial denture or an implant-supported prosthesis.

LOCATION OF THE FURCATION AND ROOT TRUNK ANATOMY

In multirooted teeth, the length of the root trunk—the distance from the cementoenamel junction (CEJ) to the root's division—determines the amount of bone that can be removed without exposing the furcation. This may cause difficulties in plaque control and increases the risk for developing caries lesions and periodontal breakdown.[17]

ADJACENT TEETH

Bone resection in order to expose sound tooth structure should not jeopardize the prognosis of the neighboring teeth.

INTEROCCLUSAL SPACE

Interocclusal space influences the extent of surgical resection of supporting periodontal tissues. Where an increase in the vertical dimension is appropriate, less of the supporting tissue will be sacrificed.

ESTHETIC CONCERNS

Surgical crown lengthening procedures in the anterior maxilla may entail esthetic risks, especially in cases with a medium or high lip line. In order to avoid an irregular gingival architecture and establish an esthetic continuity of the gingival contour, adjacent teeth in the esthetic zone should also be lengthened.[18]

Tarnow et al showed that black triangles appear interdentally when the distance from the contact point to the crest of the bone is more than 5 mm.[19] The potential risk of creating unesthetic, widened embrasure areas can be reduced or eliminated by adjusting the final prosthetic crown contours. Lengthening and widening the crown contact areas will facilitate elimination of the dark interdental spaces and accommodate the new papilla morphology. In these esthetically demanding cases, a surgical stent could be useful to the surgeon as a guide to determine the position of the new crown margins both buccally and interdentally (see Fig 9-5b). Very close communication between the restorative dentist and the surgeon is fundamental to successfully managing these demanding cases.[20]

Surgical Crown Lengthening Technique

If bone removal is not required to expose adequate tooth structure, tissue excision via gingivectomy is the technique of choice. The procedure may be carried out using a scalpel (externally beveled incisions), a round diamond bur at high speed, or a laser. In these instances care should be taken to preserve a minimum of 3 mm of attached gingiva height, especially in the presence of a subgingival restorative margin[21] (see Fig 9-1).

In cases where bone removal is needed to establish the biologic width, a flap approach should be employed. The surgical procedure begins with internally beveled sulcular or submarginal incisions (depending on the width of the keratinized gingiva). If an edentulous area is located mesial and/or distal to the involved teeth, triangular or linear wedge incisions are made following the areas of greatest attached gingiva and underlying bone. When a triangular wedge incision is selected, the base of the triangle is placed next to the tooth.[22] The distance between the tip of the triangle and the tooth or the distance between the two parallel incisions (in the linear wedge technique) is determined by the coronoapical thickness of the tissues at the edentulous area[23] (Figs 9-3a and 9-3b).

A full-thickness buccolingual mucoperiosteal flap is elevated up to the mucogingival junction, extending at least one tooth mesial and distal to the area of interest (Fig 9-3c). A partial- thickness dissection can also be performed, extending the flap apically beyond the mucogingival junction. This may facilitate apical repositioning of the flap when the apicocoronal dimension of the existing gingiva is minimal (less than 3 mm).[24] Ostectomy/osteoplasty is accomplished with burs under continuous irrigation, hand chisels, or piezoelectric cutting devices, taking care not to damage the root surfaces (Figs 9-3d to 9-3g). The amount of bone to be removed circumferentially is determined by the apical extent of the anticipated restorative margin and by anatomical factors such as the CEJ profile and bone anatomy at the adjacent sites.[25] Interestingly, Herrero et al showed that a 3-mm biologic width is not routinely achieved during crown lengthening procedures, even by experienced periodontists.[26] The physiologic form of osseous architecture must be kept in mind during osseous surgery, because the underlying osseous structure influences the overlying soft tissue. If reverse architecture remains after a crown lengthening procedure is performed to a tooth with healthy periodontium, excess gingival tissue may rebound in the healing phase, negatively affecting the surgical outcome. In the maxillary anterior area, the interproximal bone height should be coronal to the buccal/palatal bone crest, providing adequate support for the interdental papillae postoperatively. This will ensure a harmonious scalloping of the gingival margin in the esthetic zone, whereas a flatter gingival profile is acceptable in posterior areas.[27]

The postoperative flap margin should not be positioned less than 3 mm coronal to the crestal bone. When this distance is compromised, soft tissue regrowth may occur because the normal supracrestal tissue dimensions tend to re-establish themselves according to biologic width principles. If the pretreatment width of the attached gingiva is minimal (less than 3 mm), then an intrasulcular incision and an apically repositioned flap should be performed.

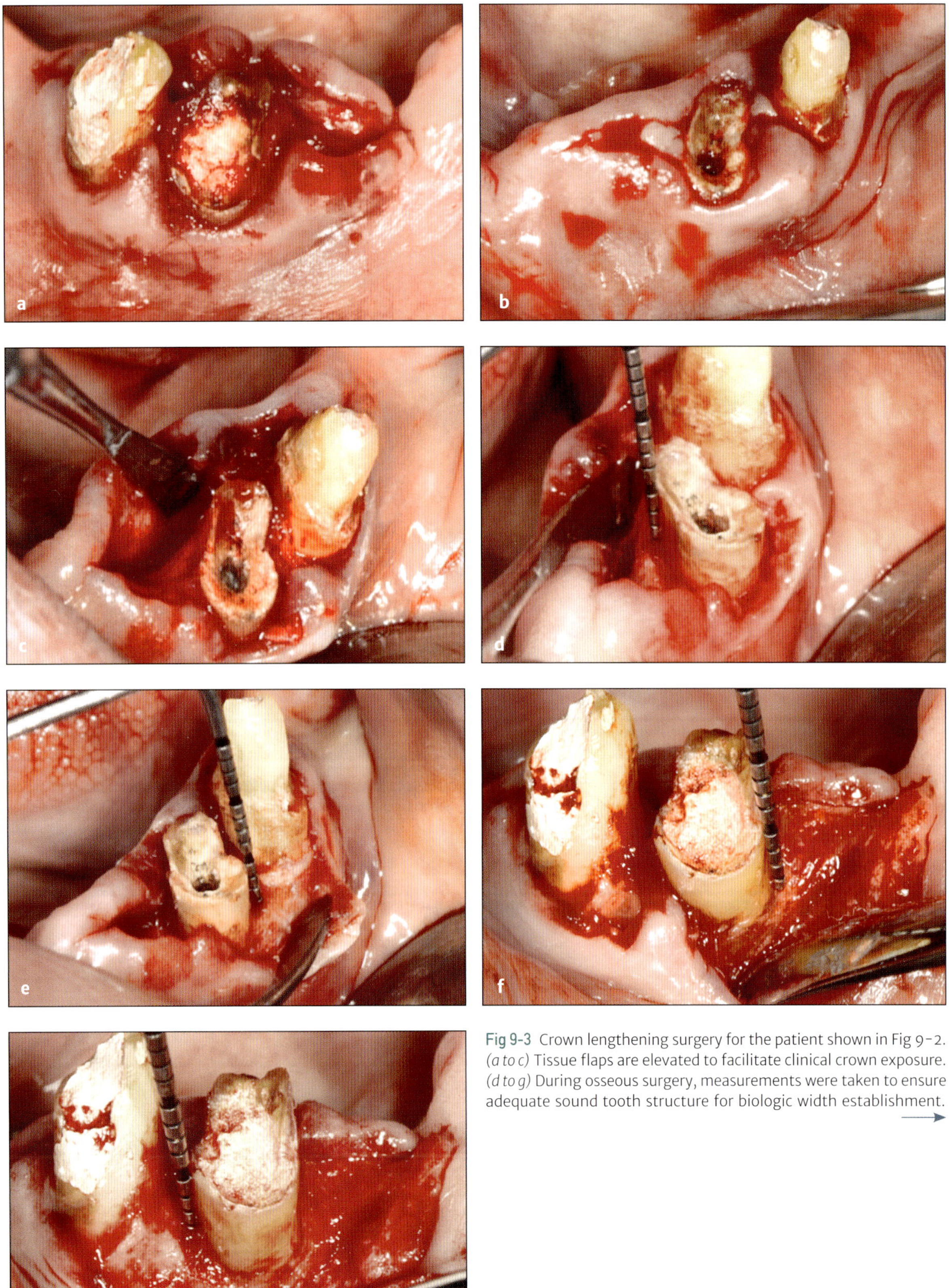

Fig 9-3 Crown lengthening surgery for the patient shown in Fig 9-2. *(a to c)* Tissue flaps are elevated to facilitate clinical crown exposure. *(d to g)* During osseous surgery, measurements were taken to ensure adequate sound tooth structure for biologic width establishment.

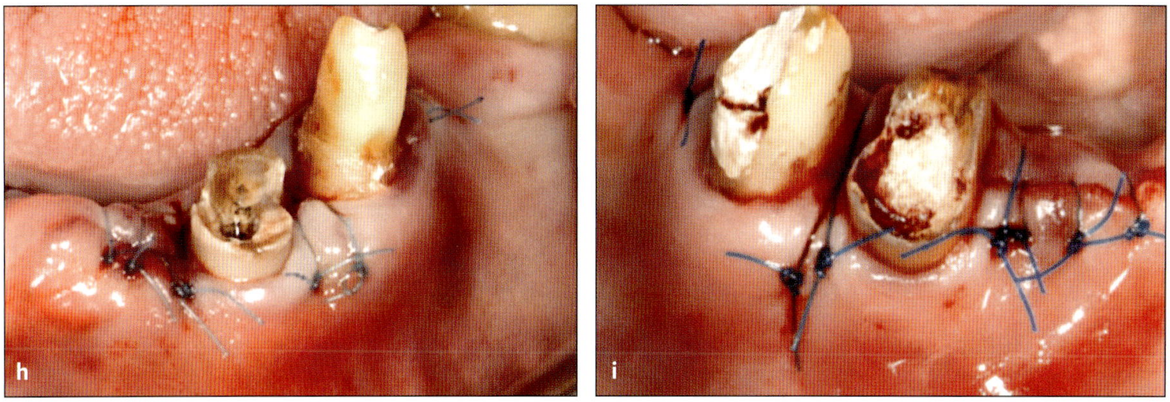

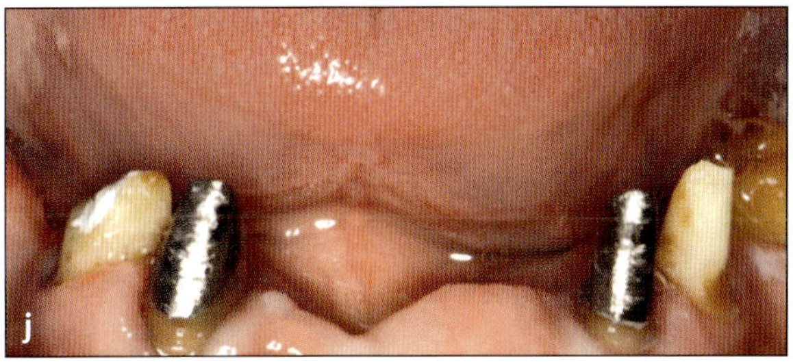

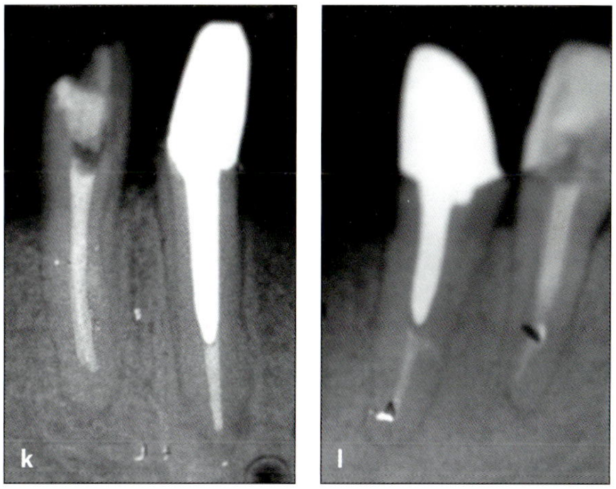

Fig 9-3 *(cont)* *(h and i)* The soft tissues are apically repositioned and sutured above the bone margin. *(j)* At 12 weeks postoperatively, the teeth are restored with post and cores. *(k and l)* Periapical radiographs of the restored teeth.

The whole gingival apparatus can be relocated apically to the osseous crest, resulting in preservation and/or a potential increase in the width of the attached gingiva after wound healing.[28]

Suturing and stabilizing the flaps in their desired locations is a primary element of crown lengthening success (Figs 9-3h and 9-3i). Different suturing techniques can be employed to achieve optimal positioning of the flaps. In case apical positioning of the flap is required, a vertical mattress suture engaging the periosteum will ensure apical placement and stabilization of the gingiva. Surgical dressings may be applied according to clinician preference. Patients are instructed to rinse daily with oral antiseptics (eg, 0.12% chlorhexidine gluconate twice daily). Dressings and sutures are removed 7 days after surgery[24,29] (Figs 9-3j to 9-3l).

Dimensional Changes During Wound Healing

Changes in gingival and alveolar bone levels during healing following crown lengthening procedures influence the final position of the gingival margin. Brägger et al followed a group of 25 patients with 85 teeth subjected to crown lengthening procedures.[30] They measured a mean apical displacement of the free gingival margin (FGM) of 1.3 mm immediately postoperatively, 1.5 mm at 6 weeks, and 1.4 mm at 6 months. Between 6 weeks and 6 months postoperatively, the FGM remained unaltered in 38% of the sites, whereas 33% demonstrated coronal displacement of 1 to 3 mm, and 29% showed further recession of 1 to 4 mm. These findings suggest

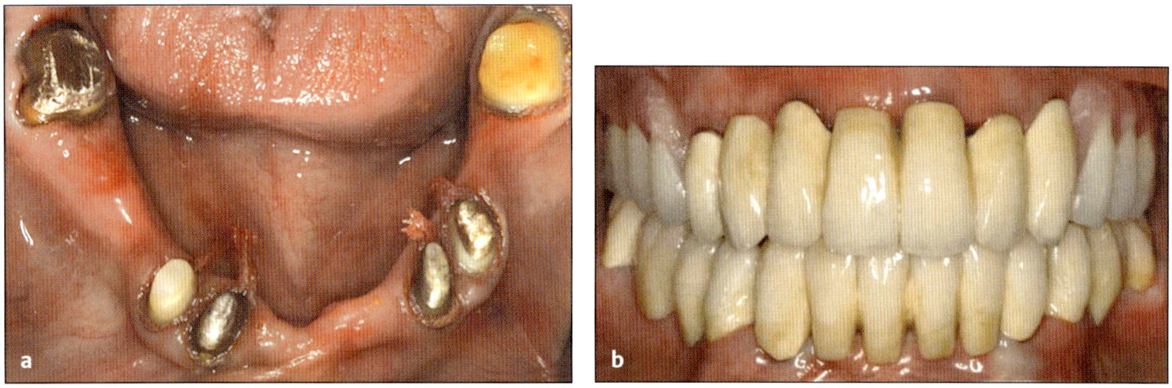

Fig 9-4 Patient shown in Figs 9-2 and 9-3. *(a)* Final preparations and impressions of the mandibular teeth (retraction cords in place) 6 months after surgery. *(b)* Definitive prostheses 1 year after surgery.

that 6 months postsurgically, one-third of the cases showed a soft tissue rebound of up to 3 mm, increasing the risk of creating subgingival restorative margins. On the other hand, almost one-third of the cases demonstrated further recession of up to 4 mm in a 6-month postoperative period, posing an elevated esthetic risk when the restorations are located in the anterior esthetic zone. Lanning et al also confirmed these results 3 months after surgery.[31] Soft tissue vertical regain may be related to the patient's periodontal biotype—the thicker the gingiva and the alveolar bone, the greater the rebounding of the FGM following standard crown lengthening surgery.[32] Positioning the flap at the level of the osseous crest often results in a vertical supracrestal soft tissue rebound (average of 3 mm) postoperatively. If the flap margin is stabilized coronal to the newly established osseous crest, less vertical gain or rebound in supracrestal soft tissues has been observed. It was concluded that surgical positioning of the soft tissue defines the future establishment of the FGM.[28,30]

Although conventional protocols require a waiting period of 4 to 6 weeks prior to definitive restoration of the teeth, in esthetic areas where crown or partial denture work is scheduled after crown lengthening procedures, this period should be prolonged to at least 6 months postoperatively[30,31] (Fig 9-4).

Esthetic Crown Lengthening for the Gummy Smile

The esthetic zone in a patient's smile is defined by the lip form and frame. A high lip line shows a large expanse of gingiva (≥ 3 mm) from the inferior border of the upper lip to the gingival margin, resulting in a "gummy" smile (see Fig 9-5a). A high lip line is not always unattractive by definition. An esthetic concern is raised only when the dimensional proportions of the teeth and their relation to the lips and the surrounding soft tissues compromise the harmony of the smile.[33]

One of the clinical criteria in diagnosing the etiology of excessive gingival display and consequently determining the therapeutic approach is the length/width proportion of the clinical crowns of the anterior teeth.[34] Table 9-1 summarizes the clinical conditions associated with the gummy smile as well as the treatment of choice. In many situations, a combination of these conditions is possible.

In adults with fully erupted and periodontally healthy teeth, the FGM is located 2 to 3 mm coronal to the CEJ. Altered eruption is an aberration in normal development where the gingival margin covers a large portion of the anatomical crown. The delayed

Table 9-1 Clinical conditions associated with the gummy smile and their treatment options

Condition	Treatment
Normal size and shape of the teeth (normal length/width proportion)	
Vertical maxillary excess	Orthognathic surgery and orthodontic treatment
Short or hypermobile upper lip	Plastic surgery, botulinum toxin injections
Clinical crown shorter than the anatomical crown (low length/width proportion)	
Excessive incisal attrition and compensatory eruption	Orthodontic treatment, and if necessary, prosthetic reconstructions and periodontal surgery (crown lengthening procedures)
Delayed/altered eruption of maxillary incisors	Surgical crown lengthening procedures (usually no necessity for restorative treatment)
Short anatomical crown (low length/width proportion)	
Short anatomical and clinical crown	Surgical crown lengthening procedures with restorative treatment

apical migration of the gingival margin results in the appearance of short and squat teeth.[35]

The amount of attached gingiva distinguishes altered eruption into two types. In type 1 there is an adequate or excessive amount of attached gingiva measured from the FGM to the mucogingival junction, while in type 2 there is an inadequate amount of gingiva. Types 1 and 2 are further subdivided into two subcategories, A and B. This subclassification denotes the relationship of the osseous crest to the CEJ of the tooth. In types 1A and 2A, the osseous crest is located more than 1 mm apical to the CEJ, which is a sufficient distance for the formation of the biologic width. Subcategory A is also referred to as *altered passive eruption*.

In types 1B and 2B, the osseous crest is at or in close proximity to the CEJ, thereby diminishing the space for the connective tissue attachment of the biologic width. Subcategory B is also referred to as *altered active eruption*.[36]

Bone sounding via transgingival probing through the sulcus, following the administration of local anesthesia, seems to be an accurate and reliable method for estimating the alveolar bone level and determining the altered eruption subclassification (see Fig 9-5h). This enables the surgeon to select the appropriate technique to expose the anatomical crown of the tooth. The primary objective is to correct irregular gingival arrangement and to establish a harmonious gingival scaffold. In the ideal esthetic situation, the gingival architecture around the two central incisors should be identical, and the most apical extent of the gingival margins in that area should be at the same level as that of the canines. The FGM at the lateral incisors is ideally located somewhat more incisally (0.5 to 1 mm) and is bilaterally symmetric. The gingival margin level at the premolar area is somewhat coronal to the line that connects the gingival margins of the central incisors and the canines (see Fig 9-5c).

In type 1A, a simple gingivectomy/gingivoplasty will sufficiently expose the anatomical crowns. Care should be taken not to compromise the interdental papillae. In type 1B, additional surgical relocation of the osseous crest 1 to 2 mm apical to the CEJ is needed. An internally beveled incision removing the appropriate soft tissue collar and elevation of a full-thickness flap are utilized for osseous recontouring procedures (ostectomy/osteoplasty), followed by flap repositioning (see Figs 9-5i to 9-5k).

In type 2A, an apically positioned flap (utilizing a split-thickness approach) is applied in order

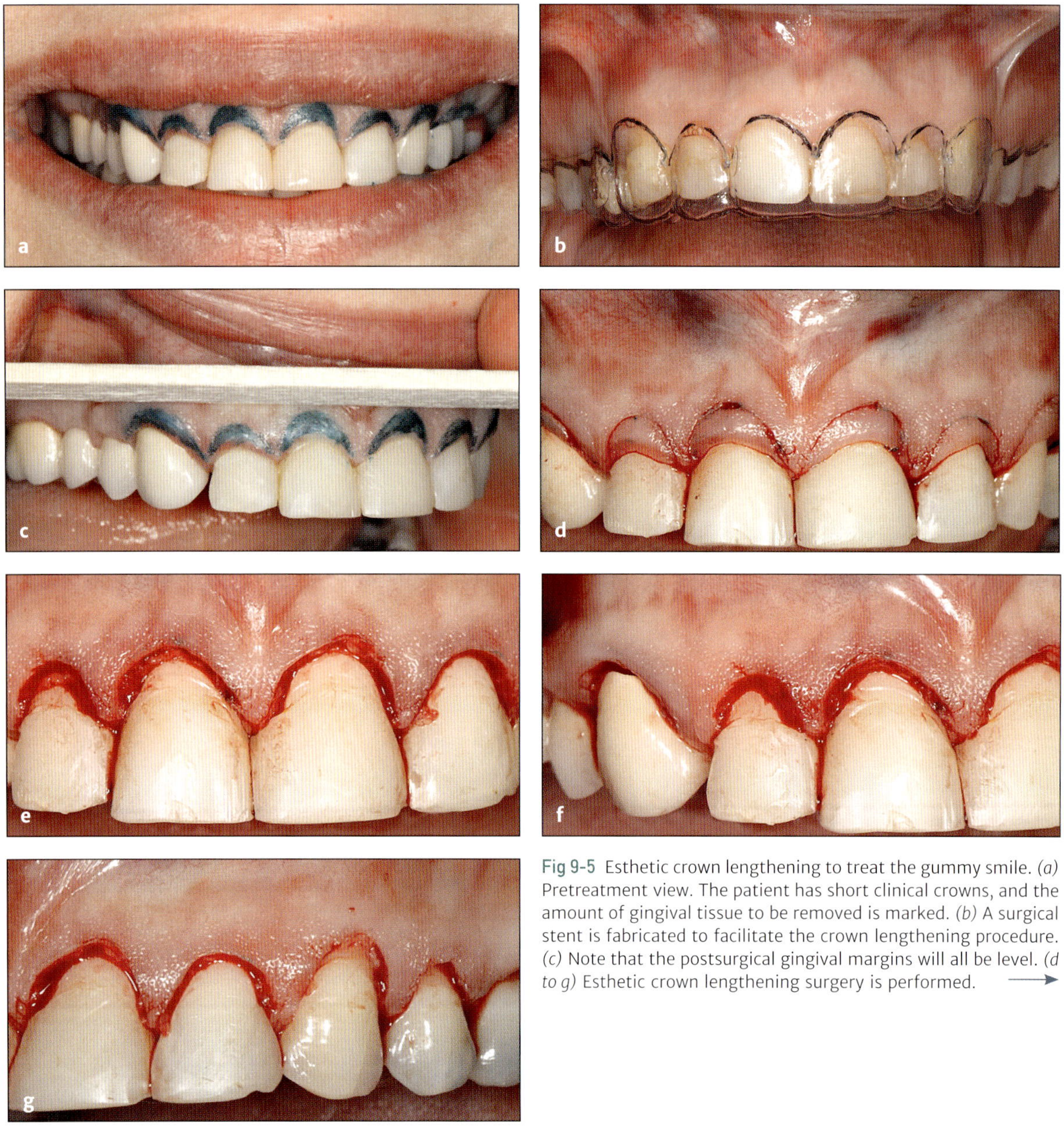

Fig 9-5 Esthetic crown lengthening to treat the gummy smile. *(a)* Pretreatment view. The patient has short clinical crowns, and the amount of gingival tissue to be removed is marked. *(b)* A surgical stent is fabricated to facilitate the crown lengthening procedure. *(c)* Note that the postsurgical gingival margins will all be level. *(d to g)* Esthetic crown lengthening surgery is performed. →

to relocate the entire dentogingival junction. No osseous surgery is needed. In type 2B, apical positioning of the gingiva is accompanied by osseous reduction.

When a mucoperiosteal flap is elevated, care should be taken to preserve the interdental papillae. After osseous surgery is completed, the parabolic form of the osseous crest should be maintained over the radicular surface and must mimic the outline of the CEJ of the teeth. It is critical to remember that the gingival tissues usually follow the shape of the underlying bone.[27]

Figure 9-5 illustrates esthetic crown lengthening in a patient with a gummy smile.

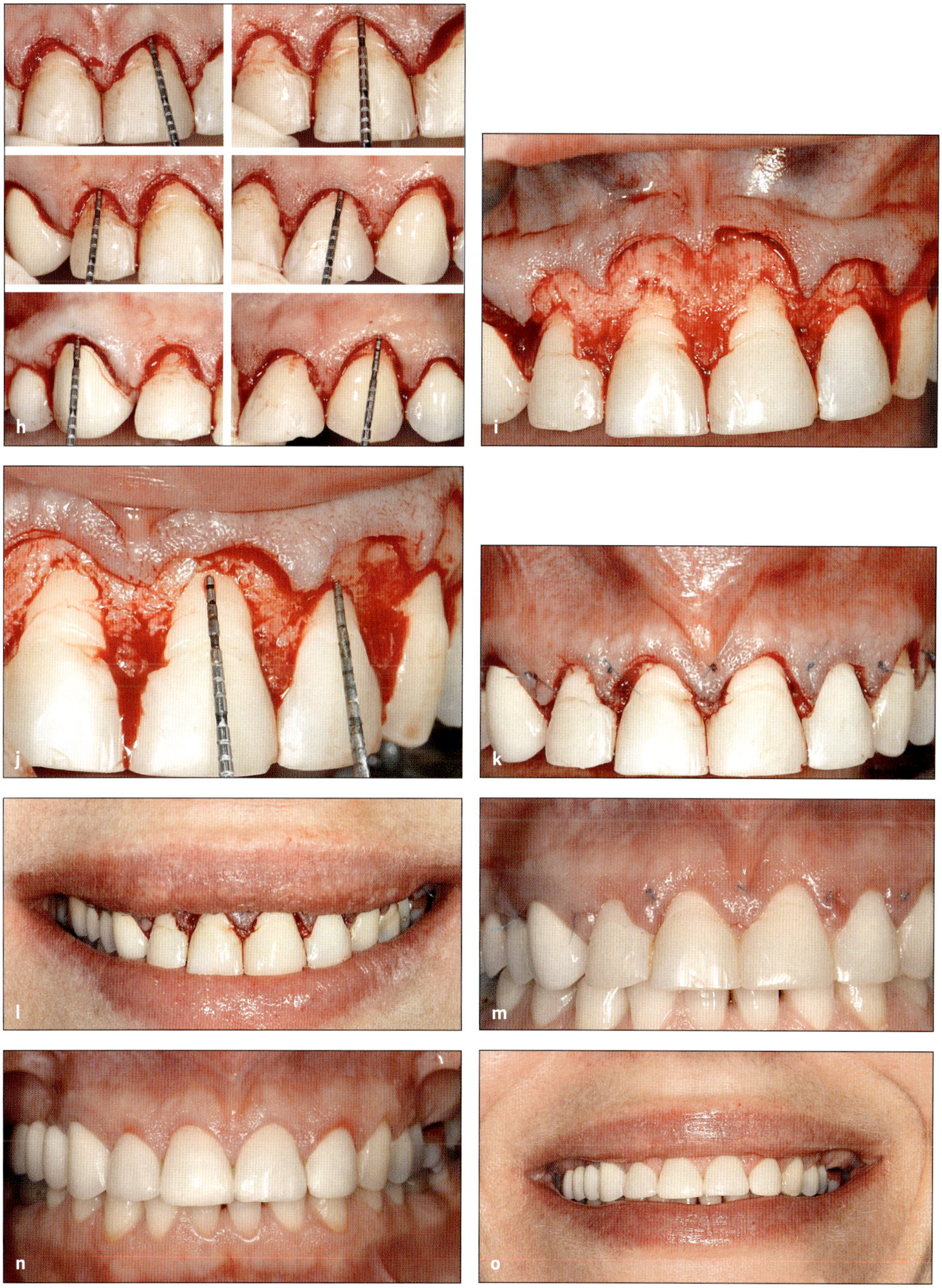

Fig 9-5 *(cont)* *(h)* Bone sounding at all sites. *(i to k)* A full-thickness flap is elevated, bone sounding is performed, and the flap is repositioned and sutured. *(l)* Smile immediately after surgery. *(m)* Intraoral view 2 weeks after surgery. Note the uneventful soft tissue healing. *(n and o)* Eight-month posttreatment view showing a much more esthetic smile.

Conclusion

Surgical lengthening of the clinical crown is a demanding and often a complicated procedure, especially in the anterior maxillary area. Single-tooth crown lengthening attempts should be avoided in esthetic areas because they jeopardize the physiologic osseous architecture and the gingival harmony of the neighboring teeth, resulting in esthetic and functional failures.

Pretreatment planning and a comprehensive approach to reconstruct the dentition are critical prior to any surgical intervention. Aside from general health contraindications, the periodontal status of the patient should be evaluated and treated successfully following the initial and definitive phases of periodontal therapy. The decision to proceed with surgical crown lengthening is made after the establishment of a periodontal-endodontic and restorative prognosis in view of clinical and radiographic re-evaluation data. The fabrication of diagnostic casts and a surgical guide are crucial because they facilitate communication between the restorative dentist and the surgeon, therefore leading to favorable long-term results.

References

1. Marzadori M, Stefanini M, Sangiorgi M, Mounssif I, Monaco C, Zucchelli G. Crown lengthening and restorative procedures in the esthetic zone. Periodontol 2000 2018;77:84–92.
2. Batista EL Jr, Moreira CC, Batista FC, de Oliveira RR, Pereira KKY. Altered passive eruption diagnosis and treatment: A cone beam computed tomography-based reappraisal of the condition. J Clin Periodontol 2012;39:1089–1096.
3. Nevins M, Skurow HM. The intracrevicular restorative margin, the biologic width, and the maintenance of the gingival margin. Int J Periodontics Restorative Dent 1984;4:30–49.
4. Gargiulo A, Wentz F, Orban B. Dimensions and relations of the dentogingival junction in humans. J Periodontol 1961;32:261–267.
5. Vacek JS, Gher ME, Assad DA, Richardson AC, Giambarresi LI. The dimensions of the human dentogingival junction. Int J Periodontics Restorative Dent 1994;14:154–165.
6. Schmidt JC, Sahrmann P, Weiger R, Schmidlin PR, Walter C. Biologic width dimensions—A systematic review. J Clin Periodontol 2013;40:493–504.
7. Al-Rasheed A, Ghabban W, Zakour A. Clinical biological width dimension around dentition of a selected Saudi population. Pakistan Oral Dent J 2005;25:81–86.
8. Novak MJ, Albather HM, Close JM. Redefining the biologic width in severe, generalized, chronic periodontitis: Implications for therapy. J Periodontol 2008;79:1864–1869.
9. Talbot TR, Briggs PF, Gibson MT. Crown lengthening: A clinical review. 1993;20:303–306.
10. Ingber JS, Rose LF, Coslet JG. The "biologic width": A concept in periodontics and restorative dentistry. Alpha Omegan 1977;7:62–65.
11. Rosenberg ES, Garber DA, Evian CI. Tooth lengthening procedures. Compend Contin Educ Gen Dent 1980;1:161–173.
12. Hempton TJ, Dominici JT. Contemporary crown-lengthening therapy: A review. J Am Dent Assoc 2010;141:647–655.
13. Eismann HF, Radke RA. Postendodontic restoration. In: Cohen S, Burns RC (eds). Pathways of the Pulp. St Louis: Mosby, 1976:640–683.
14. Libman WJ, Nicholls JI. Load fatigue of teeth restored with cast posts and cores and complete crowns. Int J Prosthodont 1995;8:155–161.
15. Sorensen JA, Engelman MJ. Ferrule design and fracture resistance of endodontically treated teeth. J Prosthet Dent 1990;63:529–536.
16. Wagenberg BD, Eskow RN, Langer B. Exposing adequate tooth structure for restorative dentistry. Int J Periodontics Restorative Dent 1989;9:322–331.
17. Ochsenbein C. A primer for osseous surgery. Int J Periodontics Restorative Dent 1986;6:8–47.
18. McGuire MK. Periodontal plastic surgery. Dent Clin North Am 1998;42:411–465.
19. Tarnow DP, Magner AW, Fletcher P. The effect of the distance from the contact point to the crest of bone on the presence or absence of the interproximal dental papilla. J Periodontol 1992;63:995–996.
20. Lee EA. Aesthetic crown lengthening: Classification, biologic rationale, and treatment planning considerations. Pract Proced Aesthet Dent 2004;16:769–778.
21. Maynard JG Jr, Wilson RD. Physiologic dimensions of the periodontium significant to the restorative dentist. J Periodontol 1979;50:170–174.
22. Robinson RE. The distal wedge operation. Periodontics 1966;4:256–264.
23. Pollack RP. Modified distal wedge procedure. J Periodontol 1980;51:513–515.
24. Becker W, Ochsenbein C, Becker B. Crown lengthening: The periodontal-restorative connection. Compend Contin Educ Dent 1998;19:239–255.
25. Kois JC. Altering gingival levels: The restorative connection. Part I:. Biologic variables. J Esthet Dent 1994;6:3–9.
26. Herrero F, Scott JB, Maropis PS, Yukna RA. Clinical comparison of desired versus actual amount of surgical crown lengthening. J Periodontol 1995;66:568–571.
27. Takei H, Yamada H, Hau T. Maxillary anterior esthetics. Preservation of the interdental papilla. Dent Clin North Am 1989;33:263–273.

28. Perez JR, Smukler H, Nunn ME. Clinical evaluation of the supraosseous gingivae before and after crown lengthening. J Periodontol 2007;78:1023–1030.
29. Kramer GM, Nevins M, Kohn JD. The utilization of periosteal suturing in periodontal surgical procedures. J Periodontol 1970;41:457–462.
30. Brägger U, Lauchenauer D, Lang NP. Surgical lengthening of the clinical crown. J Clin Periodontol 1992;19:58–63.
31. Lanning SK, Waldrop TC, Gunsolley JC, Maynard JG. Surgical crown lengthening: Evaluation of the biological width. J Periodontol 2003;74:468–474.
32. Allen EP. Surgical crown lengthening for function and esthetics. Dent Clin North Am 1993;37:163–179.
33. Garber DA, Salama MA. The aesthetic smile: Diagnosis and treatment. Periodontol 2000 1996;11:18–28.
34. Sterrett JD, Oliver T, Robinson F, Fortson W, Knaak B, Russell CM. Width/length ratios of normal clinical crowns of the maxillary anterior dentition in man. J Clin Periodontol 1999;26:153–157.
35. Miller PD Jr, Allen EP. The development of periodontal plastic surgery. Periodontol 2000 1996;11:7–17.
36. Chu SJ, Karabin S, Mistry S. Short tooth syndrome: Diagnosis, etiology and treatment management. J Calif Dent Assoc 2004;32:143–152.

CHAPTER 10

Management of Impacted Maxillary Canines

Marianna Evans
Nipul K. Tanna
Chun-Hsi Chung

The appropriate development, eruption, maturation, and final position of the canines is essential for proper occlusion, function, and esthetics. As the cornerstone of the arch, an optimally positioned canine protects the occlusion and plays a key role in the long-term stability of the dentition. When the normal eruption pattern and position come into question, diagnosis and early intervention with an appropriate interdisciplinary surgical, orthodontic, and often restorative management is critical in providing the optimal outcome.

As reported by Stones[1] in 1962 and by Bass[2] in 1967, apart from the mandibular third molar, the maxillary canine is more frequently misplaced from its rightful position in the dental arch than any other permanent tooth. The prevalence of impacted maxillary canines is 1% to 3% of the population, but there is a variation in distribution based on ethnicity.[3–5] The incidence of impaction on the palatal aspect is two to three times more frequent than on the labial aspect.[6] Numerous studies have shown that there is a sex-related factor in that the prevalence of palatally displaced canines is higher in females than in males.[7–9] Racial differences also have been reported, palatal impactions being more common in Caucasian populations[5,10] versus buccal impactions in Asian populations.[11] Bilateral occurrence is not as frequent as unilateral occurrence, and it has been reported that about 8% of canine impactions are bilateral.[12]

Maxillary canines have the longest period of development and the longest path of eruption.[13] The development of the maxillary canine begins high within the maxilla, just under the floor of the orbit, and therefore requires a long path of eruption. Mineralization of the crown begins early, between 4 to 5 months postnatal[14];

however, development of the root starts between 4 to 6 years of age and is completed late compared with the neighboring teeth, after the age of 10 to 11 years. Maxillary canines also erupt into the oral cavity after the first premolars. All of these factors may contribute to disturbances in the path of eruption.

Etiology

Some obvious pathologic conditions have been reported to interfere with maxillary canine eruption. Supernumerary teeth, odontomas, a history of trauma during early development, and cleft lip and palate may lead to canine impactions.

Outside of pathologic conditions, the etiology of buccally impacted canines has been found to be associated with a deficiency in the arch length and/or a narrow maxilla.[15] However, with palatally displaced canines, there has been an increased incidence in missing lateral incisors and/or small or malformed lateral incisors.[15] Two theories have been proposed: the guidance theory and the genetic theory.[5,16] The guidance theory has suggested that the eruption of the canine is guided by the root of the lateral incisor. Any aberrations that may occur in the normal development and eruption sequence of the maxillary incisors may impact the eruption of the maxillary canine. The genetic theory is based on the hereditary component. It suggests that there may be other anomalies such as agenesis or malformation of the permanent teeth causing canine impactions. Peck et al[17] reported that if the root of the lateral incisor is absent or abnormal, the maxillary canine may not erupt and may become impacted.

Several investigators have looked for a relationship between the width of the maxilla and the occurrence of palatally displaced canines. Langberg and Peck[18] found no significant differences in arch width between patients with palatally displaced canines versus the control group. On the contrary, Al-Nimiri and Gharaibeh[19] reported that the transverse arch dimension was significantly wider in the impaction group than in the control group. Using cone beam computed tomography (CBCT), Yan et al[20] found no correlation between the maxillary skeletal width and the palatally displaced canine; however, there was a correlation between buccal impaction and a transverse deficiency. Hong et al[21] recently studied the relationship between the maxillary transverse dimension and palatally displaced canines using CBCT. They concluded that the transverse dimension had no effect skeletally or dentally on the occurrence of palatally displaced canines. Additionally, they found a higher prevalence of permanent tooth agenesis in the palatally displaced maxillary canine group. An example of the maxillary transverse deficiency and buccal canine impactions is seen in Fig 10-1.

Diagnosis

In conjunction with the clinical examination, radiographic evaluation is essential. Traditionally, clinical palpation along with periapical, occlusal, and panoramic radiographs have been utilized to evaluate the location and position of impacted maxillary canines. Periapical radiographs utilizing Clark's[22] rule have traditionally been used to determine a labial versus a palatal impaction. Clark's rule, also referred to as the SLOB rule (same lingual opposite buccal), is based on the position of the x-ray source relative to the object and film/sensor. If the x-ray source is moved mesiodistally, the most palatal/lingual object will move in the same direction as the x-ray source, while the most labial object will move in the opposite direction (Figs 10-2 and 10-3).

Lindauer et al[23] and Ericson and Kurol[24] proposed early identification of impacted maxillary canines using a panoramic radiograph by evaluating the position of the unerupted maxillary canine crown in relation to the root of the erupted adjacent maxillary lateral incisor. Lindauer et al[23] found that when the maxillary canine cusp tip was overlapping the maxillary lateral incisor root, palatal impactions occurred. However, 22% of the impactions in his study remained undetected because they were positioned distal to the maxillary lateral incisor root,

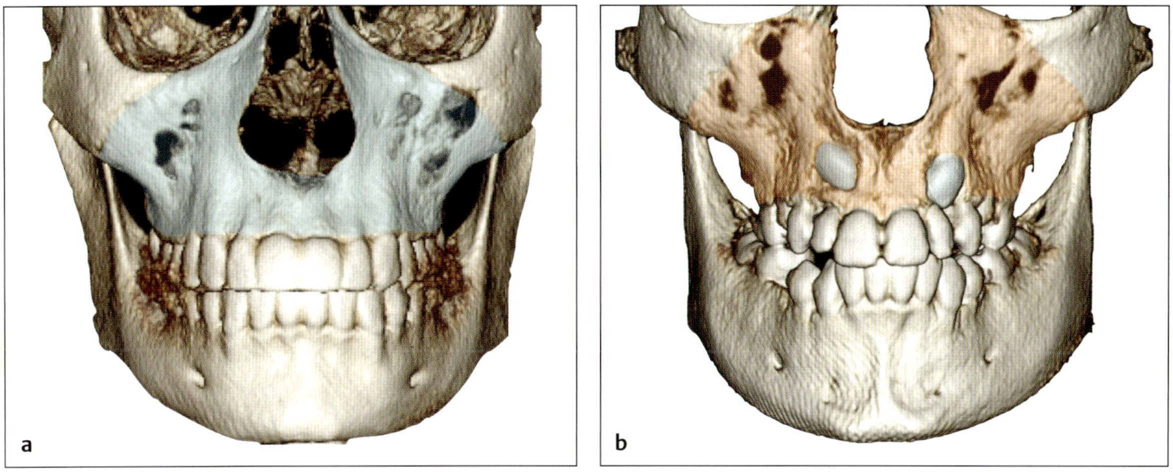

Fig 10-1 *(a)* CBCT reconstruction of a subject with normal maxillary width. *(b)* CBCT reconstruction of a subject with transverse maxillary deficiency and buccally impacted maxillary canines.

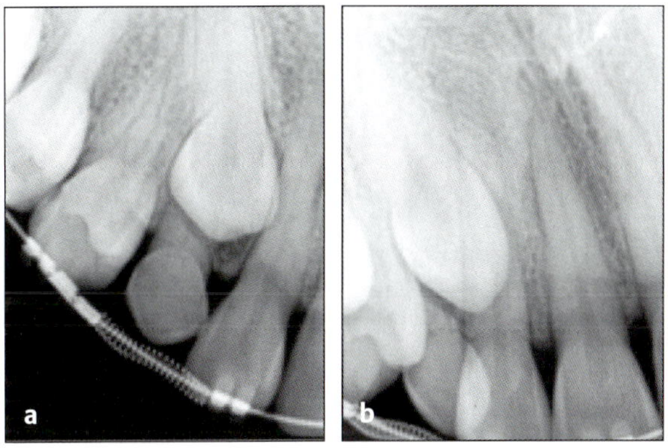

Fig 10-2 Periapical radiographs of a palatally impacted maxillary right canine. *(a)* Periapical radiograph taken with the standard parallel technique showing the impacted canine overlapping the root of the primary canine. *(b)* A second radiograph obtained by positioning the x-ray source mesially. The impacted canine has moved mesially and now overlaps most of the lateral incisor root, indicating a palatal position.

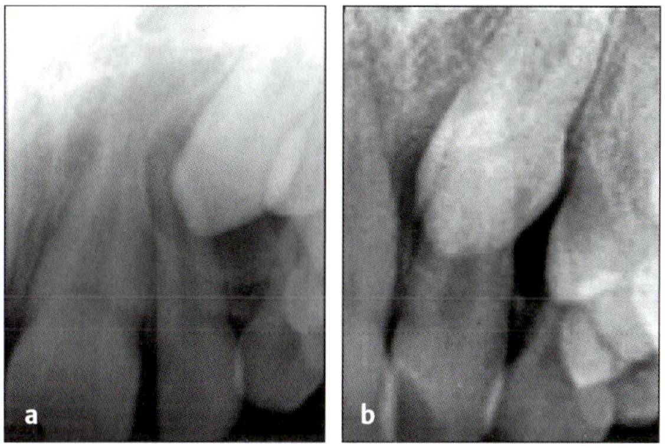

Fig 10-3 A buccally impacted maxillary left canine identified by Clark's rule. *(a)* Periapical radiograph taken with the standard parallel technique showing the impacted canine overlapping the distal half of the lateral incisor root. *(b)* Radiograph taken with the x-ray beam positioned from the distal angle showing movement of the impacted canine in the opposite direction, now completely overlapping the lateral incisor root.

leading him to conclude that we still need a more accurate method for early detection of maxillary canine impactions.

2D images have their limitations in that they may present significant distortion in the depiction of a 3D structure and can be misleading in the interpretation of the actual position and severity of the impaction, particularly along the arch curvature. In addition, 2D images present limitations in visualizing dilacerations and root resorption of teeth adjacent to the impacted canine. Advances in technology introduced the use of 3D viewing via low-radiation CBCT imaging. In a recent study, Serrant et al[25] found CBCT images to be superior to conventional radiographs in accurately locating ectopically positioned impacted maxillary canines. CBCT images allow clinicians to assess the position of the impacted maxillary canines and surrounding structures without distortion or magnification. Figure 10-4 demonstrates the advantage of using CBCT. A panoramic radiograph of a 27-year-old man showed severe horizontal impaction of the maxillary left canine, overlapping the roots of the maxillary central and lateral incisors on the ipsilateral side. On

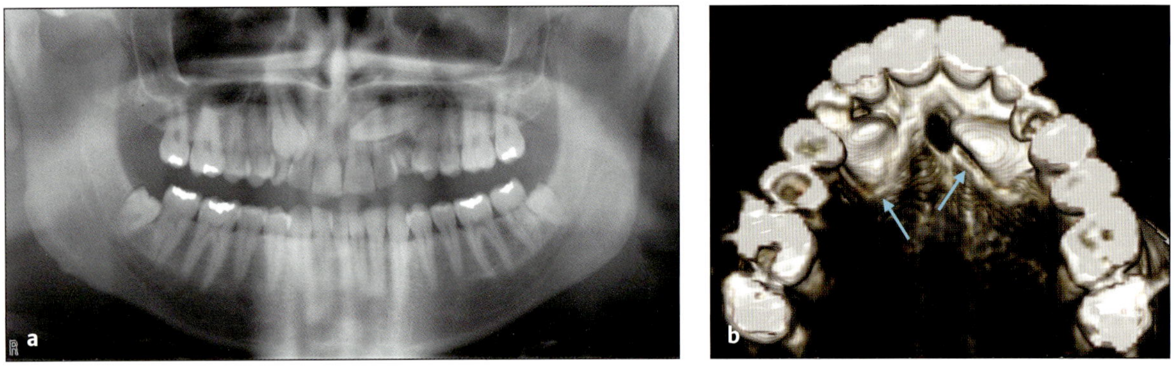

Fig 10-4 *(a)* Panoramic radiograph of a 27-year-old patient showing bilaterally impacted canines. The maxillary left canine appears horizontally impacted, overlapping the roots of the central and lateral incisors on the ipsilateral side. The maxillary right canine appears vertically impacted. *(b)* CBCT 3D reconstructed image of the same patient showing that both canines *(arrows)* are vertically impacted and are not in close proximity to the incisor roots.

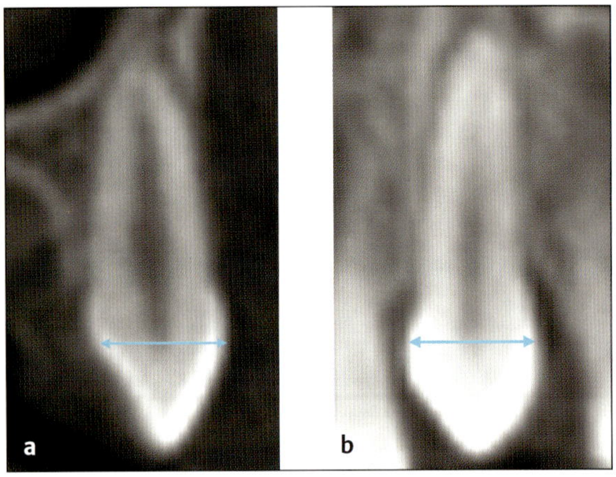

Fig 10-5 CBCT images of unerupted maxillary canines with measurements of the crown width *(arrows)*. *(a)* Buccolingual dimension. *(b)* Mesiodistal dimension.

the contrary, a 3D reconstructed CBCT image of the same patient showed a palatally displaced maxillary left canine close to its ideal position in the arch.

Diagnosis of Impacted Maxillary Canines with CBCT

3D imaging has become a critical tool not only to locate maxillary canine impactions three dimensionally but also to treatment plan surgical access and biomechanics of impactions prior to initiating orthodontic treatment. CBCT images help identify the position and morphology of the impacted maxillary canine and surrounding anatomical structures.

DETERMINING IMPACTED CANINE CROWN AND ROOT MORPHOLOGY WITH CBCT

CBCT technology also offers accuracy in determining the shape and size of the impacted maxillary canine crown prior to initiating tooth movement (Fig 10-5). This is critical in planning intra-arch space requirements and when considering canine substitution in cases with congenitally missing lateral incisors.

Root dilacerations and absence of a periodontal ligament (PDL) space observed on CBCT images may correlate with ankylosis and inability to move impacted canines into an ideal position (Fig 10-6). Having this information beforehand allows us to discuss risks and limitations of tooth movement prior to

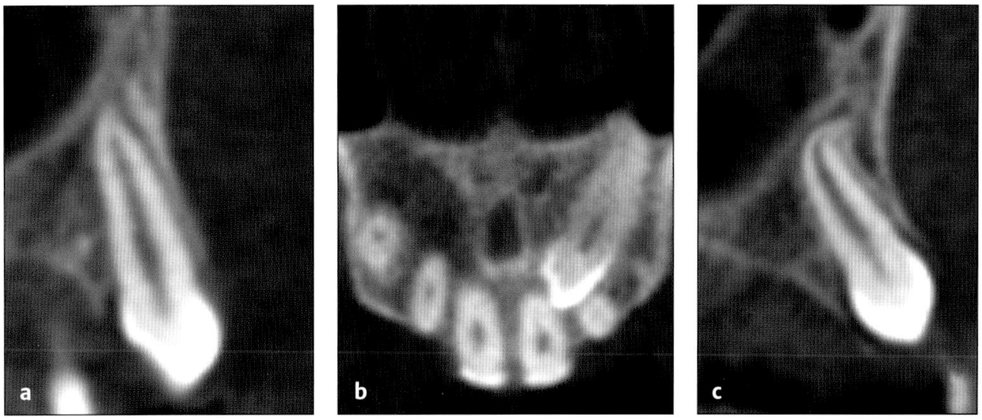

Fig 10-6 CBCT images of impacted maxillary canines with different root morphology. *(a)* Vertically positioned impacted maxillary canine with straight root form, closed apex, and identifiable PDL space, presenting a favorable prognosis for saving the tooth. *(b)* Impacted maxillary canine with no visible PDL space and root dilaceration in the apical portion, suggesting ankylosis with unfavorable prognosis for saving the tooth. *(c)* Impacted maxillary canine with visible PDL space but a dilacerated root, suggesting a questionable prognosis for tooth movement.

the start of treatment and aids in selecting the most appropriate treatment plan for an individual patient.

DETERMINING THE PROXIMITY OF AN IMPACTED CANINE TO THE ROOTS OF ADJACENT TEETH

Maxillary canine impactions present increased risk of root resorption of teeth adjacent to an impaction prior to surgical exposure and during orthodontic tooth movement. Ericson et al[26] reported an overall prevalence of root resorption related to ectopically growing maxillary canines to be 12%, with females affected four times more often than males. Although the mechanism for this pathologic resorption is not clear, it has been suggested that an enlarged or active dental follicle and pressure caused by the erupting tooth may be responsible for the resorption.[26,27] Dağsuyu et al[27] in a CT study did not find an association between the size of the dental follicle of unerupted maxillary canines and maxillary incisor root resorption, although dental follicles of the ectopically growing maxillary canines were, on average, wider and frequently asymmetric in shape when compared with normally erupting maxillary canines. He concluded that root resorption was correlated to physical contact of the crown of an unerupted maxillary canine and the roots of the neighboring maxillary incisors.

Yan et al[28] in a CBCT study found that the physical proximity (<1 mm) of the impacted canine to the neighboring roots is strongly correlated with root resorption in adjacent teeth. According to Ericson and Kurol,[29] CT increases detection of the lateral incisor root resorption related to impacted canines by almost 50%. Figure 10-7 shows the root resorption of a central incisor (see Fig 10-7a) and the root proximity between the canine and lateral incisor (see Fig 10-7b). It is important to scroll through multiple slices in sagittal and axial planes projected through the long axis of the examining tooth to accurately identify the presence and extent of root resorption (Fig 10-8). Failure to utilize this approach may lead to false diagnosis of root resorption in teeth adjacent to an impacted maxillary canine (see Fig 10-8a).

3D ORIENTATION OF THE IMPACTED MAXILLARY CANINE

Impacted maxillary canines can be positioned buccally, palatally, or in the center of the ridge, as viewed in the sagittal plane (Fig 10-9). When using CBCT imaging to locate maxillary canine impactions, a comprehensive approach requiring

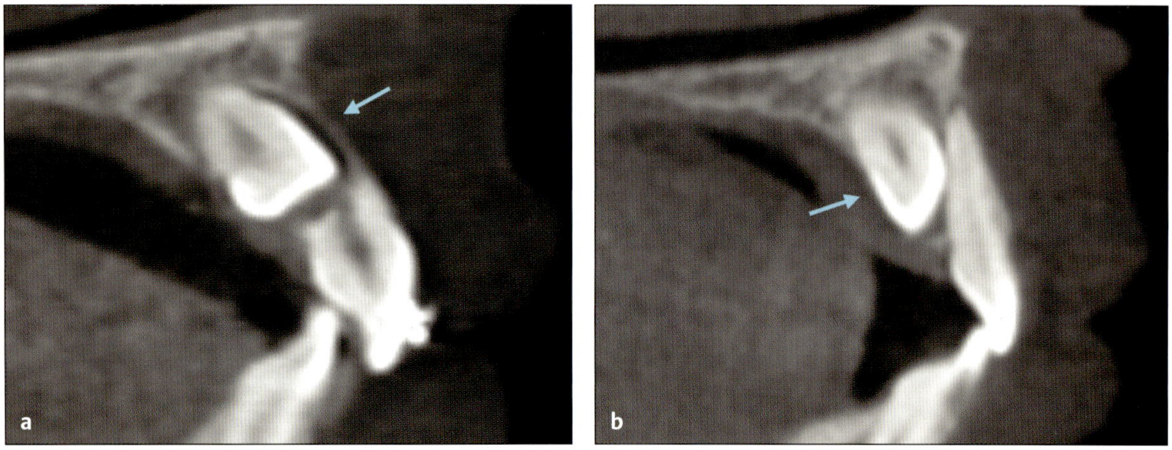

Fig 10-7 *(a)* CBCT image of a patient with severe root resorption extending almost to the cementoenamel junction of the central incisor caused by the impacted maxillary canine *(arrow)*. *(b)* CBCT image of a different patient with the sagittal slice showing close proximity of the palatally impacted maxillary canine *(arrow)* to the lateral incisor root with no evidence of root resorption in the lateral incisor.

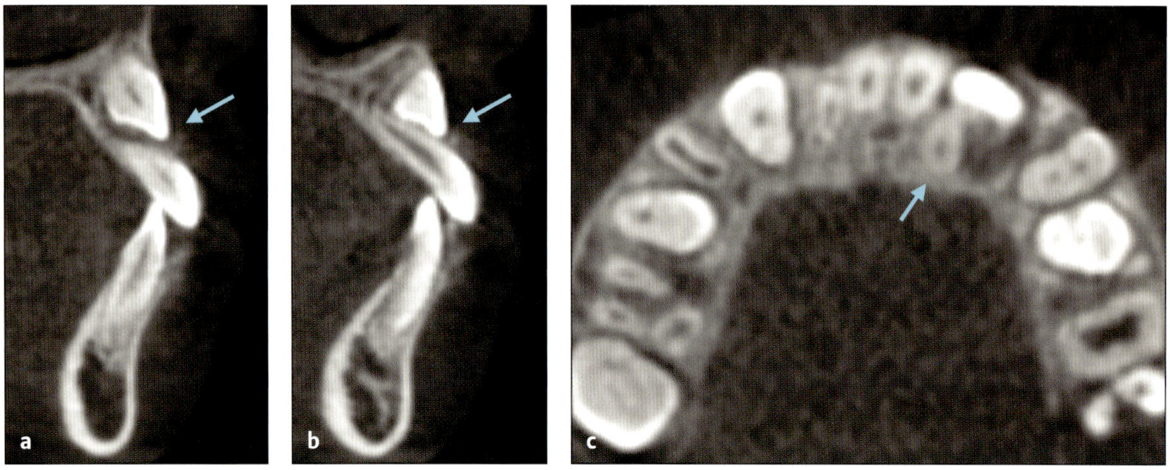

Fig 10-8 CBCT images of a 12-year-old girl with a buccally impacted maxillary left canine *(arrows)*. *(a)* A sagittal slice through the distal of the maxillary left lateral incisor root shows that the crown of the impacted maxillary canine is buccal to the root of the maxillary lateral incisor. A limited view of the maxillary lateral incisor root on this image might be mistaken for root resorption. *(b)* Another sagittal slice through the long axis of the same lateral incisor shows the buccal position of the impacted maxillary canine to the root of the maxillary lateral incisor with no evidence of root resorption. *(c)* An axial slice through the apical half of the maxillary lateral incisor root confirms its integrity with no evidence of root resorption.

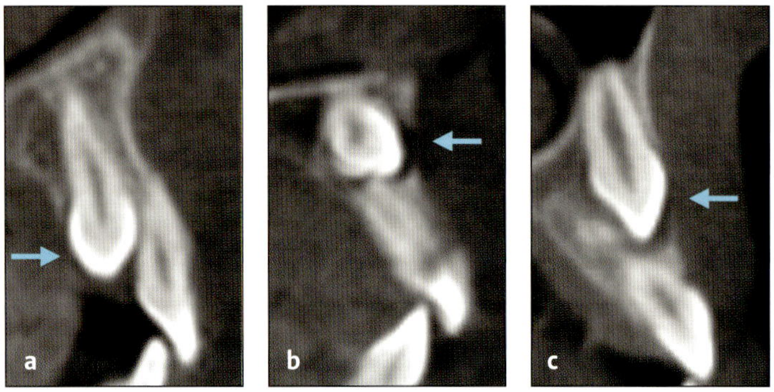

Fig 10-9 CBCT images of the buccolingual position of the impacted maxillary canines *(arrows)* in three different patients. *(a)* Palatal impaction. *(b)* Impaction in the center of the alveolus. *(c)* Labial impaction.

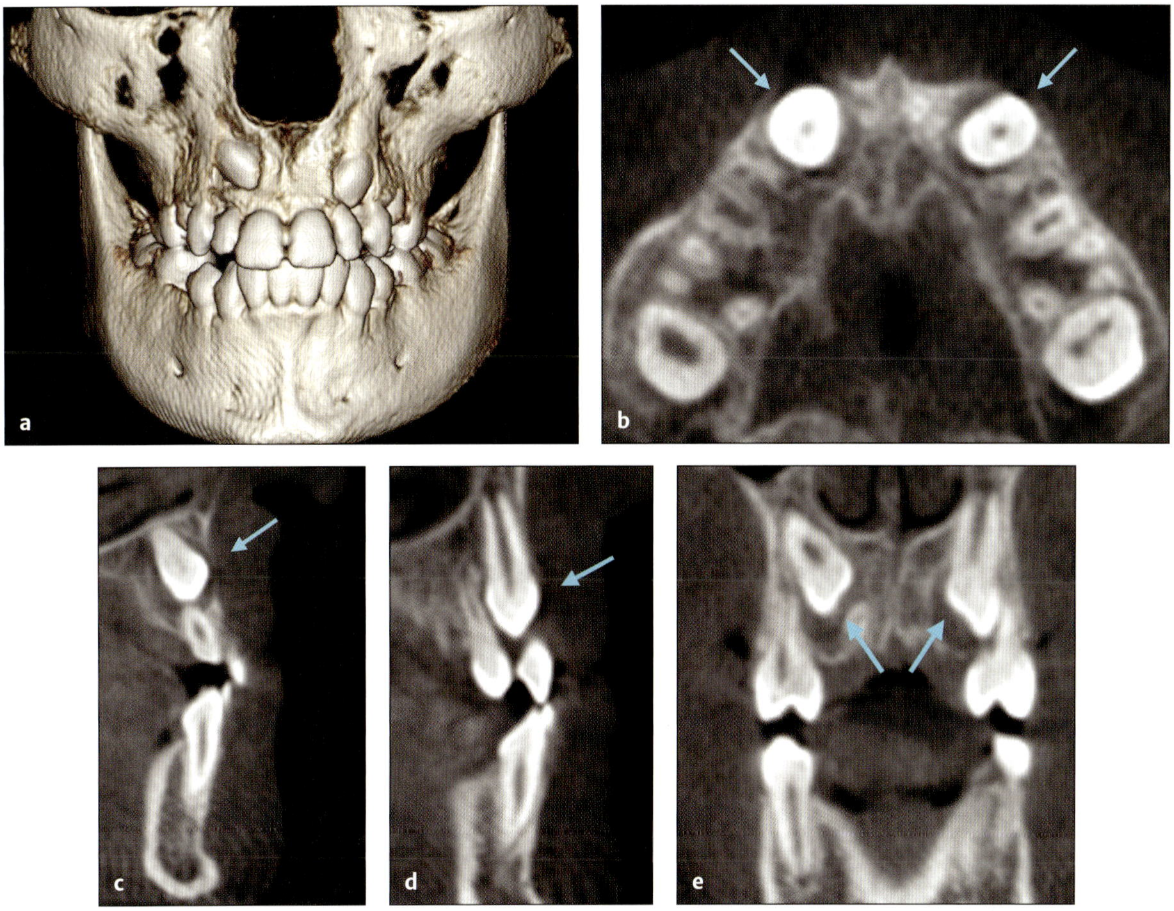

Fig 10-10 CBCT images of a 14-year-old boy with bilateral buccally impacted maxillary canines *(arrows)*. *(a)* 3D reconstructed view. *(b)* An axial slice through the cementoenamel junctions of the impacted maxillary canines. *(c)* A sagittal slice through the maxillary right canine. *(d)* A sagittal slice through the maxillary left canine. *(e)* A coronal slice through the mesial aspects of the maxillary first premolars shows a false palatal position of the buccally impacted maxillary canines.

multiplane examination of the impactions in axial, sagittal, coronal, and 3D reconstructed views should be applied. Locating impacted maxillary canines utilizing only one plane of space may present incorrect identification of the canine position. For example, the buccolingual position of the impacted maxillary canines cannot be determined from coronal slices alone. As shown in Fig 10-10, the coronal view (see Fig 10-10e) shows a palatal position of the bilaterally impacted maxillary canines. On the other hand, axial, sagittal, and 3D reconstructed views (see Figs 10-10a to 10-10d) confirm the buccal position of the same canine impactions.

CBCT images are also helpful to differentiate vertical versus horizontal position of the ectopic maxillary canines in both sagittal and transverse planes (Figs 10-11 and 10-12). This is critical for planning surgical access and biomechanics and estimating treatment duration.

DEPTH OF IMPACTION

It is essential for both the orthodontist and the surgeon to know the depth of impaction of maxillary canines prior to treatment. Impacted maxillary canines may present as superficial soft tissue impactions, partial intraosseous impactions, or deep full bony impactions (Fig 10-13). Deeper impactions will often take a longer time to be translated into the arch and may require bonding of the attachment

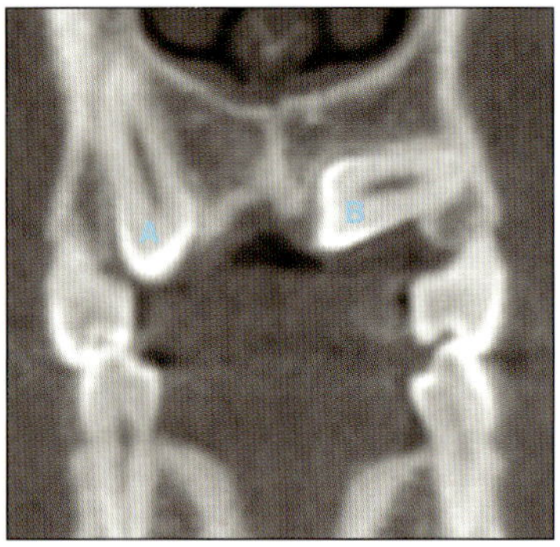

Fig 10-11 CBCT image of the coronal slice of a 14-year-old patient with a vertically impacted maxillary right canine (A) and a horizontally impacted maxillary left canine (B).

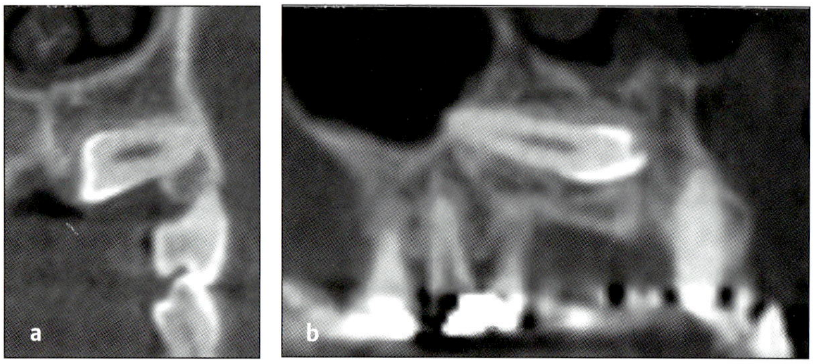

Fig 10-12 CBCT representation of horizontal maxillary canine impaction. *(a)* Coronal slice at the level of the first premolar showing a horizontal maxillary canine impaction in a buccolingual direction. *(b)* Sagittal slice representing horizontal maxillary canine impaction in the anteroposterior direction.

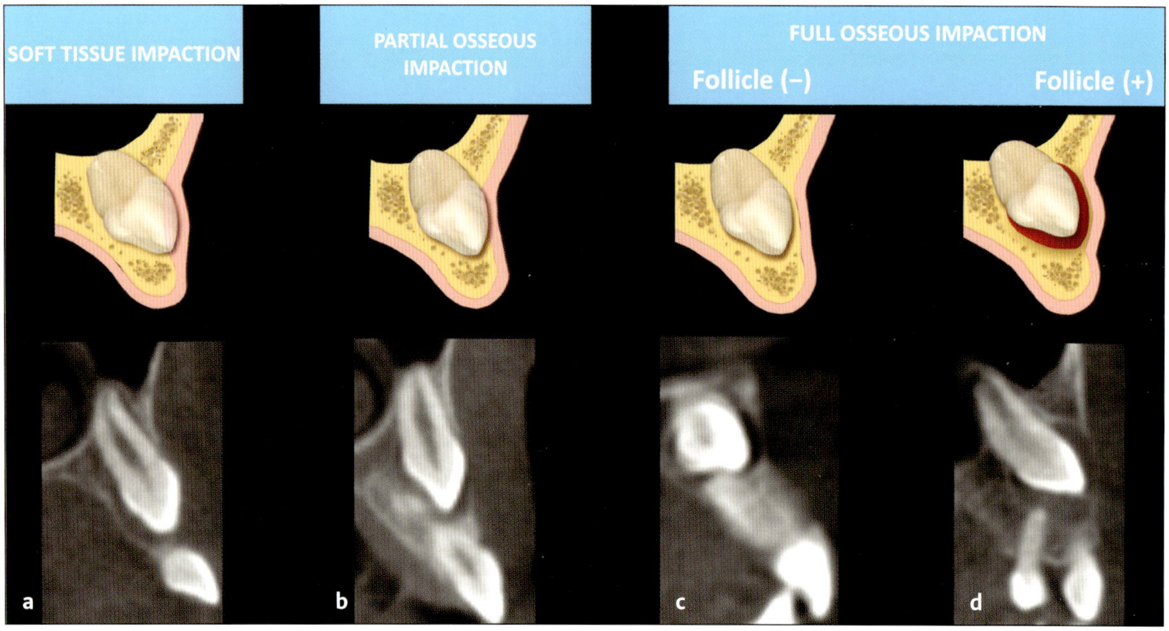

Fig 10-13 Depth of impaction. *(a)* Soft tissue impaction. *(b)* Partial osseous impaction requiring osseous recontouring during surgical exposure. *(c)* Deep intraosseous impaction without enlarged follicle (F–) requiring bone removal above the crown of the impacted tooth. *(d)* Deep osseous impaction with enlarged follicle (F+) requiring curettage of the follicular tissue and removal of the overhanging bone in the path of movement of the exposed tooth.

during surgical uncovering due to a risk of soft tissue overgrowth. Having this information prior to treatment will aid in the selection of an appropriate exposure technique and the mechanics necessary to bring an impacted tooth into the arch.

Impacted maxillary canines often present with enlarged follicles. Their size and shape can be easily determined from 3D images (Fig 10-14). Ericson and Bjerklin[30] in a CT study reported that a circular follicular shape found on conventional 2D radiographs does not always correspond to the one on 3D images. They described symmetric (see Figs 10-14a and 10-14b) and asymmetric (see Figs 10-14c and 10-14d) shapes of the dental follicle. It has been

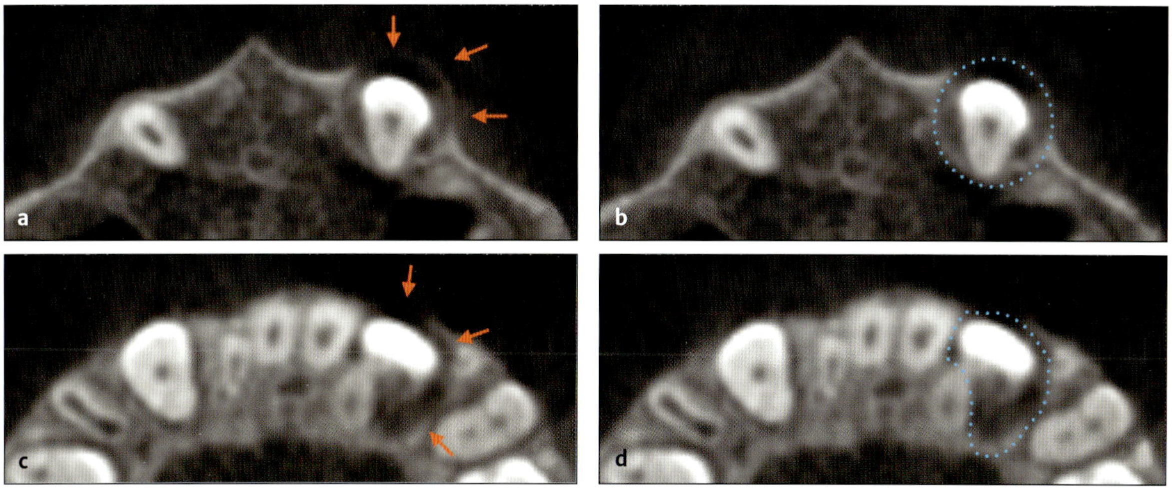

Fig 10-14 CBCT axial cross sections of impacted maxillary canines with enlarged follicles *(arrows* and *dotted lines)* that are circular and symmetric in shape *(a and b)* and asymmetric in shape *(c and d)*.

suggested that enlarged follicles may cause root resorption of the adjacent teeth.[31] Knowing follicular size prior to surgical exposure is also helpful in planning flap design for the open eruption technique. Proper surgical exposure requires not only thorough debridement of follicular soft tissue around the crown of an impacted tooth. More importantly, adequate bone recontouring of follicular walls is necessary to allow for good soft tissue flap adaptation to the exposed crown and the surrounding bone. Incomplete removal of overhanging bone walls around the impacted canines may present an obstacle during tooth movement.

3D SIMULATION OF TOOTH MOVEMENT

Recent advances in 3D reconstruction software (eg, Anatomage) allow 3D simulation of tooth movements prior to treatment. Pretreatment virtual tooth movement is very informative in situations of severely displaced impacted canines, where the decision lies between saving versus extracting the impacted tooth (Fig 10-15).

3D simulation of tooth movement is also useful in the situation of intra-arch space deficiency for a blocked-out impacted canine. It allows for the calculation of two important parameters: *(1)* the interradicular space necessary for safe traction of the impacted tooth into the arch, and *(2)* the intra-arch space necessary for optimal positioning of the impacted tooth in the arch. A virtual setup will guide the decision-making between intra-arch space opening with coils versus arch length increase with the aid of palatal expansion. Intra-arch space opening with coils may lead to the approximation of the lateral incisor and premolar roots with the impacted canine crown, increasing the risk of root resorption. Under these circumstances, palatal expansion may be a more optimal approach to create intra-arch space and an interradicular traction path for the impacted tooth (Fig 10-16).

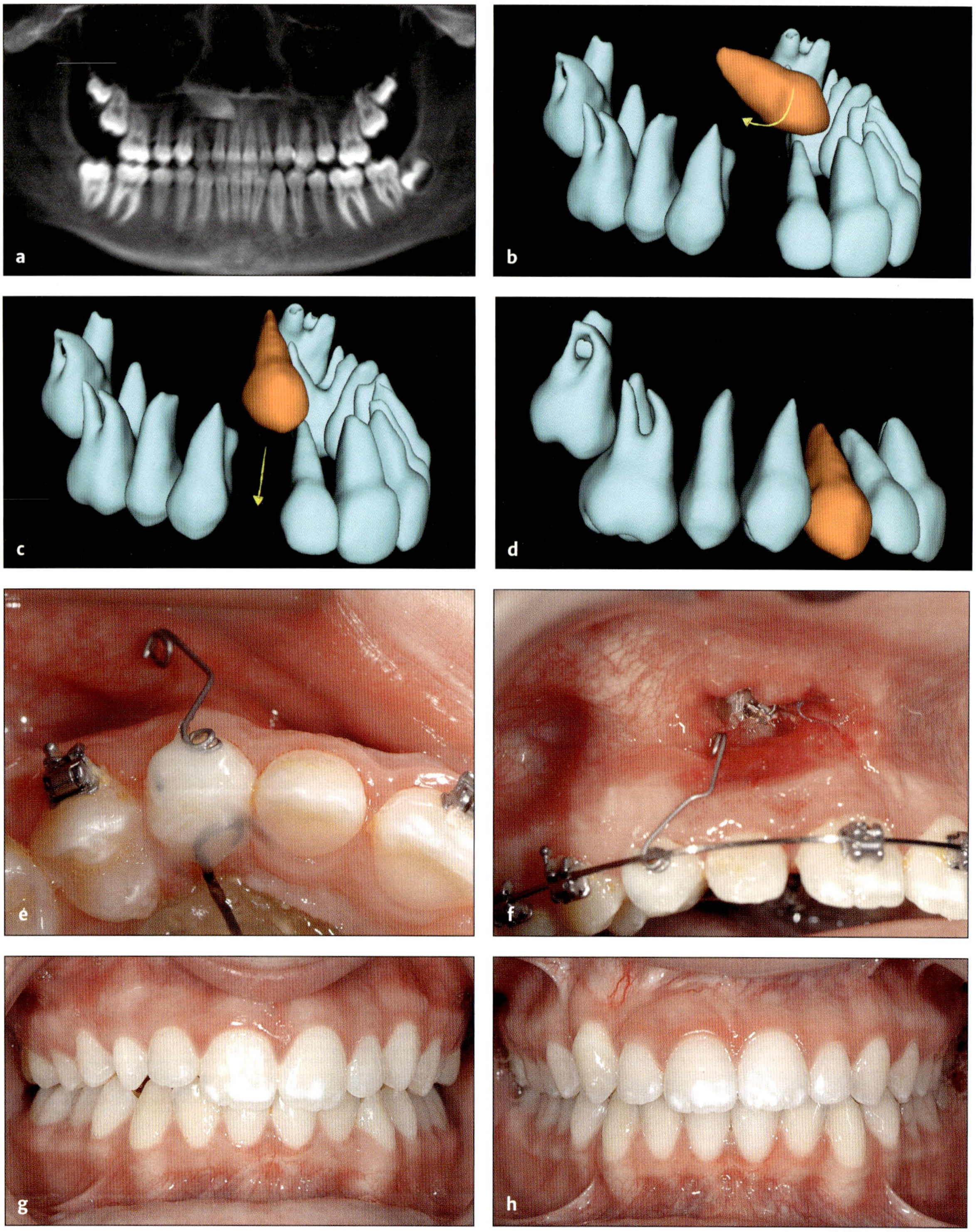

Fig 10-15 A 13-year-old girl with severe horizontal maxillary right canine impaction in the anteroposterior plane. *(a)* Panoramic radiograph showing horizontal canine impaction on the right side, with the crown of the impacted canine positioned right above the roots of the central and lateral incisors. *(b to d)* 3D simulation of the anticipated tooth movement *(arrows)*. *(e and f)* Clinical application of the simulated traction of the impacted canine utilizing a custom bent spring bonded to the primary canine with indirect anchorage to a temporary anchorage device–supported palatal expander. *(g and h)* Clinical pretreatment and posttreatment intraoral photographs demonstrating successful positioning of the previously impacted canine in the arch.

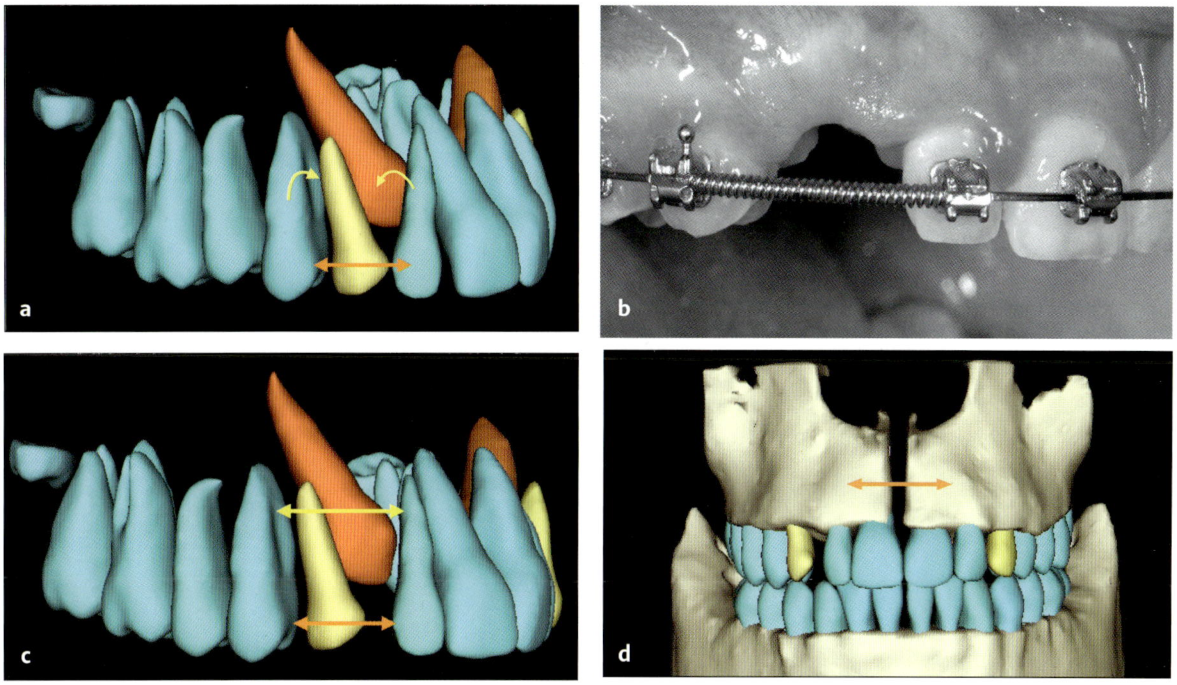

Fig 10-16 3D simulation of space opening *(arrows)* for an impacted tooth. *(a and b)* Intra-arch space opening with coils leading to root convergence of the lateral incisor and premolar toward the impacted tooth. *(c and d)* 3D simulation of space gaining with palatal sutural expansion leading to an increase of intra-arch and interradicular space for the blocked-out canine.

EARLY DETECTION AND INTERCEPTION OF ECTOPIC GROWTH OF MAXILLARY CANINES WITH CBCT

Ectopic growth of the maxillary canines in their early stages of root development (Fig 10-17) as well as maxillary hypoplasia can be identified more accurately with CBCT images.[32,33] A strong correlation has been reported between maxillary transverse deficiency and buccal canine impactions.[20] Therefore, addressing a narrow maxilla with palatal expansion prior to completion of maxillary canine root formation may be helpful in preventing labial canine impactions. Baccetti[34] et al also found early interceptive rapid palatal expansion to be effective in facilitating spontaneous eruption of palatally displaced maxillary canines. Figure 10-18 shows the case of an 11-year-old girl with severe maxillary and mandibular crowding. The CBCT evaluation confirmed maxillary transverse deficiency and ectopic growth of the maxillary left canine (Fig 10-18a). The sagittal slice (Fig 10-18b) through the long axis of the canine shows that root formation is half complete. The patient received rapid palatal expansion to address the narrow maxilla. CBCT images taken 1.5 years later show redirection of growth of the maxillary left canine into proper position without surgical intervention (Fig 10-18c) and natural eruption of the canine into the oral cavity (Fig 10-18d).

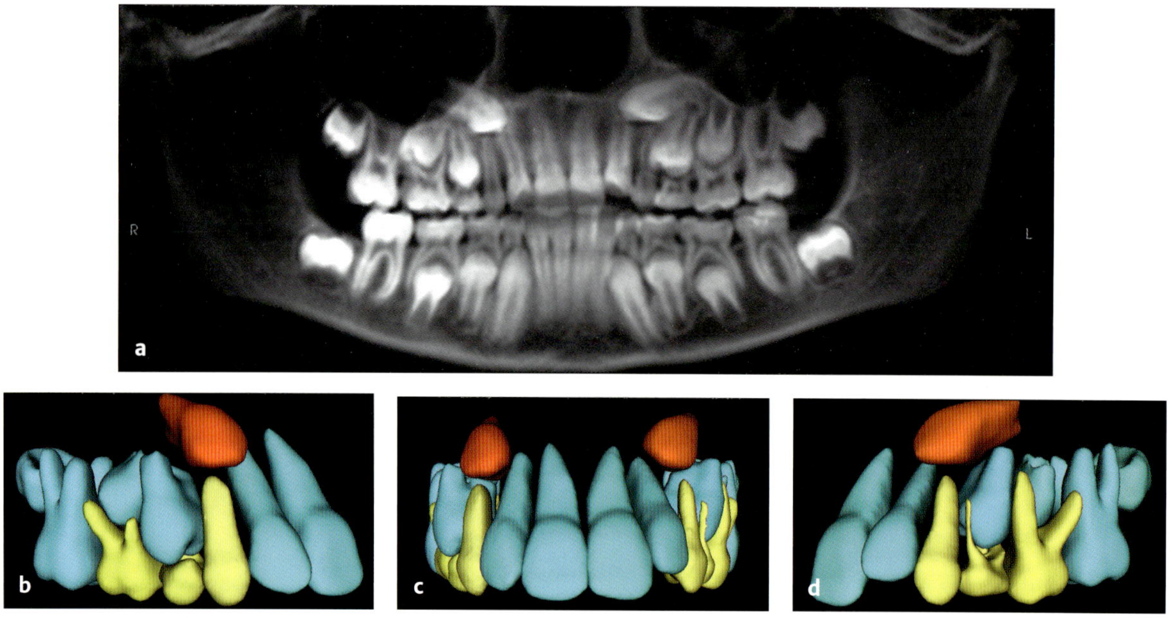

Fig 10-17 An 8-year-old girl with ectopically growing maxillary canines. *(a)* Panoramic radiograph showing horizontal position of the maxillary canines. *(b to d)* 3D reconstructed images of the same patient showing horizontal ectopic growth of the maxillary canines in an anteroposterior direction.

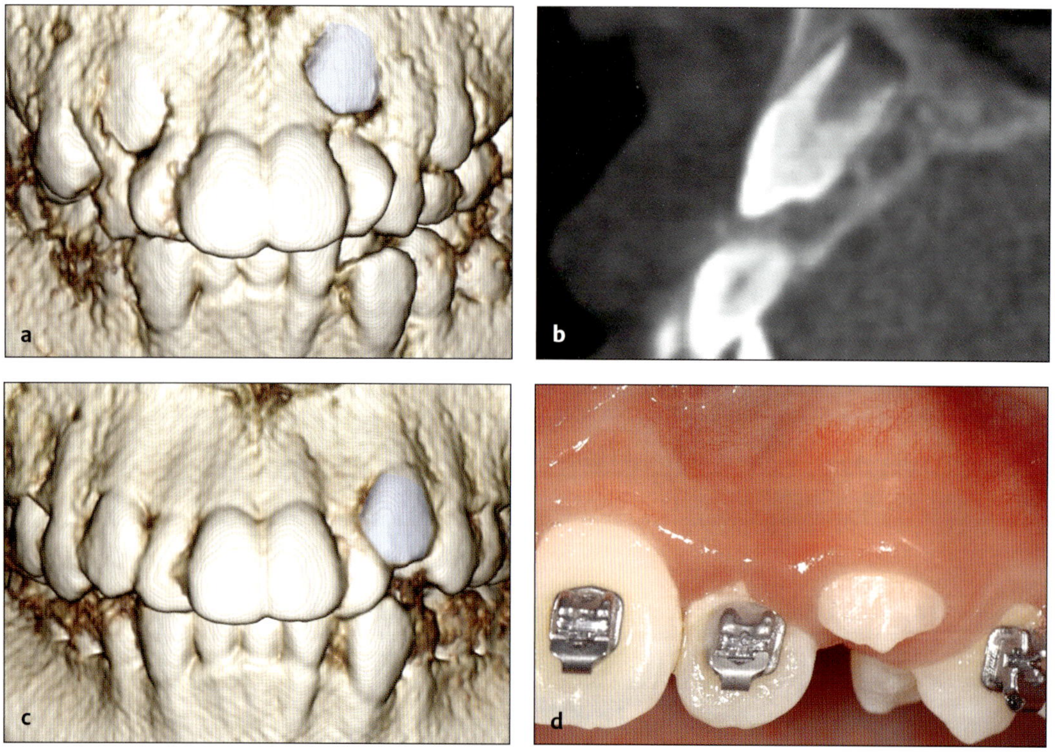

Fig 10-18 An 11-year-old girl presented with severe maxillary and mandibular crowding related to maxillary transverse hypoplasia and tooth size/arch length discrepancy. *(a)* 3D reconstructed CBCT image showing an ectopic unerupted maxillary left canine buccal to the root of the left lateral incisor. *(b)* Sagittal slice through the center of the maxillary left canine showing half root formation in the buccally positioned maxillary canine. *(c)* 3D reconstructed image of the same patient 1.5 years later showing redirection of the maxillary left canine development into the proper position. *(d)* Intraoral photograph of the naturally erupting maxillary left canine into its designated position.

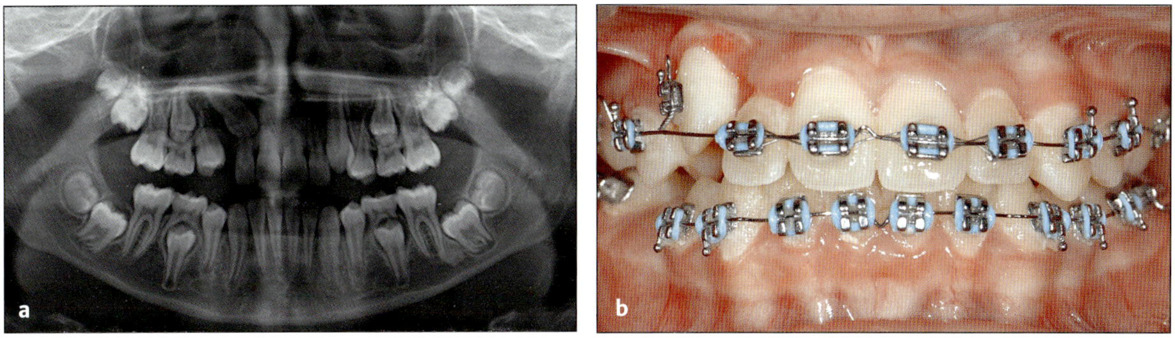

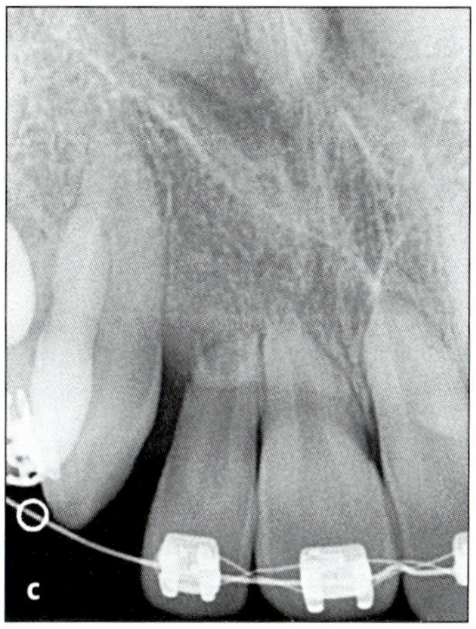

Fig 10-19 A 13-year-old girl with a history of a buccally impacted maxillary right canine. *(a)* Pretreatment panoramic radiograph showing an impacted maxillary right canine with an enlarged follicle overlapping the root of the lateral incisor and insufficient intra-arch canine space. *(b)* Clinical photograph captured several months after surgical exposure demonstrating the buccal position of the right canine and flared maxillary anterior teeth. *(c)* Periapical radiograph taken at the same visit showing root resorption and bone loss on the distal root surface of the maxillary right lateral incisor as well as root proximity between the right lateral and central incisors.

3D-Guided Classification of Maxillary Canine Impactions

CBCT imaging is an important diagnostic tool in determining the complexity of an impaction. Kau et al[35] developed the first 3D classification system for impacted maxillary canines, the KPG index. This index identifies the severity of the impacted canine crown and root tip displacement from its optimal position in the arch. KPG index is based on the deviation of canine position in three planes of space: horizontal (x), vertical (y), and axial (z). Based on this index, impacted maxillary canines are divided into four categories of treatment difficulty: easy, moderate, difficult, and very difficult. Although reliability of the KPG index was validated by several studies,[36,37] prospective studies are necessary to determine its correlation to treatment duration.

Korbendau[38] classified palatally impacted canines into three categories based on *(1)* the crown positioned within the arch near its customary position, *(2)* the crown positioned across the root of the lateral incisor, and *(3)* the crown positioned near the median palatine suture. These categories are then subdivided into deep versus superficial impactions.

Maxillary canine impactions present an increased risk of root resorption in teeth adjacent to an impaction prior to surgical exposure and during orthodontic tooth movement. It has been shown that physical proximity of less then 1 mm between the maxillary impacted canine crown and an adjacent root is correlated with root resorption.[28] In addition to root resorption during the management of maxillary canine impactions, loss of periodontal attachment may develop in exposed canines and/or neighboring teeth (Fig 10-19). The origin of periodontal attachment loss is multifactorial,[39] and it is often related to the surgical approach,[40,41] accelerated traction, heavy forces, or poor oral hygiene. It may also be observed when exposed canines or orthodontic traction devices come in contact with adjacent roots or tooth-supporting

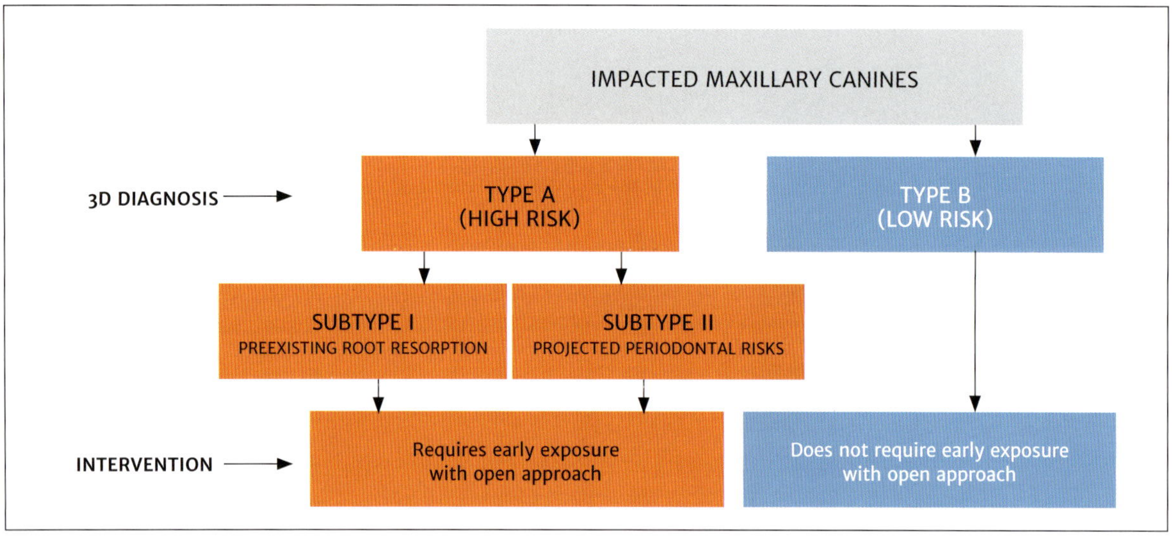

Fig 10-20 Classification of impacted maxillary canines into Type A and Type B according to Dr Marianna Evans.

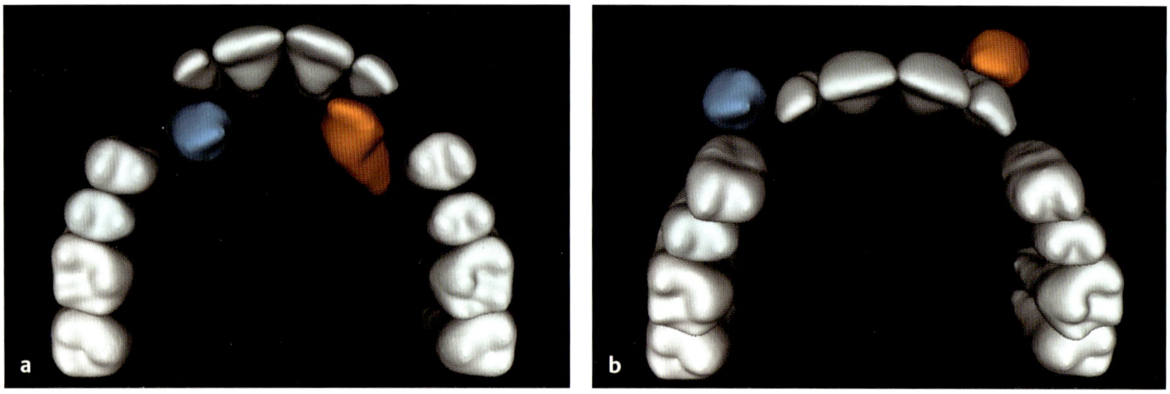

Fig 10-21 *(a)* Palatally impacted canines Type A *(orange)* and Type B *(blue)*. *(b)* Buccally impacted canines Type A *(orange)* and Type B *(blue)*. Both buccal and palatal Type A impactions are positioned in close proximity to the roots of incisors, presenting a risk of root resorption during orthodontic tooth movement. Both buccal and palatal Type B impactions are positioned a safe distance from neighboring teeth.

structures. Every effort should be made to avoid these complications. Knowing the spatial relationship of the impacted canine to the neighboring teeth prior to and during tooth movement will assist in minimizing these risks. 3D evaluation with CBCT imaging and virtual tooth movement are very helpful in identifying preexisting problems and projected risks. Avoiding these complications will often require early exposure of impacted maxillary canines with an open approach and their movement utilizing light forces away from neighboring teeth.

Thus, in order to minimize or avoid unfavorable periodontal complications, a thorough clinical examination and CBCT guidance can be used to categorize maxillary canine impactions into Type A (high risk) and Type B (low risk) groups (Figs 10-20 and 10-21).

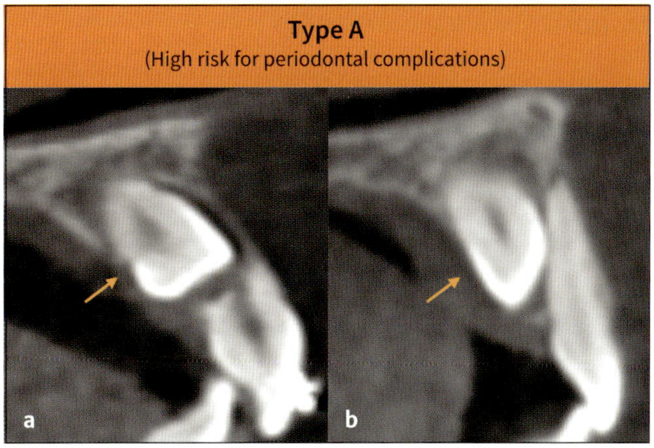

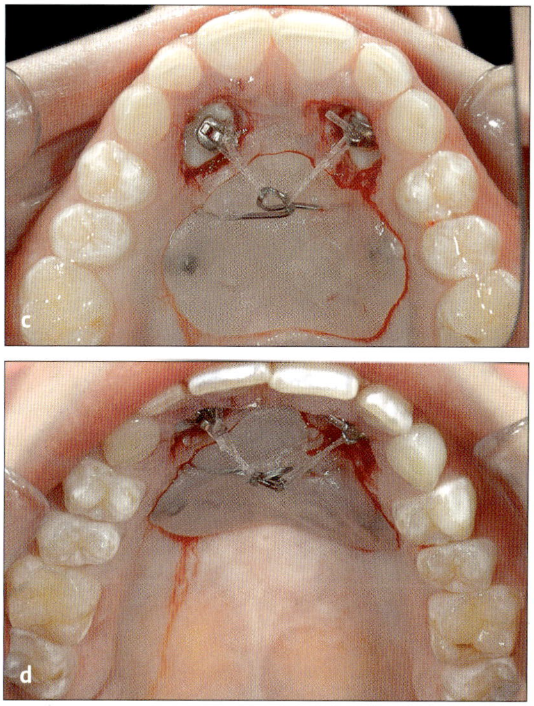

Fig 10-22 Type A impaction. *(a)* An impacted canine *(arrow)* that caused root resorption in the lateral incisor (Subtype I). *(b)* An impacted canine *(arrow)* in close proximity (less than 1 mm) to the adjacent root of the lateral incisor with no evidence of root resorption (Subtype II). *(c and d)* Type A palatally impacted canines were exposed with an open approach and activated posteriorly away from the incisors prior to the start of comprehensive orthodontic treatment.

TYPE A (HIGH RISK)

This group presents a high risk of root resorption and periodontal damage to adjacent teeth. Type A maxillary canine impactions may present with preexisting root resorption (Subtype I) or projected risks of root resorption and/or periodontal attachment loss (Subtype II).

Type A impactions include the following situations:

- Subtype I: Impacted canine that has caused root resorption in an adjacent tooth prior to treatment (Fig 10-22a)
- Subtype II:
  - Impacted canine that is positioned in close proximity to the roots of adjacent teeth (less then 1 mm) (Fig 10-22b)
  - Impacted canine that is positioned a safe distance from adjacent roots (more then 1 mm) but whose movement directly into the arch may position it in close proximity to adjacent teeth
  - Impacted canine that is initially positioned a safe distance from adjacent roots (more then 1 mm) but whose proximity to neighboring teeth will increase with orthodontic alignment
  - Impacted canines with enlarged dental follicles

Although it is controversial to link enlarged follicles around impacted canines to root resorption in adjacent teeth, follicular tissue contains cellular matter with osteoclastic and cementoclastic activity that may contribute to root and bone resorption.[42,43] Therefore, until further evidence suggests otherwise, impacted canines with enlarged follicles should be identified as high-risk Type A impactions.

Type A impactions require early (immediate) exposure and movement of the uncovered maxillary canines away from the adjacent teeth (Figs 10-22c and 10-22d). An open surgical approach will allow maximum control of the tooth movement. Maxillary teeth in close proximity to impactions

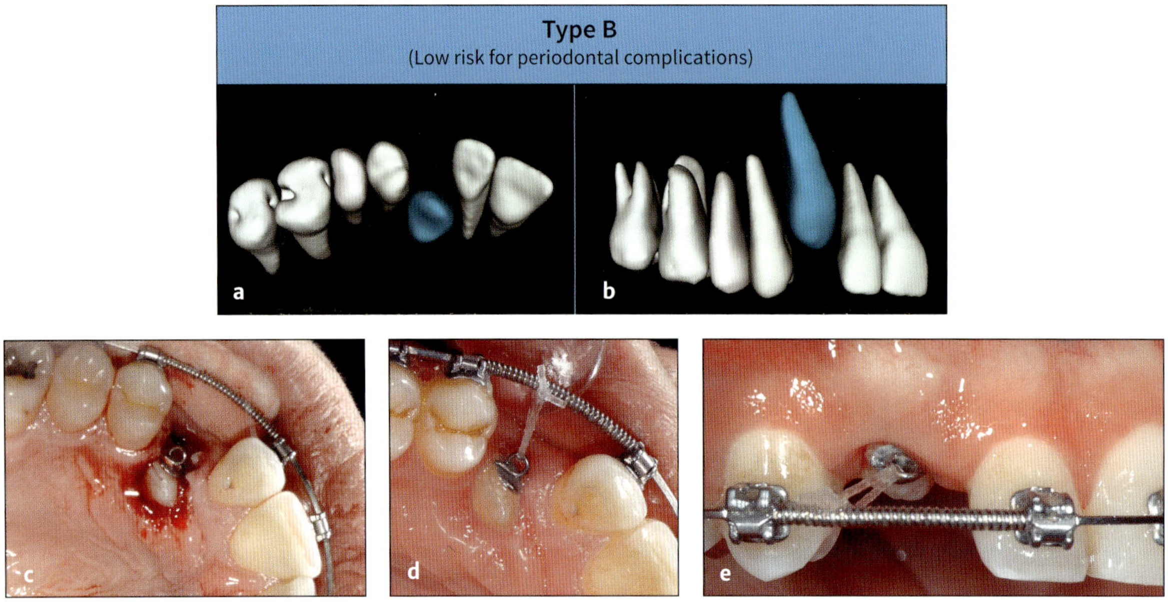

Fig 10-23 Type B impaction. *(a and b)* 3D reconstructed image of the palatally positioned impacted canine positioned a safe distance from the adjacent teeth with a cleared path in the direction of its intra-arch movement once the primary canine is extracted. *(c)* Surgical exposure with an open approach was performed once intra-arch space was created for the impacted canine. *(d and e)* The same canine activated directly into the arch after surgical exposure and extraction of the primary canine.

must be bypassed in the archwire until the crowns of the uncovered canines are positioned a safe distance from the adjacent roots. When proximity to the neighboring teeth is related to the maxillary deficiency in the intercanine area, palatal expansion may be necessary to create sufficient interradicular and intra-arch space to allow healthy traction and positioning of the impacted canine in the arch.

TYPE B (LOW RISK)

This group presents a low risk of root resorption and periodontal damage to adjacent teeth prior to or during orthodontic tooth movement. In Type B cases, the impacted maxillary canine can be safely moved directly into its designated position once it is surgically exposed (Fig 10-23). Under these circumstances, anchorage preparation will determine the optimal timing for canine exposure.

Preventive Intervention

Providing an environment that is most favorable for natural eruption is the first treatment of choice. In some situations, intra-arch space creation will allow physiologic eruption of the maxillary canines without a need for surgical intervention. Ericson and Kurol[24] originally suggested extraction of the primary canine in selected cases to allow natural eruption of the ectopically growing maxillary canines. According to their findings, when the crown of an ectopically growing maxillary canine does not cross the midline of the lateral incisor on the panoramic radiograph, extraction of the primary maxillary canine before the age of 11 years will allow redirection and natural eruption of the permanent maxillary canine in 91% of cases. However, there is only a 64% success rate of spontaneous eruption when the crown of an ectopically growing maxillary canine crosses the midline of the maxillary lateral incisor on the panoramic radiograph. They also reported that if the crown of the impacted maxillary canine is positioned past the mesial root surface of the maxillary lateral incisor, then extraction of the primary maxillary canine will not allow for self-correction, and surgical intervention will be required. Alessandri Bonetti et al[44] found extractions of the primary maxillary canines and first molars to be more effective in preventing palatal and central canine impactions than extractions of primary canines alone.

As demonstrated earlier in Fig 10-18, in cases where the maxilla is narrow in the intercanine area or an arch length deficiency with anterior crowding is present, palatal expansion may also allow for self-correction and natural eruption of ectopically growing maxillary canines.

In general, while cases have variations, once the ectopically positioned maxillary canine does not respond to preventive measures, surgical intervention becomes necessary.

Surgical and Orthodontic Treatment

First and foremost, a thorough review of the patient's medical history along with a clinical and radiographic examination is essential. After an appropriate diagnosis, in the majority of cases, surgical exposure and orthodontic eruption into the arch is the treatment of choice. Providing adequate periodontal support with maintenance of hard and soft tissue integrity has to be considered with this method. Other factors to consider include but are not limited to patient age, patient motivation, adequate hygiene, evaluation of adequate space, position of the canine, and whether the dentition is favorable for orthodontic manipulation.

If factors exist that would limit surgical exposure or the time of treatment to achieve an acceptable result, the options of maxillary canine extraction and maxillary premolar substitution, possible retention of the primary maxillary canine, autotransplantation, and future implant placement may also have to be considered. Horizontal impactions with full root formation, ankylosis, and root dilacerations often present poor treatment prognoses and will require extractions with alternative treatment options. In some situations, ankylosed maxillary canines may be mobilized with luxation during surgical exposure and immediate application of orthodontic traction. Incorrect surgical exposure and orthodontic movement will often lead to attachment loss on the exposed maxillary canine or on adjacent teeth, root resorption, and prolonged treatment time.[40]

Conventionally, the arch is first leveled and aligned, adequate space is created, and the appropriate anchorage is established before surgical intervention. Providing adequate anchorage requires placement of a rigid stainless steel base archwire sufficient enough to support the orthodontic traction. In Type A impactions where there is an increased risk of root resorption or attachment loss in adjacent teeth, surgical intervention must precede orthodontic tooth movement. In these situations, temporary anchorage devices (TADs) may be utilized for anchorage. The size and location of the TAD can be determined as part of the 3D orthodontic and surgical treatment planning.

Kokich and Mathews[45] proposed an alternative method for the management of palatally impacted and displaced maxillary canines in which the surgical exposure precedes the initiation of orthodontic treatment. With this method, a full-thickness mucoperiosteal flap is elevated on the palate, and bone is removed from all areas covering the enamel surface up to the cementoenamel junction (CEJ). The flap is repositioned, and the portion of the flap covering the maxillary canine is excised. This method essentially allows the impacted canine to self-erupt. Figure 10-24 shows the self-eruption of a palatally impacted maxillary canine in a 12-year-old boy.

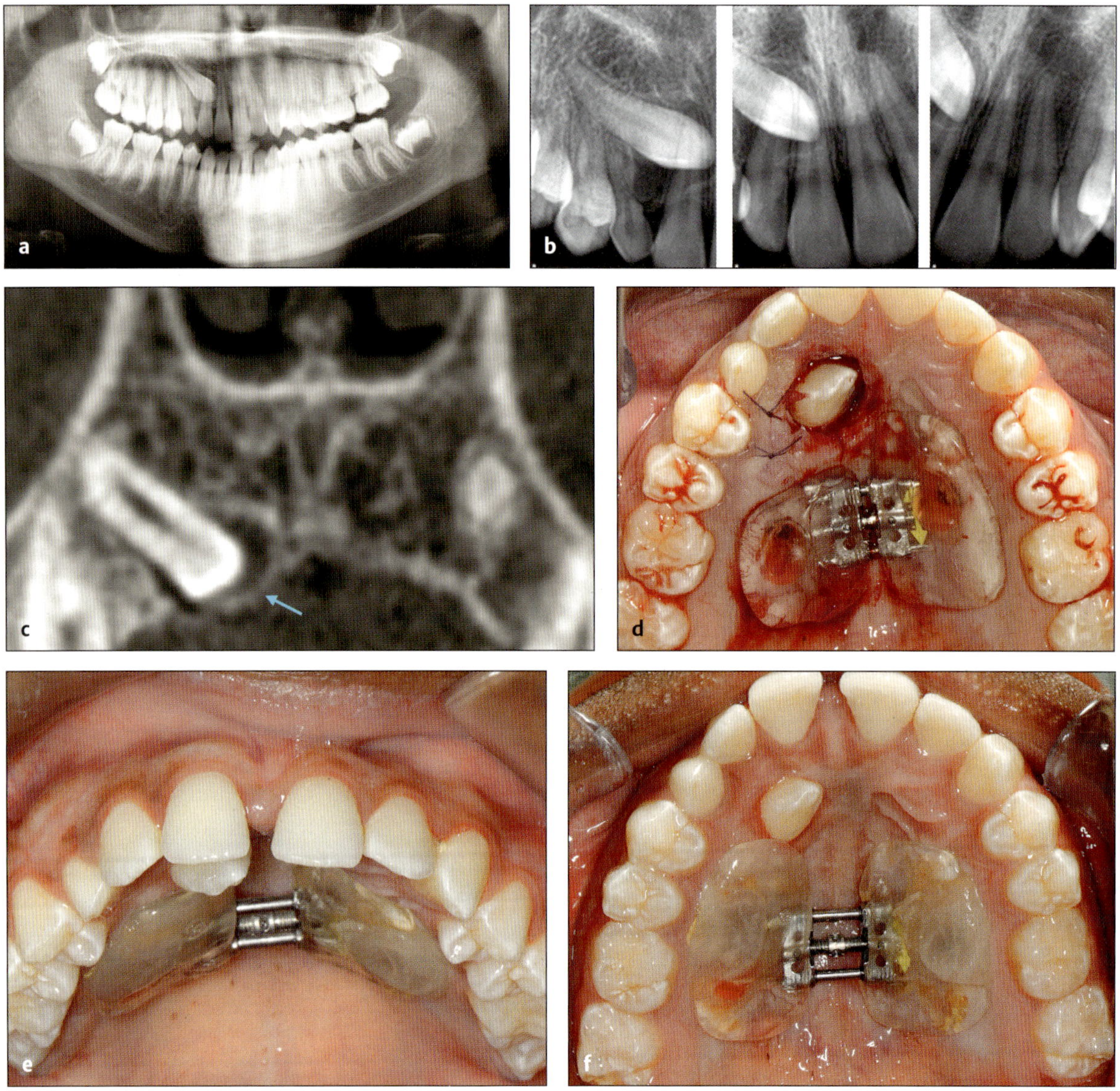

Fig 10-24 A 12-year-old boy presented with an impacted maxillary right canine. *(a)* Panoramic radiograph of the impacted maxillary right canine. *(b)* Periapical radiographs of the impacted tooth. Utilizing Clark's rule on the periapical radiographs, the canine is found to be positioned palatally. *(c)* A CBCT coronal slice shows the palatal position of the impacted canine *(arrow)*. *(d)* The impacted canine was exposed with an open approach during delivery of a TAD-supported expander before the start of tooth movement. *(e and f)* Frontal and occlusal views taken 2 months after surgical exposure show vertical self-eruption of the maxillary right canine into the oral cavity. (Courtesy of Dr Philip Josephs.)

Surgical Management of Labial Impactions

For labially impacted maxillary canines, there are three surgical techniques available: *(1)* gingivectomy/excision, *(2)* apically positioned flap (APF), and *(3)* closed eruption.[12] Each of these techniques has its indications, benefits, and limitations. In a systematic review, Incerti-Parenti et al[41] found the excisional approach to result in less favorable periodontal outcomes compared to an APF. A systematic review by Cassina et al[46] reported a smaller risk of

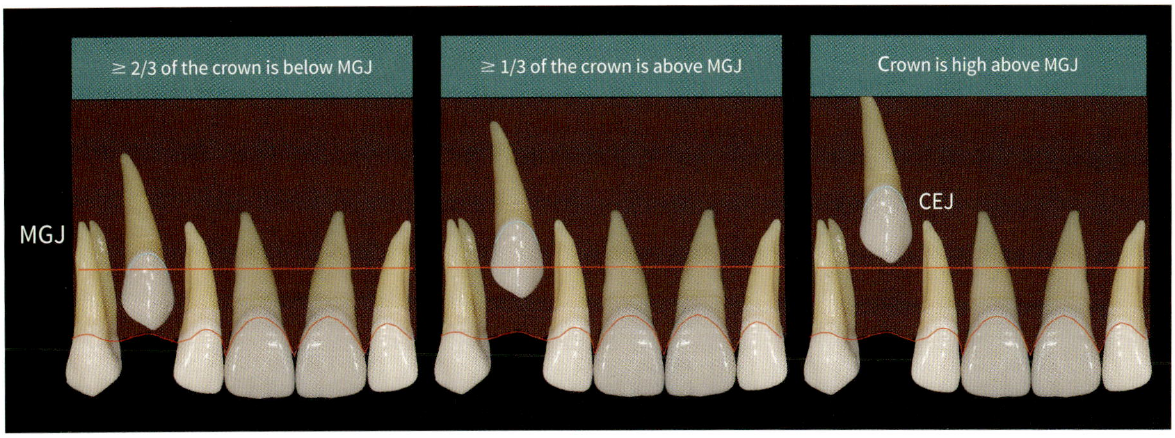

Fig 10-25 Modified Kokich classification of labially impacted maxillary canines based on their relationship to the MGJ.

ankylosis and shorter treatment times with the open versus closed surgical technique.

An adequate zone of attached gingiva is necessary to prevent the detachment of marginal periodontal tissues by labial and buccal musculature.[47] Orban and Sicher[48] were the first to describe a clear distinction between alveolar mucosa and masticatory mucosa. The structural feature of submucosa that is present in areas that undergo mechanical stress (masticatory mucosa) differs greatly from those areas that, under normal conditions, are not exposed to the same level of mechanical stress (lining mucosa). Masticatory mucosa is tightly bound to the underlying tissue and has a uniform network of dense connective tissue extending from bone to the epithelium with a minimal presence of elastic fibers, while alveolar mucosa generally has a rather thin layer of dense connective tissue that is not tightly bound but rather mobile and rich in elastic fibers. It has been well reported in the literature that alveolar mucosa does not serve well as marginal tissue and always presents with some level of inflammation.[47,49] Orthodontic movement in the presence of inflammation poses great risks of attachment loss.[47] The mucogingival junction (MGJ) separates the attached masticatory and alveolar mucosa. Labially impacted maxillary canines may be positioned at a different height in relationship to the MGJ (Fig 10-25). Surgical exposure of the labially impacted maxillary canine must be performed with strong consideration of its position relative to the MGJ in order to avoid mucogingival problems around exposed teeth.[45] To help achieve this objective, Levin and D'Amico[50] and Vanarsdall and Corn[47] proposed the APF for uncovering labially impacted teeth.

TECHNIQUE TO PROJECT THE MGJ ON CBCT IMAGES

To identify the precise position of the impacted maxillary canine to the MGJ, a combined technique utilizing clinical and 3D evaluation must be applied (Fig 10-26). First, the MGJ is identified adjacent to the maxillary impacted tooth during the intraoral clinical examination. A periodontal probe is used to measure the distance from the center of the crown tips of the adjacent maxillary teeth to the MGJ (Figs 10-26a and 10-26c). The MGJ is marked on the adjacent teeth at point X and point Y. These measurements are then transferred to the 3D reconstructed image (Figs 10-26b and 10-26d). A line connecting points X and Y is the projected MGJ at the level of the maxillary impaction. The last step is to determine the position of the maxillary impacted tooth in relation to the projected MGJ. Once that position is determined, the most appropriate surgical access is selected.

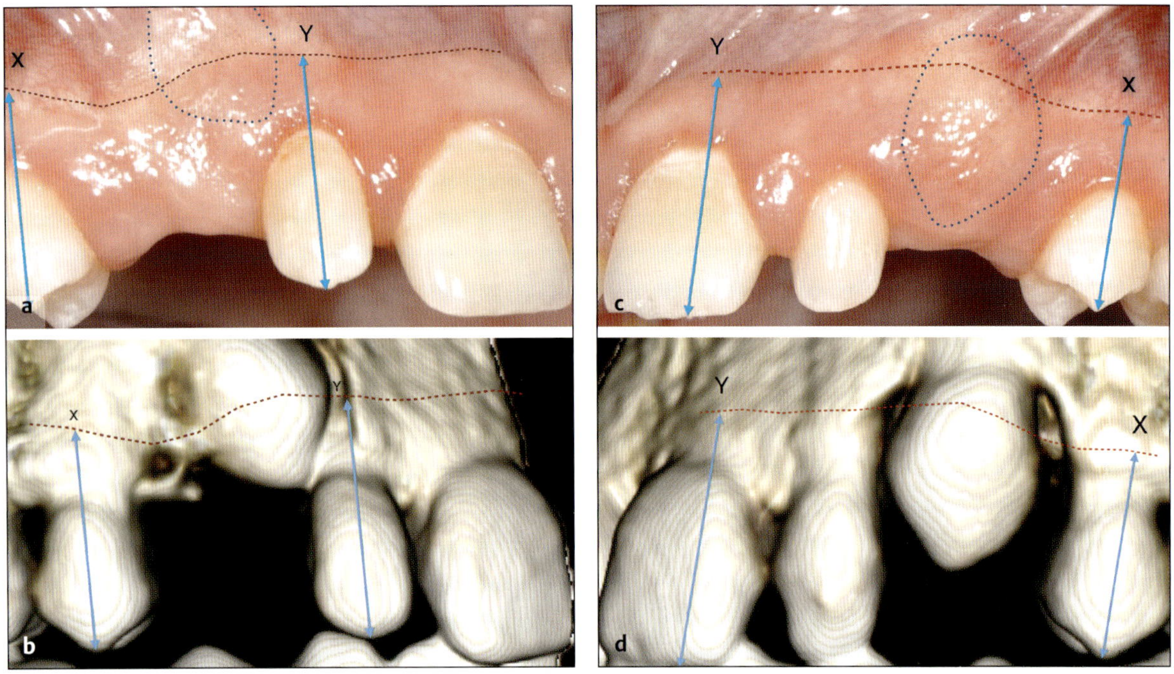

Fig 10-26 Projection of the MGJ in the CBCT 3D reconstructed images utilizing linear clinical measurements. *(a and b)* Buccally impacted maxillary right canine is identified to be positioned halfway below the MGJ. *(c and d)* Buccally impacted maxillary left canine is identified to be positioned two-thirds below the MGJ.

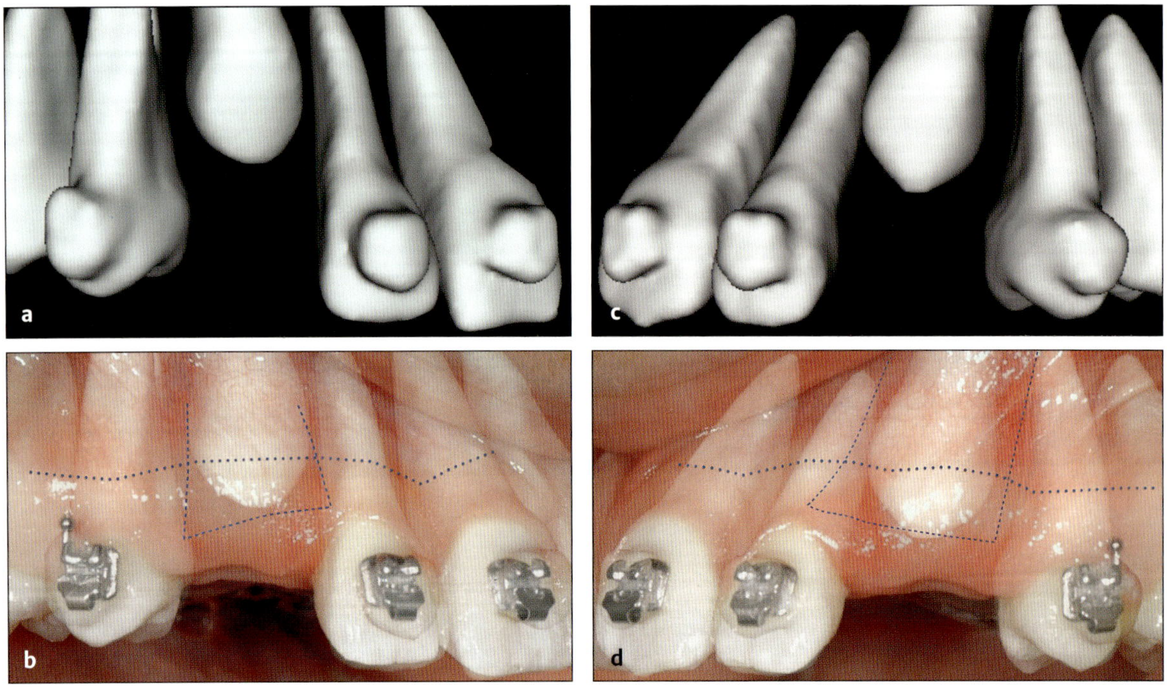

Fig 10-27 *(a to d)* 3D superimposition of the 3D CBCT model over the clinical photographs with outlined MGJ used in planning the apically positioned flap.

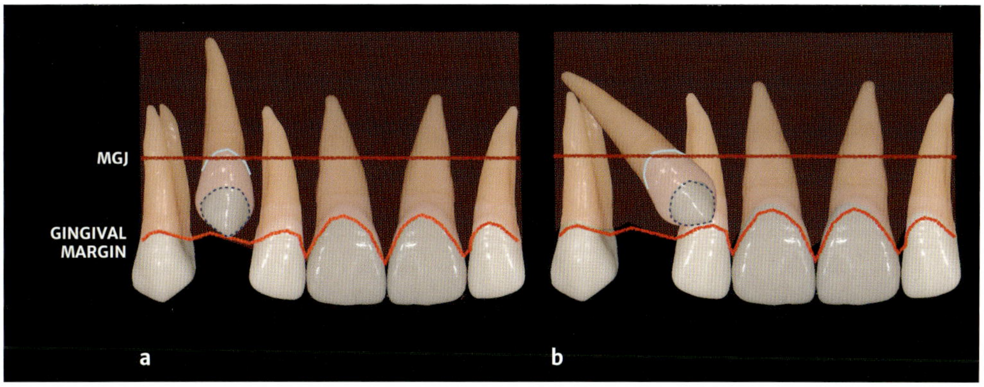

Fig 10-28 *(a)* Vertical impaction. *(b)* Angulated impaction. Both have more then two-thirds of the crown of the impacted maxillary canine positioned coronal to the MGJ. Gingivectomy should be performed in the area outlined with the *blue dotted line*, which leaves 3 to 4 mm of keratinized gingiva apical to the incision line.

Another technique to project the MGJ over a labially positioned impacted canine is to utilize 3D superimposition of the intraoral scans or photographs over the CBCT scan (Fig 10-27). This technique simplifies communication between the orthodontist and the surgeon and offers precision in planning of the incision design.

GINGIVECTOMY/EXCISION

Gingivectomy/excision is a simple technique whereby the gingiva over an impacted maxillary canine is excised. Although this technique is considered to be the least invasive, it is technique sensitive. Improper identification of the impacted maxillary canine and the incision design might compromise the uncovered tooth periodontally.

Indications

This technique is indicated in soft tissue impactions only when no bone is covering the crown of the impacted tooth and at least two-thirds of the crown is positioned coronal to the MGJ. This technique may be performed for labially impacted maxillary canines in both upright and angulated positions when an adequate band of gingiva is present to allow for preservation of keratinized apical gingiva of 3 to 4 mm in width on the exposed crown (Fig 10-28).

Contraindications

Gingivectomy/excision is contraindicated when more than one-third of the crown of the impacted maxillary canine is positioned apical to the MGJ and when any bone removal overlying this crown is required. In these situations, flap reflection is mandatory to complete proper exposure.

Procedure

Every precaution has to be made to prevent exposure of the CEJ of the impacted canine with this technique. Precise identification of the CEJ of the impacted maxillary canine in relation to the MGJ is required prior to excising any gingiva. This may be done with the aid of 3D images and a clinical periodontal examination. Adequate gingival width of at least 3 to 4 mm must be preserved apical to the exposure area to prevent development of mucogingival problems. Although this technique may be accomplished with a surgical blade (Fig 10-29), laser, or electrosurgical unit (Fig 10-30), the use of a blade will allow minimal tissue damage and remodeling. Due to the superficial position of the maxillary

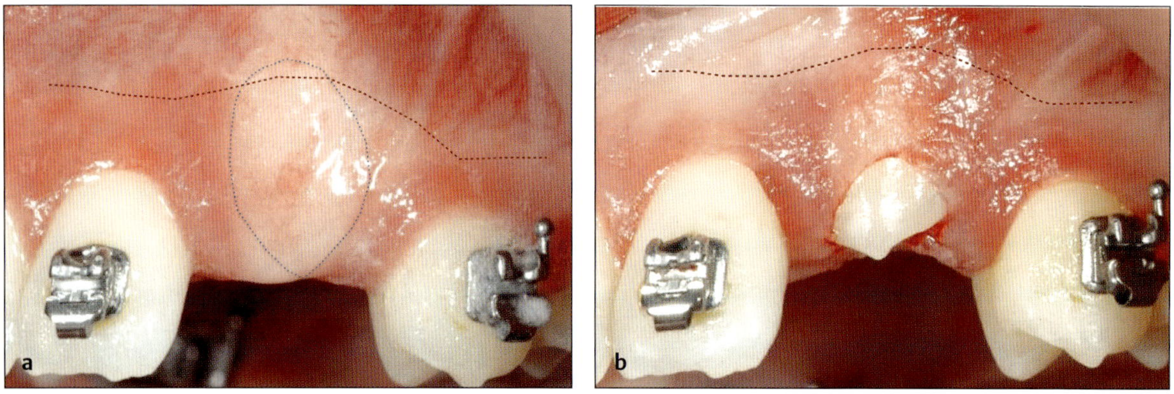

Fig 10-29 A 15-year-old patient presents with an impacted maxillary left canine and a thin gingival biotype. *(a)* The projected crown of the impacted maxillary left canine with the CEJ slightly apical to the MGJ. *(b)* Surgical exposure with a gingivectomy/excisional approach performed with a 15C blade. Only one-third of the anatomical crown was exposed surgically, leaving 4 mm of keratinized gingiva apical to the incision line.

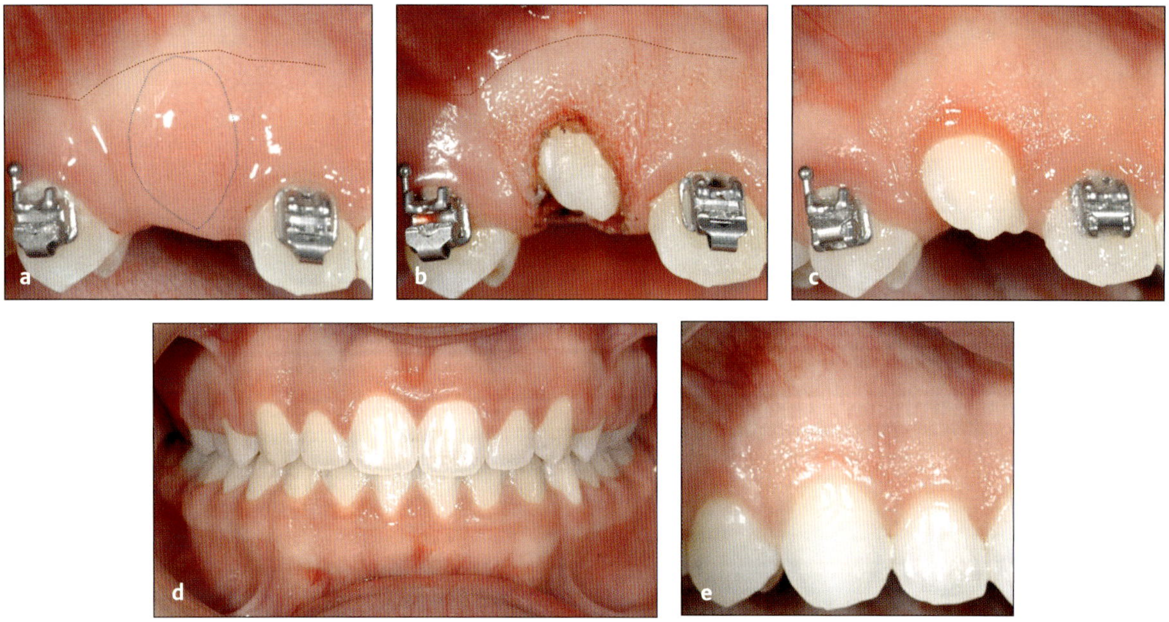

Fig 10-30 A 13-year-old girl with an impacted maxillary right canine and a thick gingival biotype. *(a)* The projected crown of the impacted maxillary right canine with the CEJ slightly coronal to the MGJ. *(b)* Surgical exposure with an excisional approach performed with an electrosurge. Observe the irregular contour of the gingival margins on this partially exposed maxillary canine crown. Only one-third of the anatomical crown was exposed surgically, leaving 4 mm of keratinized gingiva apical to the incision line. *(c)* Healing at 1 month. *(d)* At the 1-year follow-up, the marginal gingiva on the maxillary right canine is at the same level as that on the contralateral canine. *(e)* Follow-up at 3 years.

canine, minimal crown exposure is required with this technique, especially when performed with a laser or an electrosurgical unit. The thinner the gingiva, the less crown exposure is necessary, as some of the marginal gingiva will remodel and shrink apically during the healing process (Fig 10-31). Excessive removal of tissue may cause gingival shrinkage to the MGJ that will lead to recession and absence of attached gingiva (Fig 10-32). Blade incision is performed with an internal bevel to allow optimal soft tissue adaptation to the exposed crown. When the maxillary canine is positioned in the center of the ridge, removal of gingiva is also required from the palatal surface of the cusp tip.

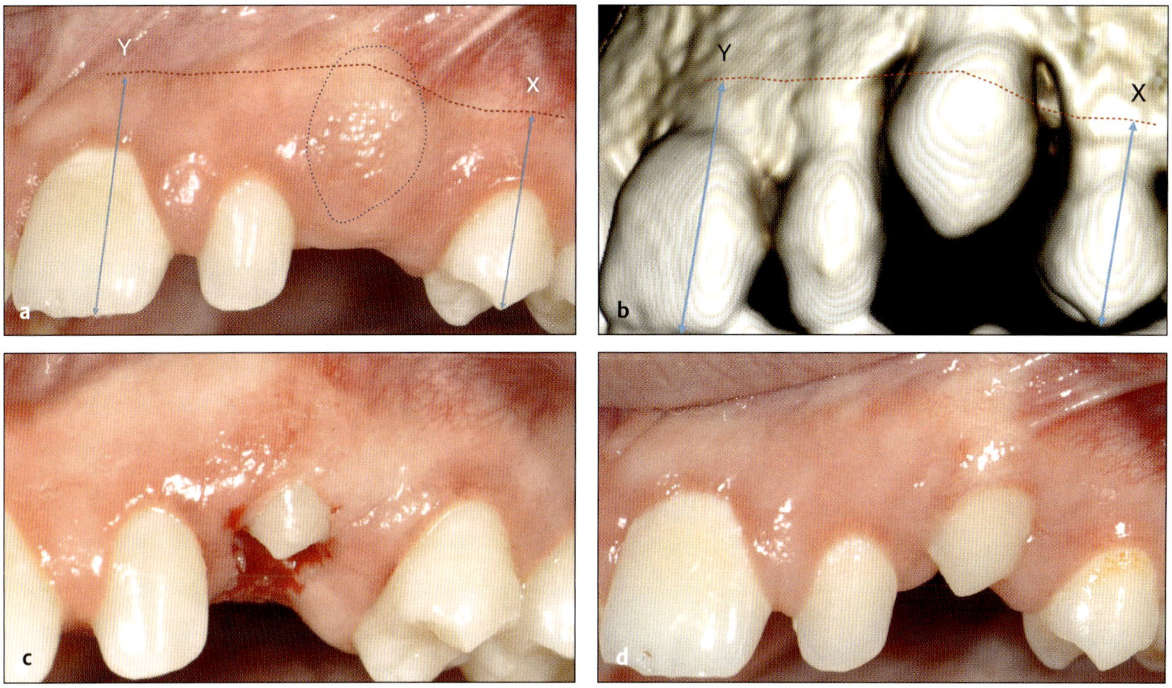

Fig 10-31 A 12-year-old boy with a buccally impacted maxillary left canine and a thin gingival biotype. *(a)* The projected crown of the impacted maxillary left canine with the CEJ slightly apical to the MGJ. *(b)* 3D reconstructed image of the impacted canine with the projected MGJ. *(c)* Surgical exposure with an excisional approach performed with a 15C blade. Only one-fourth of the anatomical crown was exposed surgically, leaving 5 mm of keratinized gingiva apical to the incision line. *(d)* At 2 weeks postsurgically, observe the significant remodeling of the gingival tissue apical to the incision line, leaving only 3 mm of keratinized gingiva apical to the gingival margin.

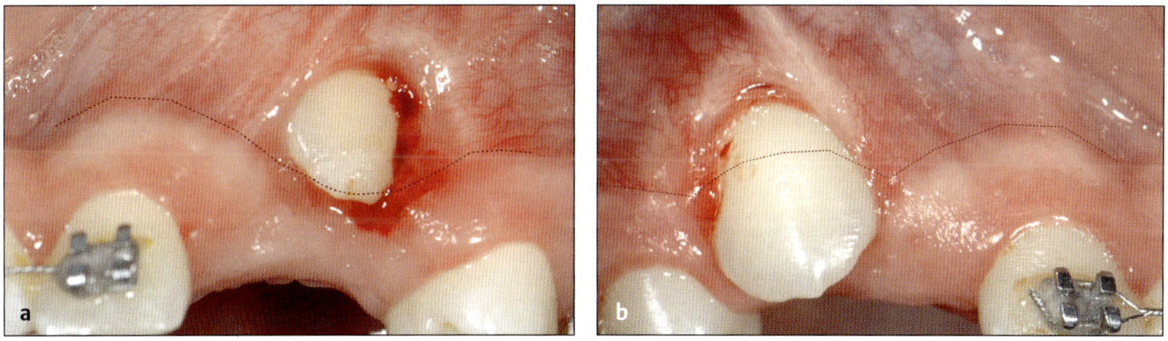

Fig 10-32 *(a and b)* A 25-year-old woman with ectopically positioned maxillary canines with the CEJ located apical to the MGJ. Both canines present with mucosa as marginal tissue with signs of inflammation and bleeding due to the lack of keratinized attached gingiva 2 months after improper surgical exposure with an excisional approach.

Bonding of the attachment

Bonding of the attachment to the exposed crown and initiation of traction may be done at the time of exposure or after completion of soft tissue healing.

APICALLY POSITIONED FLAP

In order to provide an adequate band of masticatory mucosa around the exposed maxillary canine, this technique utilizes the concept of a soft tissue pedicle graft where the coronal portion of the keratinized gingiva is released from the incisal, mesial, and distal

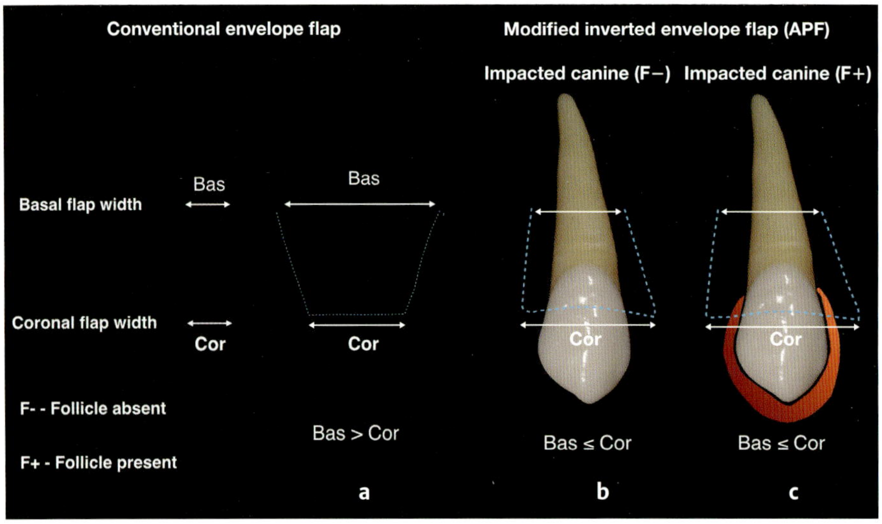

Fig 10-33 *(a)* Diagram of the conventional flap utilized in ridge augmentation surgery showing a basal flap width that is wider than the coronal aspect of the flap. *(b and c)* Diagrams of the modified reverse flap utilized to expose buccally impacted maxillary canines with an apically positioned flap. *(b)* An impacted maxillary canine without an enlarged follicle requires the coronal flap width to be slightly wider than the crown width, line angle to line angle. *(c)* An impacted maxillary canine with an enlarged follicle requires the coronal flap width to be slightly wider then the widest portion of the follicle.

aspects but remains attached at the apical base. The pedicle flap is then repositioned apically to cover the cervical third of the exposed crown. It is probably the most technique-sensitive exposure procedure and requires thorough knowledge of periodontal anatomy and skills in periodontal plastic surgery. Improperly applied or performed APF may lead to unesthetic outcomes and gingival recession.[39,51]

Indications

This technique is indicated when at least half of the crown of the impacted canine is positioned apical to the MGJ. APF may be performed for labially impacted maxillary canines in both Type A and Type B categories as well as for soft tissue and osseous impaction situations.

Contraindications

This technique essentially has no contraindications. However, it becomes very challenging when performed in the situations of high vestibular impactions or deep osseous impactions, when good flap adaptation to the canine becomes difficult. In these scenarios, thorough planning is required with 3D images to identify exact tooth position in relation to the MGJ. Additional parameters determined from CBCT images such as tooth width, crown tip in the buccolingual direction, rotation, angulation, and follicular size are critical in planning flap angulation and width.

Procedure

Success of the APF is strongly dependent on the blood supply in the dissected marginal keratinized gingiva and relates to the pedicle thickness and incision design. In order to achieve optimal flap adaptation and esthetics when uncovering buccally positioned impacted canines, a modification to the conventional envelope flap design should be considered. Unlike in conventional surgery for ridge augmentation when the flap is wider at the base (Fig 10-33a), with the modified APF technique, it is the author's (ME) recommendation that the flap should be either equal in width at the base and at the coronal portion or narrower at the base (Fig 10-33b), with a minimum basal width of 4 to 5 mm. It is essential that the pedicle flap is wide enough mesiodistally to at least cover the crown of the exposed tooth 1.5 mm beyond the line angles (see Fig 10-33b). When the impacted tooth presents with an enlarged follicle, the coronal width of the flap should be wider than the width of the follicle to ensure good flap adaptation to the crown and adjacent bone walls (Fig 10-33c). This design allows free rotation, apical displacement, and passive adaptation of the flap to the exposed crown (Fig 10-34). When impacted maxillary canines are in an angulated position, the flap may be elevated from the edentulous ridge and rotated toward the exposed crown or outlined parallel to the angulated tooth position based on the 3D superimposition.

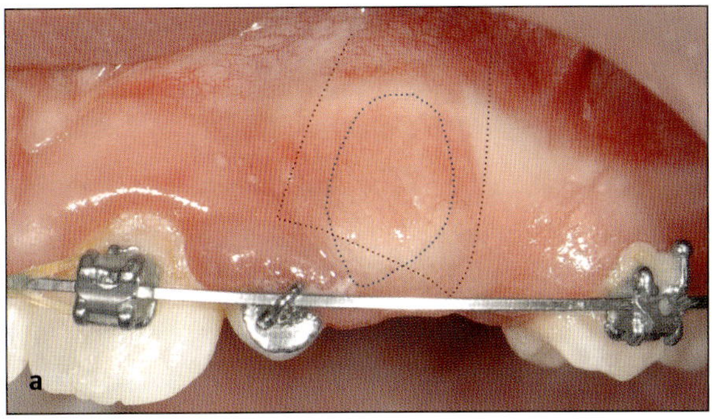

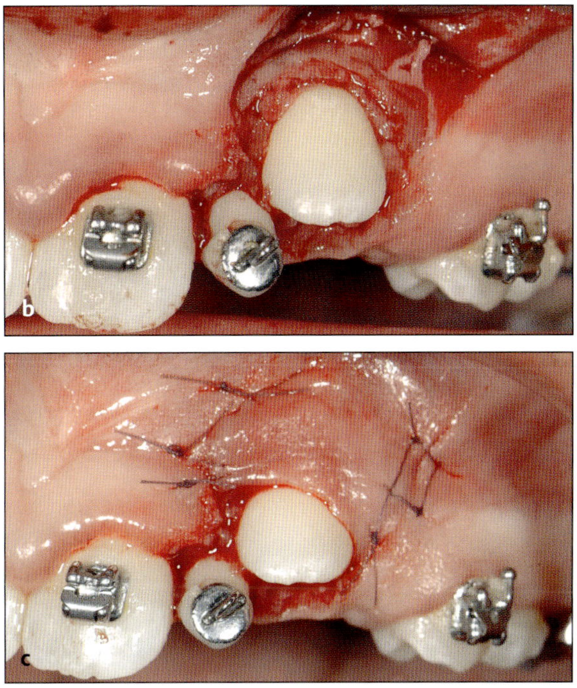

Fig 10-34 A 13-year-old boy with a buccally impacted maxillary left canine. *(a and b)* Outline of the buccal flap with the coronal portion of the flap wider than the apical portion to allow passive apical flap displacement and adaptation around the crown of the exposed tooth. *(c)* Apically displaced flap secured with interrupted vicryl sutures. Gingival tissue was also partially excised from the peg-shaped left lateral incisor and the palatal portion of the impacted canine with the goal to expose the cusp tip.

If there is sufficient width of keratinized tissue on the maxillary lateral and central incisors, it may be elevated right below the impacted tooth and then apically repositioned.

Based on the 3D findings of the impacted tooth position and size, the incision line is outlined with a 15C blade in the coronal, mesial, and distal aspects. The split partial-thickness flap is gently dissected apically, leaving periosteum attached to the bone. Once the flap is released completely from the three sides, soft tissue and bone removal is completed with a surgical curette and burs to uncover the enamel portion of the impacted maxillary canine. In situations of enlarged follicles or deep osseous impactions, any bone ledges around the exposed crown, particularly in the area of the cusp tip, must be removed to avoid impingement on tooth movement and flap adaptation. Every precaution has to be taken not to expose the root surface of the impacted maxillary canine. The graft is then positioned apically approximately 2 to 3 mm coronal to the CEJ and sutured. A pedicle flap that is well-adapted to the exposed crown will not move with lip movement and often does not require suturing. Every precaution needs to be taken to prevent hematoma formation between the flap and the root surface. Placement of a dressing will protect the newly grafted area and allow a good seal between the flap and the tooth surface.

Bonding of the attachment

With this technique, generally a bracket or other attachment is not placed at the time of the surgery. Initial healing allows time for epithelialization and for reattachment of the soft tissue before orthodontic forces are applied. An orthodontic attachment can be bonded a week to 10 days postsurgery, and light forces can be applied at that time. In the situations of deep high impactions, it is advised to bond the attachment on the day of surgery due to risk of soft tissue overgrowth that might compromise bonding at later appointments (Fig 10-35).

CLOSED ERUPTION

Closed eruption is a surgical exposure technique whereby the flap is repositioned back to cover the surgically accessed tooth after an attachment (gold chain) is bonded to it.

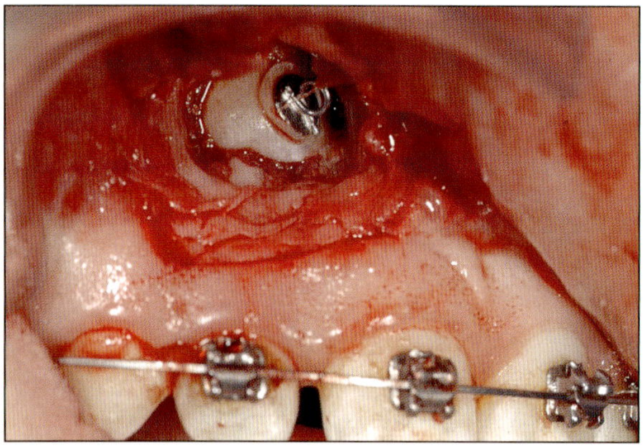

Fig 10-35 Bonding of the bracket to the deeply positioned impacted maxillary right canine at the time of surgery.

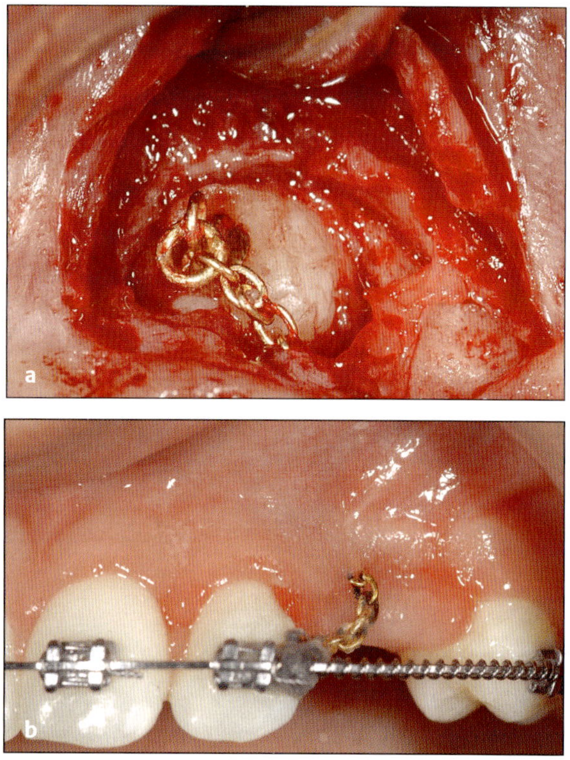

Fig 10-36 *(a)* Bonding of the attachment during surgical uncovering. *(b)* A gold chain extending from the healed incision line attached to the wire.

Indications

This technique is indicated for high vertically positioned maxillary canines that do not overlap the roots of adjacent teeth (Type B) and can be erupted by tracking directly into the arch. It has been reported by Vermette et al[51] that if an impacted canine is positioned significantly apical to the MGJ, there exists the possibility of instability and reintrusion of the impacted canine exposed with APF. These authors also suggested using the closed eruption technique in cases of deep alveolar impactions.

Contraindications

This technique is contraindicated in Type A impactions where the impacted maxillary canine is angulated and positioned over the roots of the adjacent teeth. In these cases, direct traction into the arch is contraindicated due to the risk of root resorption or bone loss in adjacent teeth. In these situations, the impacted maxillary canine has to be exposed with an open approach, moved away from adjacent roots in the labial direction, and then directed down into the arch.

Procedure

A crestal incision is made in keratinized gingiva, and the buccal flap is reflected. Unlike with the APF, when partial dissection is utilized, the closed eruption technique requires full-thickness flap reflection to access the crown of the impacted maxillary canine. Any overlying bone over the impacted canine has to be removed in a similar way as was described for the APF. Attachment with a gold chain is bonded to the crown of the impacted maxillary canine once it has been exposed. The flap is repositioned back over the impacted canine and sutured with the gold chain extending through the incision line to allow for application of orthodontic traction.

Debonding of the attachment is a concern with this approach and may result in a second surgery to gain access to rebond the attachment. Vanarsdall and Corn[47] also reported that closed eruption may cause soft tissue scarring, which may slow down orthodontic movement. Connective tissue may also in-grow into the gold chain, causing pain during activation.

Bonding of the attachment

With this technique, the attachment is bonded at the time of surgery (Fig 10-36).

Surgical Management of Palatal Impactions

Maxillary palatal impactions are encountered more frequently than maxillary labial impactions. Surgical intervention of palatal impactions can be managed via two techniques: excision and closed eruption. According to a recent randomized controlled study[52] and systematic reviews,[46,53] both techniques present with similar esthetic and periodontal outcomes; however, the open approach offers a shorter treatment time and a smaller risk of ankylosis.[46]

EXCISION

Indications

This approach is indicated for Type A and Type B impactions.

Contraindications

There are no contraindications to this approach.

Procedure

With the excisional technique, a semilunar incision is placed 3 mm away from the gingival margins of adjacent teeth, extending 5 mm anteriorly and posteriorly to the area of impaction. Then a full-thickness mucoperiosteal flap is elevated; all bone covering the enamel portion of the crown is removed up to the CEJ. Once the flap is repositioned, any soft tissue covering the crown portion of the impacted maxillary canine is removed with an external bevel incision to prevent tissue overgrowth. Interrupted sutures are used to secure the flap and to prevent postoperative bleeding. A periodontal dressing is recommended to cover the palatally exposed canine, which will allow for better flap adaptation, help to prevent tissue overgrowth, and provide for patient comfort during the healing process (Fig 10-37).

Bonding of the attachment

An attachment may be bonded during the surgical exposure or after completion of soft tissue healing. Due to the risk of tissue overgrowth in situations of deep intraosseous impactions and also in cases when the exposed tooth presents with minimal to no mobility and requires immediate activation, the attachment should be bonded during the surgical exposure. In all other situations, bonding of the attachment may be performed after soft tissue healing approximately 2 weeks after exposure. This will allow optimal isolation during the bonding procedure.

Palatally exposed canines, once moved closer to the arch, often require a secondary gingivectomy procedure to remove compressed palatal gingiva on the path of the crown movement into the arch. This is more common for maxillary canines positioned further away from their designated position (mesial to the paramidpalatal line).

Modifications

In situations when the primary maxillary canine is retained and the permanent maxillary canine is palatally impacted, it is critical to determine the proximity between the two with CBCT images. When the impacted maxillary canine is positioned in close proximity to the primary maxillary canine (distal to the paramidpalatal line), extraction of the primary maxillary canine should be performed during surgical exposure of the impacted maxillary permanent canine. In addition to the palatal exposure procedure described above, soft and hard tissue separating the extraction socket and the crown of the impacted canine should be excised to free up the path of eruption of the exposed canine into the arch. This approach will allow for efficient tooth movement and might eliminate the need for a secondary gingivectomy procedure. In situations of Type B palatal

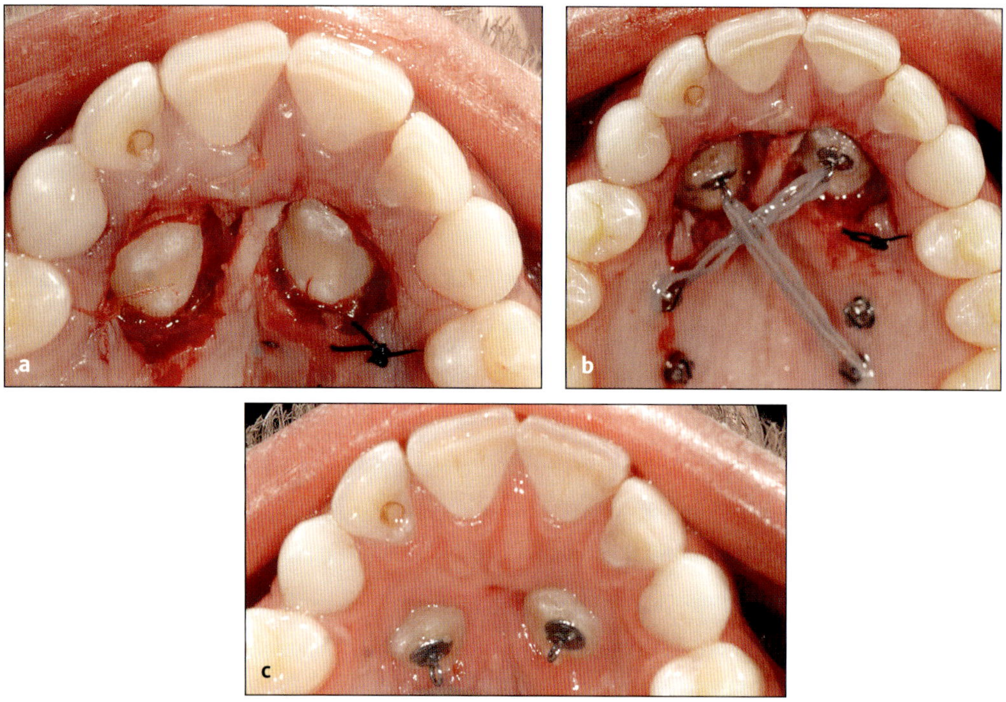

Fig 10-37 *(a)* Palatally exposed impacted maxillary canines with an open approach. The excision line was recontoured circumferentially with an external bevel to prevent tissue regrowth. *(b)* Both canines were activated immediately after exposure with TADs. *(c)* One month after the surgical exposure. Both canines present with healthy gingival margins with no evidence of soft tissue regrowth.

impactions where the primary maxillary canine is absent and the exposed maxillary canine may be activated directly into the arch without causing damage to the adjacent teeth, the gingiva should be excised and any bone removed that is in the path of tooth movement into the arch. This is more likely to be indicated for impacted maxillary canines positioned distal to the paramidpalatal line.

CLOSED ERUPTION

Indications

This approach is indicated in Type B impactions only, when the tooth can be moved directly into the arch without risk of attachment loss or root resorption in adjacent teeth.

Contraindications

This approach is contraindicated in Type A impactions, where there is a risk of root damage to adjacent teeth.

Procedure

This technique requires elevation of a full-thickness mucoperiosteal flap and removal of bone over the enamel up to the CEJ. However, no soft tissue is excised. An attachment with a wire or chain is bonded to the crown of the impacted maxillary canine, the flap is reapproximated, and the chain or wire emerges from the soft tissue at the incision line (Fig 10-38). Orthodontic traction is initiated via activation of the chain or wire. As the maxillary canine erupts, excess links can be removed from the chain as needed and the activation continued. If debonding occurs with this method, a second surgery is required to gain access to rebond the attachment.

Bonding of the attachment

With closed eruption, the attachment is bonded at the time of surgery.

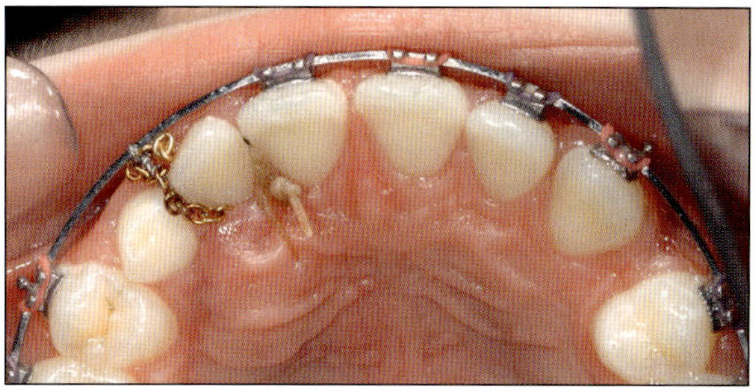

Fig 10-38 Image of the palatally impacted maxillary canine exposed with the closed approach.

Postsurgical Orthodontic Management of Impacted Maxillary Canines

Orthodontic movement of the exposed maxillary canine is impossible without an intact PDL. It is critical to evaluate the presence of a PDL space around the root of the impacted canine as well as the root morphology from CBCT images prior to the start of treatment. Impacted maxillary canines with a lack of PDL space on radiographs might be ankylosed. Dilacerated roots also may not respond to orthodontic traction. Canine mobility should also be checked during every surgical exposure. Maxillary canines that are lacking mobility and are confirmed to be ankylosed during surgical exposure need to be luxated and activated immediately. Exposed canines require activation with continuous light force. This is achieved by activation intervals every 2 to 3 weeks utilizing elastic threads or elastomeric chains.

Orthodontic management of maxillary canine impactions is complex and requires proper intra-arch space opening, adequate anchorage control, and utilization of special auxiliaries for continuous activation.

SPACE-OPENING CONSIDERATIONS

Maxillary canine impactions often present with insufficient intra-arch space. This is often caused by maxillary transverse skeletal deficiency with or without crowding or migration of the adjacent teeth into the canine space. Intra-arch canine space should be created by addressing causative factors. Transverse skeletal discrepancy needs to be addressed with orthopedic maxillary expansion. On the other hand, teeth that have migrated into the canine space should be moved back to their proper positions with conventional intra-arch and interarch mechanics. In some situations, adjacent teeth (usually maxillary first premolars) might present an obstacle for movement of the impacted canine into the arch and therefore may require extraction. In these situations, the benefits of premolar extractions should outweigh the risks. Extraction of premolars should be postponed until the impacted maxillary canine is exposed and confirmed not to be ankylosed. Final movement of the exposed canine into the arch should be delayed until sufficient space is created for it. In Type A impactions, where proximity between the impacted canine and the adjacent roots poses a risk of root resorption or attachment loss, space opening should be delayed until the exposure is completed and the canine is moved away from the adjacent roots.

ANCHORAGE CONSIDERATIONS

Ectopic position as well as prominent root anatomy of the maxillary canines can present significant resistance to orthodontic traction. When orthodontic anchorage is not set properly to withstand this resistance, unfavorable tooth movement may take place. This will present clinically as arch distortion, bite opening, anchorage loss, and intrusion of the teeth adjacent to the impacted canine (Fig 10-39).

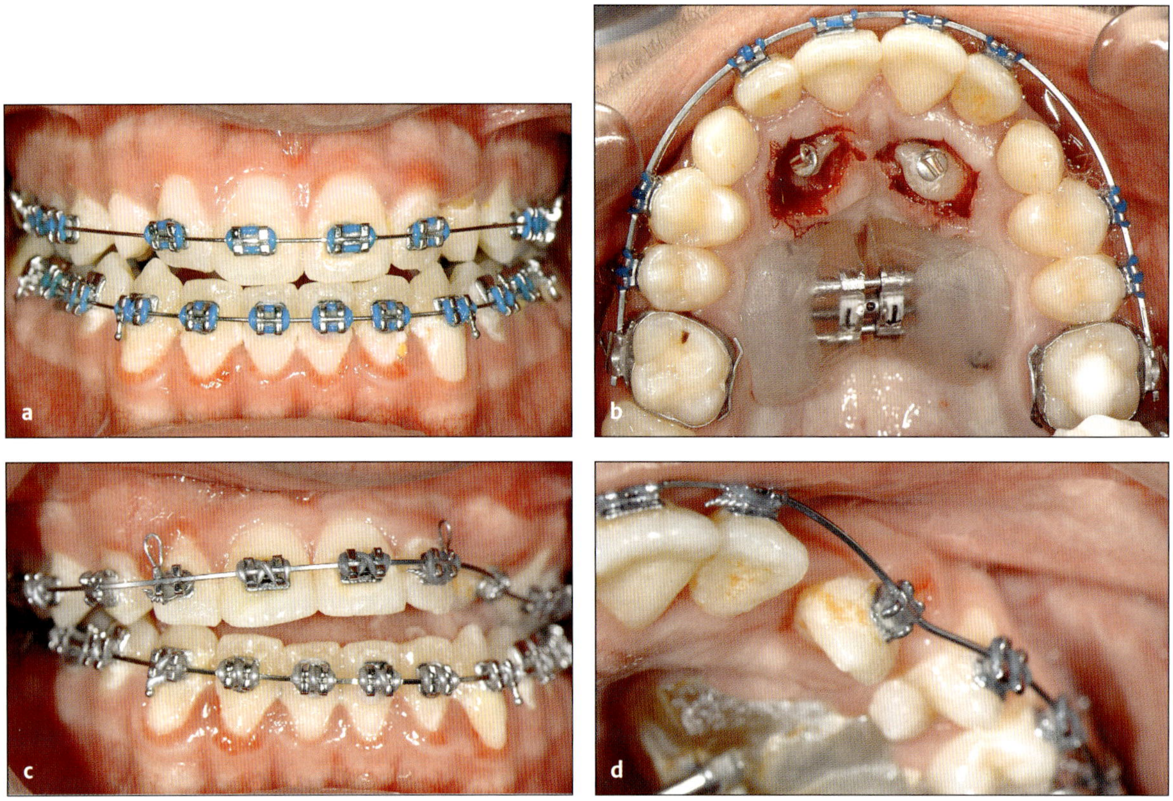

Fig 10-39 *(a and b)* A 21-year-old man with a narrow maxilla presented immediately after surgical exposure of palatally impacted canines and placement of a TAD-supported palatal expander. *(c and d)* Eight months after orthodontic traction of the palatally positioned canines, the patient developed an anterior open bite and a maxillary occlusal plane cant due to ankylosis of the maxillary left canine.

Orthodontic anchorage for the management of impacted canines can be classified as tooth-supported, tooth-free appliances, or a combination of both (Fig 10-40). Tooth-supported appliances include rigid stainless steel archwires, transpalatal bars and ligature twisted wires (Fig 10-41), Nance appliances, and tooth-supported rapid palatal expanders (Hyrax, bonded rapid palatal expanders [RPEs] and Haas RPEs). When orthodontic treatment is rendered with a 022 bracket slot size, it is suggested that a stainless steel archwire of 0.019 × 0.025 or larger be used for anchorage control. In cases when treatment is rendered with an 018 bracket slot size, a stainless steel archwire may not be rigid enough to offer sufficient anchorage. In these situations, additional means of anchorage are required to avoid undesired tooth movement. Tooth-free appliances include TADs and TAD-supported appliances such as TAD-supported RPEs, which offer optimal anchorage for Type A impactions when surgical exposure and orthodontic traction are performed in the beginning of orthodontic treatment before intra-arch anchorage preparation is completed (Fig 10-42). Combination appliances include the use of indirect anchorage, when exposed maxillary canines are activated to the archwire or directly to the teeth that have been reinforced with TADs to prevent unnecessary tooth movement (Fig 10-43).

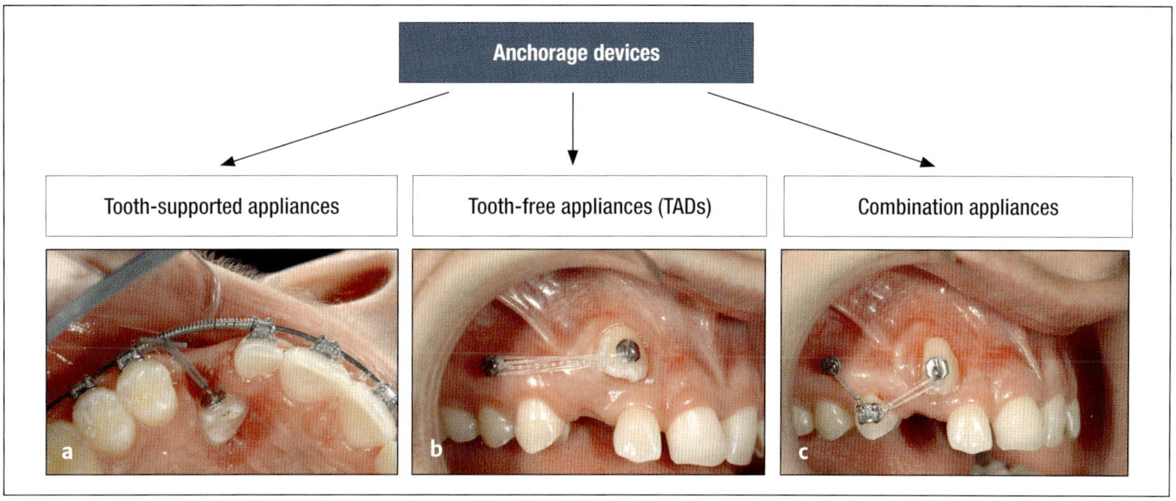

Fig 10-40 Types of orthodontic anchorage in the management of impacted canines. *(a)* Tooth-supported anchorage. Activation of the palatally positioned canines to the rectangular 0.019 × 0.025 stainless steel archwire. *(b)* Tooth-free anchorage. Activation of the buccally positioned canine directly to the TAD. *(c)* Combination anchorage. Activation of the buccally positioned canine to the premolar reinforced by attachment to the TAD.

Fig 10-41 Palatal view of Type A palatally impacted canines shortly after surgical exposure with an open approach activated to the transpalatal twisted ligature wire in the posterior downward direction away from the maxillary incisor roots.

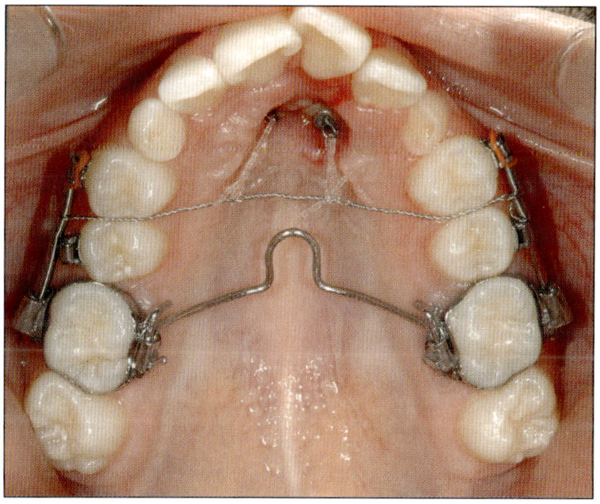

ACTIVATION CONSIDERATIONS

When planning activation of the force applied to impacted maxillary canines, it is critical to understand the direction of the required tooth movement. In Type A impactions, exposed maxillary canines first have to be moved away from neighboring teeth. Deeply positioned canines need to be erupted into the oral cavity before being moved into their designated position in the arch. Several auxiliaries are available to move the exposed canines, including elastomeric chains, elastomeric threads, nickel-titanium (NiTi) coils, and custom-made auxiliary springs such as a swinging gate and ballista

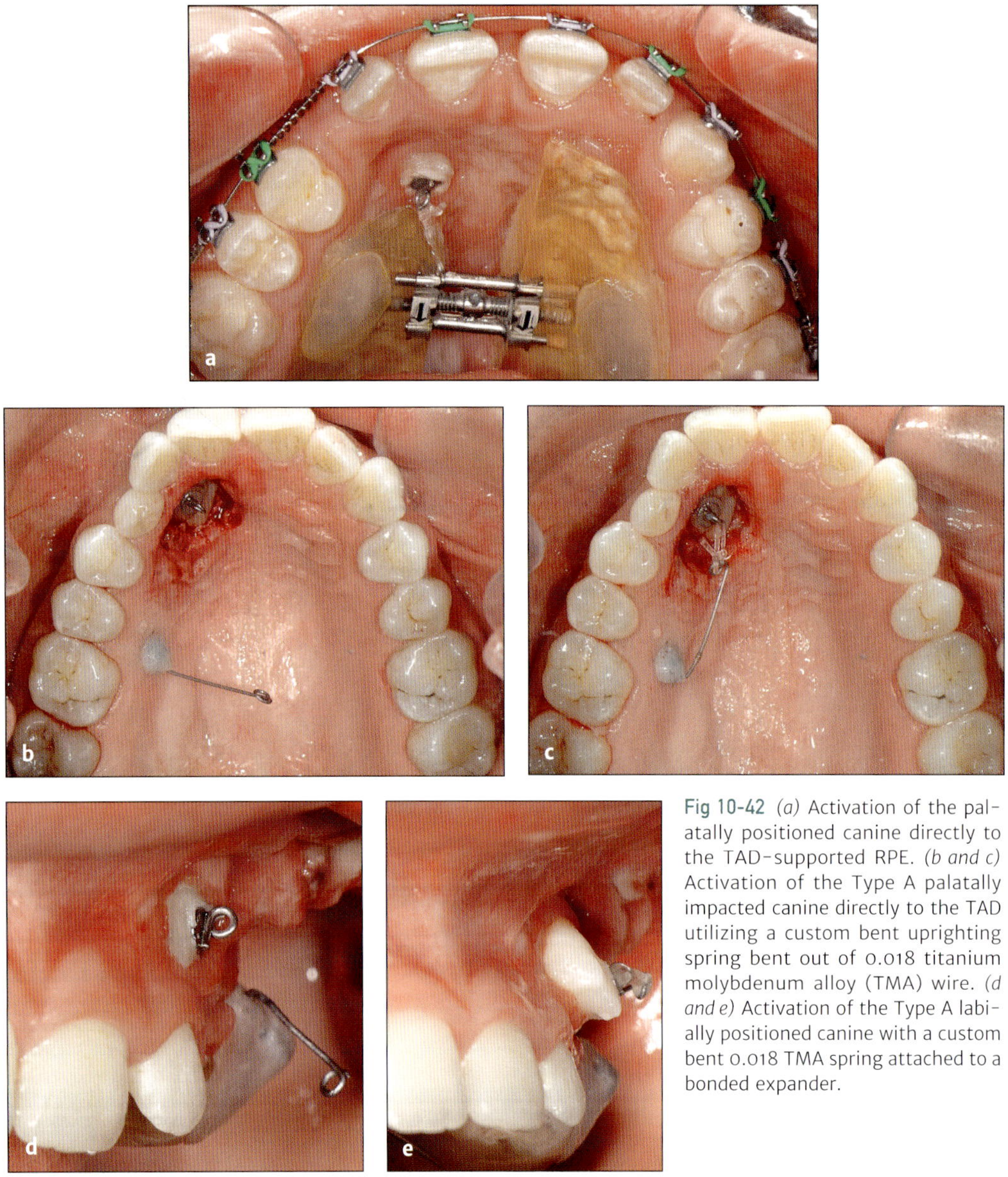

Fig 10-42 *(a)* Activation of the palatally positioned canine directly to the TAD-supported RPE. *(b and c)* Activation of the Type A palatally impacted canine directly to the TAD utilizing a custom bent uprighting spring bent out of 0.018 titanium molybdenum alloy (TMA) wire. *(d and e)* Activation of the Type A labially positioned canine with a custom bent 0.018 TMA spring attached to a bonded expander.

spring. Different attachments are available for activation of the impacted teeth, including islets and brackets. Exposed canines may be activated directly to the archwires, a transpalatal auxiliary wire, or to TADs.

LABIAL IMPACTION CONSIDERATIONS

For a low-positioned labial impaction, it is possible to piggyback a light NiTi wire onto the base arch and extrude the canine into the arch (Fig 10-44). If the

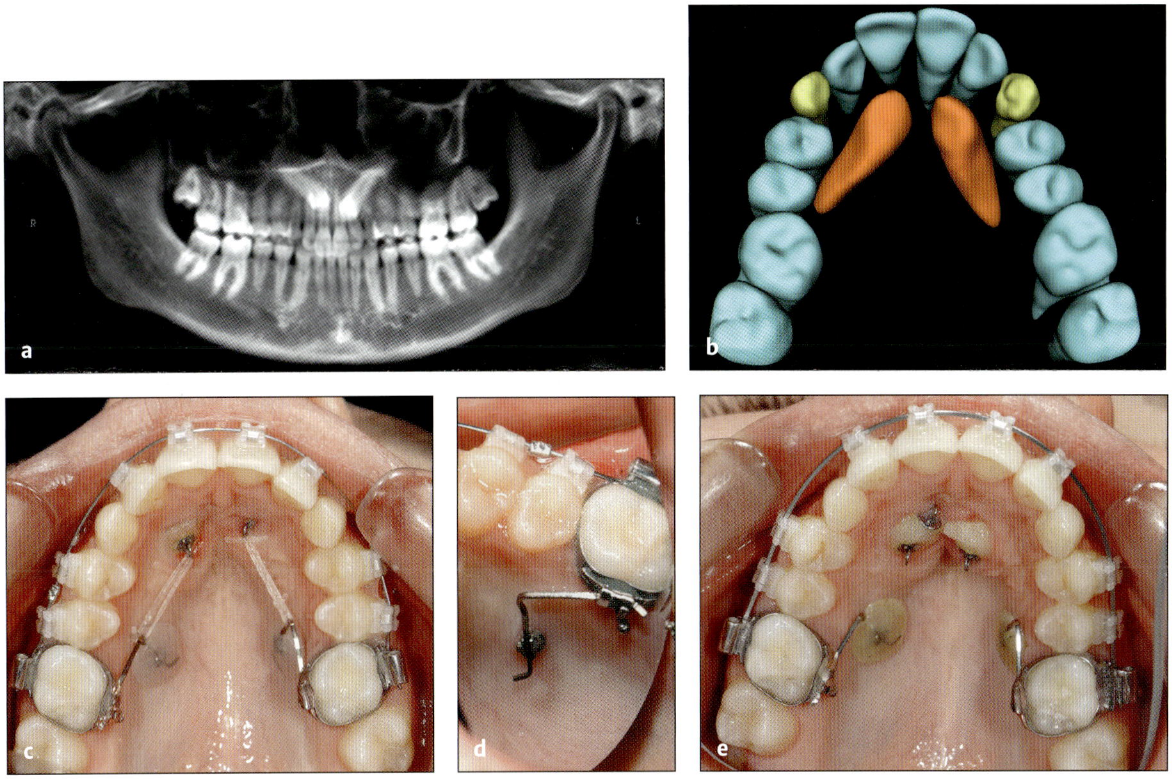

Fig 10-43 A 22-year-old woman with bilateral palatal canine impactions. *(a and b)* Panoramic radiograph and 3D reconstructed images showing the angular position of the palatally impacted canines. *(c and d)* Combination indirect anchorage device designed to introduce a posterior vertical eruption vector to the deep canine impactions. *(e)* Palatal view after 5 months of activation showing vertical eruption of the canines into the oral cavity.

position is too apical, vertical traction via an attachment and a power thread tied directly to the base arch is needed. If the canine is positioned directly over the lateral incisor, distal force may be appropriate in conjunction with a labial vector guiding the canine away from the lateral incisor. This may be accomplished via a swinging gate (Fig 10-45) fabricated from 0.018 titanium molybdenum alloy.[41] Once the canine is guided away from the lateral incisor, it can be guided further distally and, once low enough, moved directly into the arch.

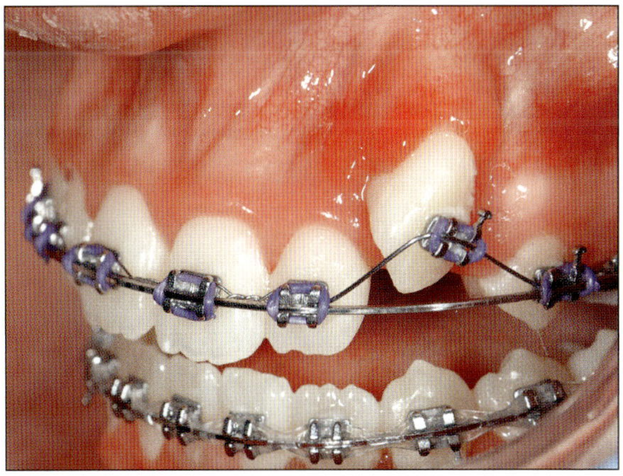

Fig 10-44 Labially positioned (exposed with APF) maxillary left canine in a 15-year-old girl. Traction was initiated with a piggyback light 0.014 nickel-titanium wire.

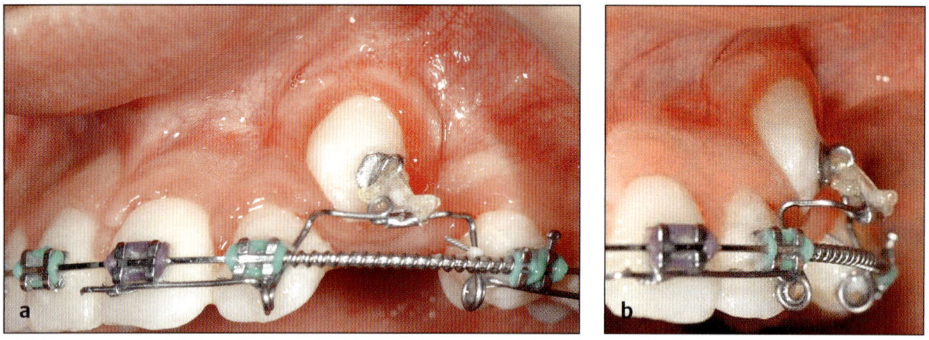

Fig 10-45 *(a and b)* Buccal traction of the maxillary left canine with a swinging gate approach in a 15-year-old girl.

PALATAL IMPACTION CONSIDERATIONS

Based on the depth of the impaction and the distance from the optimal position in the arch, palatally impacted maxillary canines may be activated either directly to the archwire or to anchorage devices positioned on the palate. The position of the palatally impacted canine can be related to the paramidpalatal line in the axial plane. This line is parallel to the midpalatal suture and is projected through the contact between the lateral and central incisors (Fig 10-46a). A palatally impacted canine positioned distal to the paramidpalatal line (right canine in Fig 10-46b) may be directly activated to the archwire due its close proximity to the ideal position in the arch. On the other hand, palatally impacted canines positioned mesial to the paramidpalatal line indicate their further displacement and need for vertical activation to anchorage auxiliaries positioned on the palate (left canine in Fig 10-46b).

Vertical eruption can be accomplished by attaching an elastomeric thread from the maxillary canine to the transpalatal ligature wire (0.010-inch twisted; see Fig 10-46b) or a ballista spring (0.018 Australian), as shown in Fig 10-47. Kokich[12] reported the use of a ballista loop, which directs forces over the alveolar housing and thereby minimizes the labial component of force. If a gold chain is bonded to the impacted maxillary canine, activation via an elastic thread tied to the chain link can be utilized. During vertical eruption, close monitoring is important. With an activated ballista spring, regular follow-up visits every 2 to 3 weeks are critical due to the possibility of overeruption of the canine out of the palate with increased risk of attachment loss.

CONSIDERATIONS FOR TIMING OF EXTRACTION OF OVERRETAINED PRIMARY CANINES

Patients with impacted maxillary canines often present with overretained primary canines. While extractions of the primary maxillary canines may be helpful in preventing impactions in the early stages of permanent maxillary canine root development, their extraction in the beginning of orthodontic treatment may be an esthetic concern in older patients. When maxillary canines are positioned further away from their ideal location in the arch, extraction of the overretained primary canines may be postponed until the exposed canines are moved closer to their optimal position, as demonstrated in Fig 10-48.

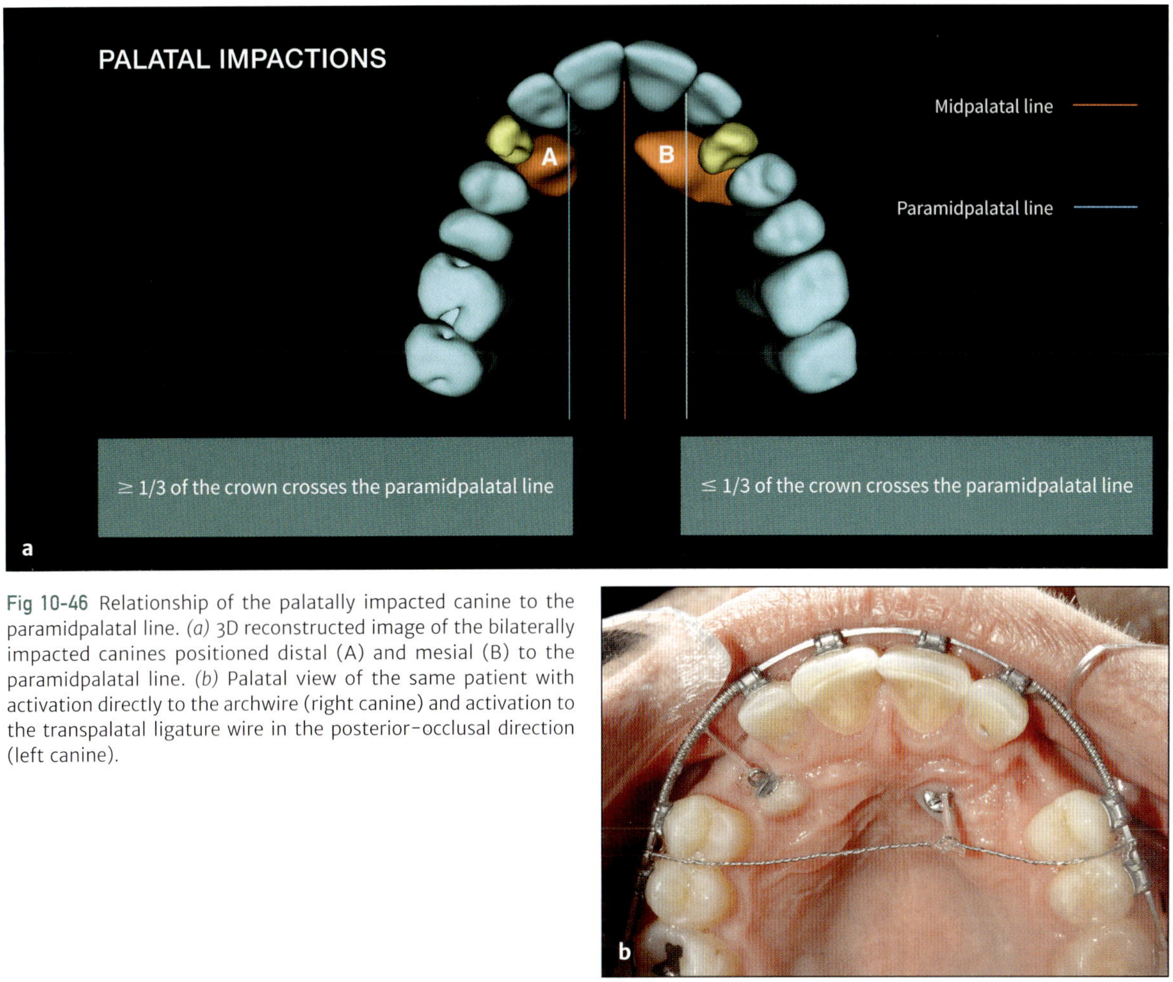

Fig 10-46 Relationship of the palatally impacted canine to the paramidpalatal line. *(a)* 3D reconstructed image of the bilaterally impacted canines positioned distal (A) and mesial (B) to the paramidpalatal line. *(b)* Palatal view of the same patient with activation directly to the archwire (right canine) and activation to the transpalatal ligature wire in the posterior-occlusal direction (left canine).

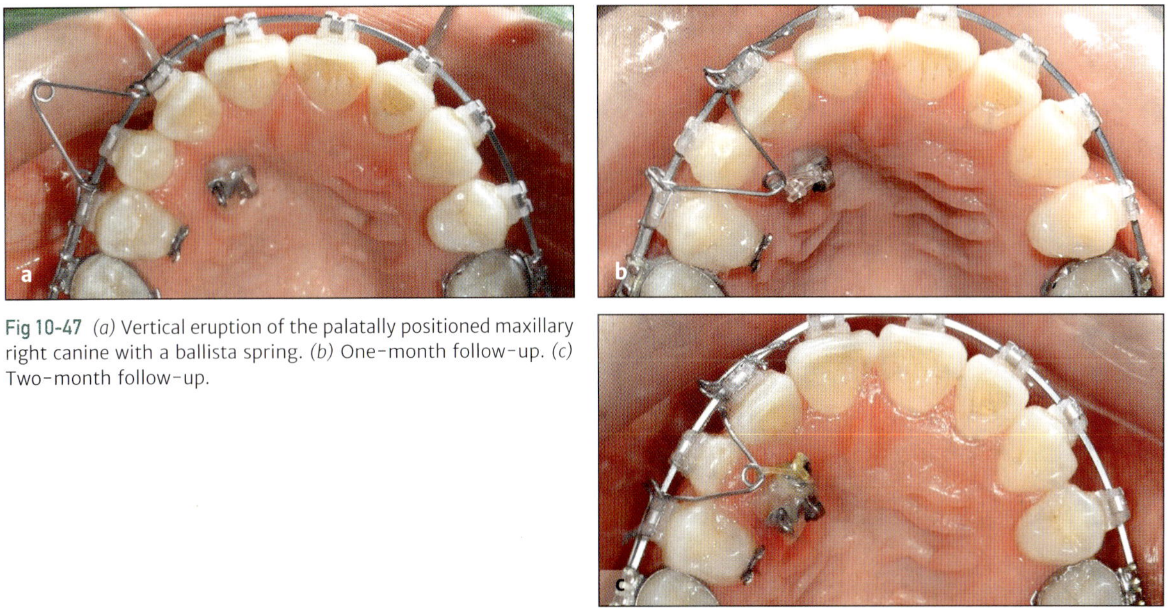

Fig 10-47 *(a)* Vertical eruption of the palatally positioned maxillary right canine with a ballista spring. *(b)* One-month follow-up. *(c)* Two-month follow-up.

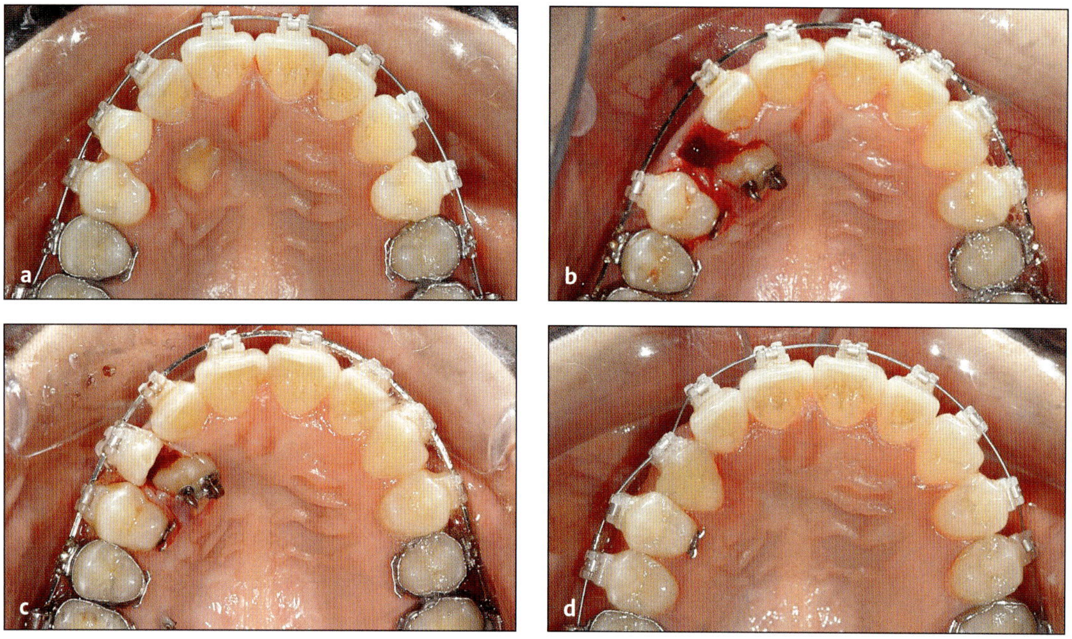

Fig 10-48 A 25-year-old woman presented with a palatally impacted maxillary right canine and an overretained primary right canine. *(a)* The primary canine was kept for esthetic reasons and was engaged in the initial archwire. *(b)* The primary canine was extracted when the permanent canine was moved closer to the optimal position in the arch. *(c)* The crown of the primary canine was preserved and remained engaged in the archwire until the permanent canine was moved into the arch *(d)*.

Conclusion

Traditional 2D images have been greatly enhanced with advanced 3D CBCT technology. The latest computer-guided software and CBCT imaging have opened the doors to accurate diagnosis and treatment planning. Virtual planning after a thorough and accurate diagnosis has become a reality and allows for improved treatment among clinicians in an interdisciplinary approach. This allows us to further fine-tune our parameters so that we may continue to improve treatment outcomes for the benefit of patients.

References

1. Stones HH. Oral and Dental Diseases: Aetiology, Histopathology, Clinical Features and Treatment, ed 4. Edinburgh: E & S Livingstone, 1962.
2. Bass TB. Observations on the misplaced upper canine tooth. Dent Pract Dent Rec 1967;18:25–33.
3. Becker A. The Orthodontic Treatment of Impacted Teeth, ed 2. Oxford: Informa Healthcare, 2007.
4. Kokich V, Mathews D. Surgical and orthodontic management of impacted teeth. Dent Clin North Am 1993;37:181–204.
5. Peck S, Peck L, Kataja M. The palatally displaced canine as a dental anomaly of genetic origin. Angle Orthod 1994;64:249–256.
6. Bishara SE. Impacted maxillary canines: A review. Am J Orthod Dentofacial Orthop 1992;101:159–171.
7. Cooke J, Wang HL. Canine impactions: Incidence and management. Int J Periodontics Restorative Dent 2006;26:483–491.
8. Proffitt WR, Fields HW Jr, Sarver DM. Contemporary Orthodontics, ed 4. St. Louis: Mosby, 2007.
9. Bedoya MM, Park JH. Diagnosis and management of impacted canines. J Am Dent Assoc 2009;140:1485–1493.
10. Ericson S, Kurol J. Radiographic examination of ectopically erupting maxillary canines. Am J Orthod Dentofacial Orthop 1987;9:483–492.
11. Kim Y, Hyun HK, Jang KT. The position of maxillary canine impactions and the influenced factors to adjacent root resorption in the Korean population. Eur J Orthod 2012;34:302–306.
12. Kokich V. Surgical and orthodontic management of impacted maxillary canines. Am J Orthod Dentofacial Orthop 2004;126:278–283.
13. Dewel BF. The upper cuspid: Its development and impaction. Angle Orthod 1949;19:79–90.
14. McConnell TL, Hoffman DL, Forbes DP, Janzen EK, Weintraub NH. Maxillary canine impaction in patients with transverse maxillary deficiency. ASDC J Dent Child 1996;63:190–195.

15. Becker A, Smith P, Behar R. The incidence of anomalous maxillary lateral incisors in relation to palatally-displaced cuspids. Angle Orthod 1981;51:24–29.
16. Sajnani AK, King NM. The sequential hypothesis of impaction of maxillary canine: A hypothesis based on clinical and radiographic findings. J Craniomaxillofac Surg 2012;40:e375–e385.
17. Peck S, Peck L, Kataja M. Concomitant occurrence of canine malposition and tooth agenesis: Evidence of orofacial genetic fields. Am J Orthod Dentofacial Orthop 2002;122:657–660.
18. Langberg BJ, Peck S. Adequacy of maxillary dental arch width in patients with palatally displaced canines. Am J Orthod Dentofacial Orthop 2000;118:220–223.
19. Al-Nimri K, Gharaibeh T. Space conditions and dental and occlusal features in patients with palatally impacted maxillary canines: An aetiological study. Eur J Orthod 2005;27:461–465.
20. Yan B, Sun Z, Fields H, Wang L, Luo L. Etiologic factors for buccal and palatal maxillary canine impaction: A perspective based on cone-beam computed tomography analyses. Am J Orthod Dentofacial Orthop 2013;143:527–534.
21. Hong WH, Radfar R, Chung CH. Relationship between the maxillary transverse dimension and palatally displaced canines: A cone-beam computed tomographic study. Angle Orthod 2015;85:440–445.
22. Clark CA. A method of ascertaining the relative position of unerupted teeth by means of film radiographs. Proc R Soc Med 1910;3:87–90.
23. Lindauer SJ, Rubenstein LK, Hang WM, Andersen WC, Isaacson RJ. Canine impaction identified early with panoramic radiographs. J Am Dent Assoc 1992;123:91–97.
24. Ericson S, Kurol J. Early treatment of palatally erupting maxillary canines by extraction of the primary canines. Eur J Orthod 1988;10:283–295.
25. Serrant PS, McIntyre GT, Thomson DJ. Localization of ectopic maxillary canines—Is CBCT more accurate than conventional horizontal or vertical parallax? J Orthod 2014;41:13–18.
26. Ericson S, Bjerklin K, Falahat B. Does the canine dental follicle cause resorption of permanent incisor roots? A computed tomographic study of erupting maxillary canines. Angle Orthod 2002;72:95–104.
27. Dağsuyu IM, Okşayan R, Kahraman F, Aydın M, Bayrakdar IS, Uğurlu M. The relationship between dental follicle width and maxillary impacted canines' descriptive and resorptive features using cone-beam computed tomography. Biomed Res Int 2017;2938691:1-5.
28. Yan B, Sun Z, Fields H, Wang L. Maxillary canine impaction increases root resorption risk of adjacent teeth: A problem of physical proximity. Am J Orthod Dentofacial Orthop 2012;142:750–757.
29. Ericson S, Kurol J. Resorption of incisors after ectopic eruption of maxillary canines: A CT study. Angle Orthod 2000;70:415–423.
30. Ericson S, Bjerklin K. The dental follicle in normally and ectopically erupting maxillary canines: A computed tomography study. Angle Orthod 2001;71:333–342.
31. Ericson S, Kurol J. Incisor resorption caused by maxillary cuspids. A radiographic study. Angle Orthod 1987;57:332–346.
32. Alqerban A, Jacobs R, Fieuws S, Willems G. Radiographic predictors for maxillary canine impaction. Am J Orthod Dentofacial Orthop 2015;147:345–354.
33. Miner RM, Qabandi SA, Rigali PH, Will LA. Cone-beam computed tomography transverse analyses. Part 2: Measures of performance. Am J Orthod Dentofacial Orthop 2015;148:253–263.
34. Baccetti T, Mucedero M, Leonardi M, Cozza P. Interceptive treatment of palatal impaction of maxillary canines with rapid maxillary expansion: A randomized clinical trial. Am J Orthod Dentofacial Orthop 2009;136:657–661.
35. Kau CH, Gallerano RL, English JD. A novel classification system for canine impactions – The KPG index. Int J Med Robotics Comput Assist Surg 2009;5:291–296.
36. Dalessandri D. Migliorati M, Rubiano R. Reliability of a novel CBCT-based 3D classification system for maxillary canine impactions in orthodontics: The KPG index. Sci World J 2013;2013:921234.
37. Kau CH, Lee JJ, Souccar NM. The validation of a novel index assessing canine impactions. Eur J Dent 2013;7:399–404.
38. Korbendau JM, Patti A. Clinical Success in Surgical and Orthodontic Treatment of Impacted Teeth. Paris: Quintessence, 2006.
39. Vanarsdall RL. Efficient management of unerupted teeth: A time-tested treatment modality. Semin Orthod 2010;16:212–221.
40. Woloshyn H, Artun J, Kennedy DB, Joondeph DR. Pulpal and periodontal reactions to orthodontic alignment of palatally impacted canines. Angle Orthod 1994;64:257–264.
41. Incerti-Parenti S, Checchi V, Ippolito DR, Gracco A, Alessandri-Bonetti G. Periodontal status after surgical-orthodontic treatment of labially impacted canines with different surgical techniques: A systematic review. Am J Orthod Dentofacial Orthop 2016;149:463–472.
42. Cahill DR, Marks SC Jr. Tooth eruption: Evidence for the central role of the dental follicle. J Oral Pathol 1980;9:189–200.
43. Matejka M, Porteder H, Ulrich W, Watzek G, Sinzinger H. Prostaglandin synthesis in dental cyst. J Oral Maxillofac Surg 1985;23:190–194.
44. Alessandri Bonetti G, Zanarini M, Incerti Parenti S, Marini I, Gatto MR. Preventive treatment of ectopically erupting maxillary permanent canines by extraction of deciduous canines and first molars: A randomized clinical trial. Am J Orthod Dentofacial Orthop 2011;139:316–323.
45. Kokich VG, Mathews DP. Impacted teeth: Surgical and orthodontic considerations. In: McNamara JA (ed). Orthodontics and Dentofacial Orthopedics. Ann Arbor, MI: Needham, 2001:395–422.
46. Cassina C, Papageorgiou SN, Eliades T. Open versus closed surgical exposure for permanent impacted canines: A systematic review and meta-analysis. Eur J Orthod 2018;40:1–10.
47. Vanarsdall RL, Corn H. Soft-tissue management of labially positioned unerupted teeth. Am J Orthod 1977;72:53–64.
48. Orban B, Sicher H. The Oral Mucosa. J Dent Educ 1946;10:163.

49. Lang NP, Löe H. The relationship between the width of keratinized gingiva and gingival health. J Periodontol 1972;43:623–627.
50. Levin MP, D'Amico RA. Flap design in exposing unerupted teeth. Am J Orthod 1974;65:419–422.
51. Vermette ME, Kokich VG, Kennedy DB. Uncovering labially impacted teeth: Apically positioned flap and closed-eruption techniques. Angle Orthod 1995;65:23–32.
52. Parkin NA, Milner RS, Deery C, et al. Periodontal health of palatally displaced canines treated with open or closed surgical technique: A multicenter, randomized controlled trial. Am J Orthod Dentofacial Orthop 2013;144:176–184.
53. Sampaziotis D, Tsolakis I, Bitsanis E, Tsolakis AI. Open versus closed surgical exposure of palatally impacted canines: Comparison of the different treatment outcomes—A systematic review. Eur J Orthod 2018;40:11–22.

SECTION III

Orthodontic Considerations for the Periodontic Patient

CHAPTER 11

Clinical Evidence on the Effect of Orthodontic Treatment on the Periodontal Tissues

Spyridon N. Papageorgiou
Theodore Eliades

Orthodontic treatment with fixed appliances has become an integral part of contemporary orthodontics. However, it has been associated with certain adverse effects to the periodontium, which are generally thought to be transient and not related to any lasting tissue damage.[1,2] These include increased clinical plaque and bleeding indices,[3] enlargement of gingival pockets,[3] marginal bone loss,[3,4] and quantitative or qualitative changes in the oral microbiota.[5] Orthodontic treatment-induced microbial changes[6,7] can be attributed to the plaque-retentive characteristics of orthodontic appliances,[8] while deepening of the gingival crevice through hyperplasia might additionally offer a favorable environment for periodontopathogenic anaerobic bacteria.[9] Overall, these conditions contribute to the fixed appliance treatment phase, posing a potential threat to the health of the periodontal tissues.

This chapter summarizes the data from high-quality clinical studies in humans on the effect of orthodontic treatment with fixed appliances on periodontal health. It is based on existing systematic reviews with meta-analyses that fulfill the PRISMA guidelines[10] (Preferred Reporting Items for Systematic Reviews and Meta-Analyses). These meta-analyses were updated by manual searches for this chapter, whenever possible, and reanalyzed with random-effects meta-analyses with the improved Paule-Mandel algorithm,[11] contour-enhanced forest plots,[12] and the GRADE approach[13] (Grading of Recommendations, Assessment, Development, and Evaluations) to judge the overall quality of evidence. Randomized clinical trials are preferred over nonrandomized studies, and prospective nonrandomized studies are preferred over retrospective nonrandomized studies, whenever possible, according to the research scope, in order to provide the most robust existing evidence in each case.

Microbiologic Changes

Treatment-induced microbial changes[6,7] during fixed appliance treatment can be attributed to the plaque-retentive characteristics of the orthodontic appliances. Brackets, bands, wires, and orthodontic auxiliaries present a unique challenge for oral hygiene, as their complex geometry encourages plaque accumulation and creates food/plaque traps.[8] Indeed, an increase in the plaque index of orthodontic patients has been documented in the first 3 months after appliance placement.[14,15] However, it is important to note that even though orthodontic appliances might be associated with increased plaque accumulation, children with malocclusion might still have higher plaque index values than children with orthodontic appliances in situ.[16] At the same time, the observed deepening of the gingival crevice through gingival enlargement that is often seen during fixed appliance treatment[17] might offer a favorable environment for the proliferation of periodontopathogenic anaerobic bacteria.[9] This gingival enlargement is generally mild, and proper cases of hyperplastic or hypertrophic gingivitis occur in only about 10% of orthodontic patients.[8] Also, as the burden of increased intraoral plaque communities exists, a microbial shift occurs in the first weeks after appliance placement from aerobic to anaerobic bacteria, reflecting a parallel shift from periodontal health to periodontal disease, including spirochetes, fusiform bacteria, facultative anaerobes, lactobacilli, and *Prevotella intermedia*.[6,18] Around 2 to 3 months after appliance placement, the previously increased amount of cocci decreases, while the amount of spirochetes and motile rods increases, and subsequently bacteria associated with the red and orange complexes are established.[7]

As far as cariogenic bacteria are specifically concerned, the results of numerous studies suggest that the placement of a fixed orthodontic appliance leads to an increase in plaque volume[7] and total bacterial count[19] and a disproportionate increase in *Streptococcus mutans* and lactobacilli[20] that consequently leads to increased caries risk.

As far as periodontopathogenic bacteria are concerned, it is important to note that considerable differences exist between the supragingival and subgingival intraoral microbial populations in both health and disease.[21] At the same time, a direct correlation has been observed between microbial changes and the transition from periodontal health via gingivitis to periodontal disease.[22] These changes have been shown to be more pronounced in subgingival rather than supragingival plaque.[21] Additionally, members of the red or orange complex, specifically *Tannerella forsythia*, *Porphyromonas gingivalis*, *Aggregatibacter actinomycetemcomitans*, and *P intermedia*, have been found more frequently in patients with inflammation and periodontal pockets than in healthy subjects.[23]

A recent systematic review summarized clinical evidence on the qualitative changes of the subgingival microbiota induced by orthodontic treatment with fixed appliances[24] and found that considerable changes were seen. After insertion of the orthodontic appliances, there was a tendency for increased subgingival identification of many species, including *A actinomycetemcomitans*, *Campylobacter rectus*, *P intermedia*, *Treponema denticola*, and *T forsythia*. There was only scarce evidence of low quality from controlled studies with untreated patients, indicating that 3 to 6 months after appliance insertion, *A actinomycetemcomitans* was more likely to be found in the sulcus of orthodontic patients than in the sulcus of untreated patients (relative risk [RR] = 15.49; 95% confidence interval [CI] = 3.17 to 75.76) (Fig 11-1). Conversely, a tendency was seen for normalization of the microbiota after removal of the appliances, but still significant differences to untreated patients were found up to 6 months after removal for *A actinomycetemcomitans* (RR = 3.97; 95% CI = 1.23 to 12.88) and *T forsythia* (RR = 2.25; 95% CI = 1.40 to 3.60) (see Fig 11-1). This indicates that a longer period might be needed until the microbiota can completely revert to before-treatment levels. Similar findings have also been reported for supragingival changes in the oral microbiota, where a systematic review[5] found moderate evidence that the presence of fixed appliances has a transitional effect on

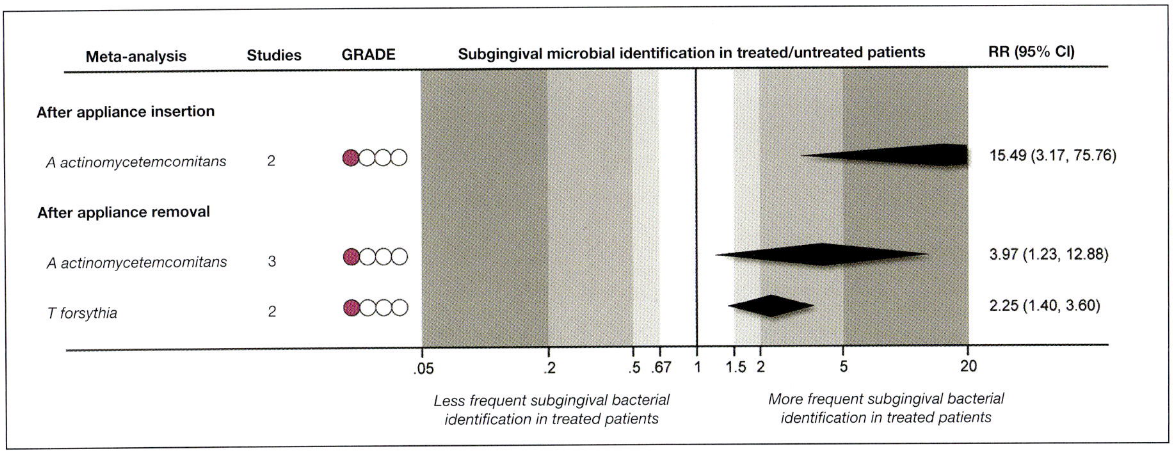

Fig 11-1 Summary of meta-analyses on the identification of periodontopathogenic bacteria subgingivally among treated and untreated patients. The forest plot has been enhanced with contours of effect magnitude, and the data used stems from the systematic review by Papageorgiou et al.[24]

oral microbiota depending on oral hygiene control. Furthermore, orthodontic appliances increase the likelihood that yeast is found in subgingival biofilms, with one study reporting a threefold increase in the prevalence of yeast in patients with orthodontic appliances compared to those without.[25] The most frequent yeast observed was *Candida albicans* (47.2%) in both gingivitis and periodontitis patients, and other yeasts included *Candida parapsilosis*, *Candida dubliniensis*, *Candida tropicalis*, *Candida guilliermondii*, *Candida sake*, and *Rhodotorula* species.[25]

Clinical Effects of Orthodontic Treatment on the Periodontium

Orthodontic fixed appliances make maintenance of proper oral hygiene more difficult, resulting in increased plaque accumulation and a subsequent mild inflammation of the oral tissues. It has been documented that fixed appliances have a significant impact on periodontal conditions,[26] which can vary according to patient-, site-, and appliance-specific characteristics.[8] This impact is generally characterized as increased pocket probing depth, increased bleeding on probing, increased crevicular fluid volume, and a shift from aerobic to anaerobic microbial species.[8,26] Other clinical changes concomitant to appliance insertion include increases in the gingival index and gingival bleeding index,[14,15,23,27,28] although these generally decrease after the first 3 to 6 months in treatment as the patient adapts the oral hygiene regimen to the presence of fixed appliances. It is believed that these treatment-induced changes are mostly transient,[29] are normalized (at least partly) after removal of the orthodontic appliances,[28] and are not associated with any lasting detrimental effect on the surrounding periodontal tissues.[29]

The effect of orthodontic treatment on pocket probing depth was assessed in the systematic review by Bollen et al.[3] Reanalysis of the review's data for this chapter indicated that patients treated orthodontically experienced an average increase in pocket probing depth of 0.35 mm (95% CI = −0.03 to 0.72) compared with untreated patients (Fig 11-2), which is of minimal clinical importance by any account. It has been documented that gingival enlargement occurs after the placement of fixed orthodontic appliances and might subsequently be eliminated after appliance removal, when proper oral hygiene can again be exercised by the patient.[17] This inflammatory gingival enlargement can partly explain the increased probing depth at initial examination and thus its reduction after treatment.[17,30,31] This reduction in pocket depth after removal of the appliances

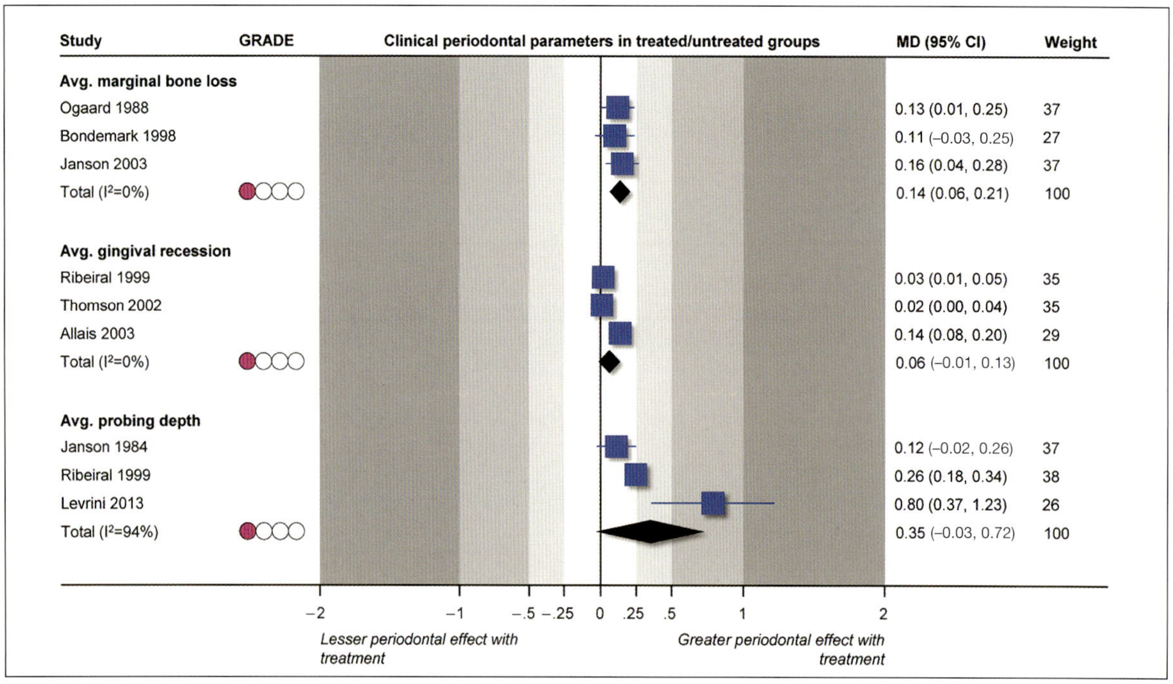

Fig 11-2 Meta-analyses of nonrandomized studies on the clinical periodontal parameters among treated and untreated patients. The forest plot has been enhanced with contours of effect magnitude, and the data used stems from the systematic review by Bollen et al[3] and an added study from the manual update of the review.

can also contribute to the normalization of the subgingival microbiota that is generally seen.

As far as periodontal clinical attachment loss with regard to comprehensive orthodontic treatment is concerned, a recent systematic review[4] indicated that there was a small difference in average clinical attachment loss between treated and untreated patients (mean difference [MD] = 0.14 mm; 95% CI = −0.17 to 0.45 mm), which was neither statistically nor clinically significant (Fig 11-3). However, only a couple of studies contributed to this comparison with an overall very low quality of evidence, which means that additional studies are needed to robustly assess this matter. It must also be noted that there is a risk that the measured clinical attachment loss has been overestimated, because all studies report attachment loss during treatment or up to the first 3 to 4 months after appliance removal. At these time points, the existing gingival enlargement might have made identification of the cementoenamel junction (which is necessary to measure attachment loss) difficult, while the periodontal connective tissue is probably still lightly inflamed, and that might lead on its own to deeper penetration by the periodontal probe and increased measured attachment loss.[32] In summary, observed amounts of clinical attachment loss during or after orthodontic treatment with fixed appliances are by all accounts minimal and do not correspond to the observed pocket probing depths, which might be explained by pseudopockets or measuring artifact due to tissue inflammation.

Contrary to the case of comprehensive orthodontic treatment, intrusion of maxillary anterior teeth seems to be associated with a minimal attachment gain compared with untreated patients (MD = −0.49 mm; 95% CI = −0.35 to -0.63 mm)[4] (see Fig 11-3). This is supported by other researchers reporting moderate clinical attachment gains attained through low-magnitude intrusive forces,[33] but caution is warranted in the interpretation of this finding because only one study with a limited sample and moderate risk of bias contributed to it.

In general, it seems that orthodontic treatment with fixed appliances exerts only a minimal effect on clinical periodontal parameters that is mostly transient and does not cause irreversible harm to

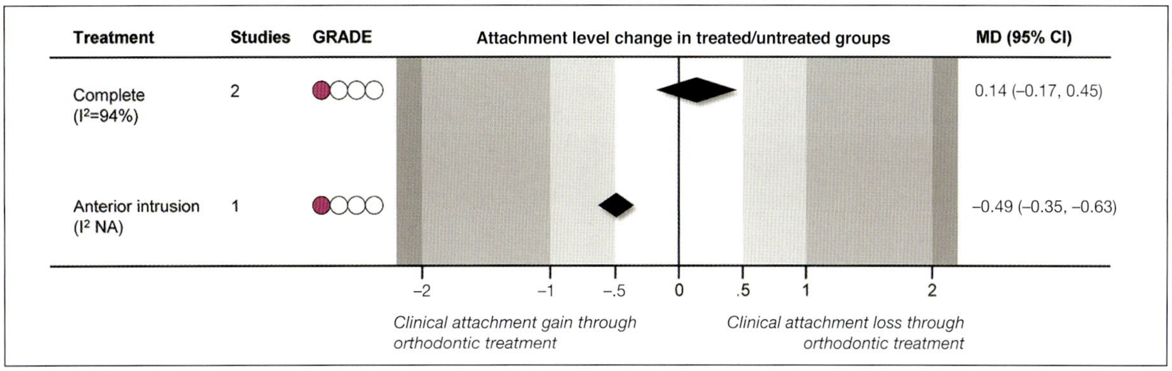

Fig 11-3 Summary of meta-analyses of nonrandomized studies on the differences in periodontal clinical attachment loss among treated and untreated patients. The forest plot has been enhanced with contours of effect magnitude, and the data used stems from the systematic review by Papageorgiou et al.[4]

the periodontium. There is a small subset of patients that might be more prone to orthodontic adverse effects in terms of attachment loss,[34] and careful risk assessment prior to treatment (including factors like high plaque index, subgingival encroachment of the cervical margins of bands, deep probing depths, and length of orthodontic treatment[35]) as well as meticulous monitoring during treatment might be needed to identify high-risk patients in a timely manner and minimize harms.

Radiographic Marginal Bone Loss

The biologic mechanism of orthodontic tooth movement has been described as a form of aseptic inflammation, mediated by a variety of inflammatory cytokines, neuropeptides, and vasoactive molecules, that relies on the coordinated resorption and apposition of bone. At the same time, the increased microbial load due to plaque accumulated around the orthodontic appliances can lead to periodontal inflammation, which in turn can have adverse effects on the periodontal tissues during tooth movement, including marginal bone loss. Bollen at al,[3] in one of the few systematic reviews on the subject, assessed the average amount of marginal bone loss after orthodontic treatment from controlled clinical evidence. Reanalysis of their data for this chapter (see Fig 11-2) indicated that orthodontic treatment was associated with statistically higher marginal bone loss (MD = 0.14 mm; 95% CI = 0.06 to 0.21 mm) compared with untreated patients, which is however of little clinical relevance. This is in agreement with Bondemark,[36] who reported that both orthodontically treated and untreated patients suffered from minimally relevant marginal bone loss that was in all cases less than 2 mm, although treated maxillary molars did indeed suffer from some marginal bone loss.

Existing studies on marginal bone loss as a result of orthodontic treatment with fixed appliances report contradictory results as to the magnitude of the effect, due to the fact that they employ bitewing and periapical radiography, which might be problematic in accurately assessing proximal bone surfaces.[37] Research using computerized tomography reported a relatively high incidence of dehiscences and fenestrations at the mandibular anterior region after orthodontic treatment,[38] indicating a potential use of such imaging modalities in assessing treatment-induced marginal bone changes. Consequently, a number of studies were conducted on the subject using cone beam computed tomography (CBCT).[37,39,40] Lund et al[37] reported that large amounts of marginal bone loss (> 2 mm) could be seen during the course of orthodontic treatment with extractions at the buccal and palatal/lingual surfaces of the anterior teeth. These were most often seen at the palatal side of the maxillary anterior teeth (in

15.8% to 21.4% of the cases) and especially the lingual side of the mandibular anterior teeth (in 25.4% to 83.5% of the cases), although these might not be necessarily attributed to orthodontic treatment per se. On the contrary, Castro et al[40] found that both the labial and palatal/lingual sides of all teeth experienced statistically significant marginal bone loss during nonextraction treatment, which was however less than 1 mm in all cases. Therefore, evidence from CBCT on this matter remains inconclusive.

It must be noted that the marginal bone loss as a function of orthodontic treatment is not uniform, and a wide array of factors have been suggested as having a possible influence. It has been suggested that marginal bone loss as a result of fixed appliance treatment is greater in patients over 30 years old than in younger patients, and therefore pretreatment CBCTs might be useful for such patients.[41] Also, evidence suggests that the inclusion of extractions in the orthodontic treatment might be associated with increased marginal bone loss, as well as the appearance of intraosseous defects, particularly in the mandibular arch.[39] Additionally, pretreatment thin mandibular symphyses and thin cortical bone zones seem to be associated with greater treatment-induced marginal bone loss.[42] However, it must be noted that most existing studies employing CBCT for treatment-related marginal bone loss are small pilot cohort studies, and evidence from them has not been appraised systematically in order to gauge their clinical relevance and the justification of the additional radiation; therefore, these data should be viewed with caution.

Gingival Recessions

Gingival recessions are a common manifestation in many populations, with prevalence varying from 3% to 100% depending on the sample or analysis methods[43] and incidence increasing as a function of age.[44] Gingival recessions can be localized or generalized and lead to exposure of the root surface and subsequently increased esthetic impairment,[45] risk of tooth loss,[45] susceptibility to root caries,[46] and dentin hypersensitivity.[47]

The development of gingival recessions might be influenced by several factors, the most prominent being recessions as a result of periodontal diseases, mechanical trauma, age, bone dehiscences, and smoking.[43,45,48–52] Orthodontic tooth movement has also been proposed as a possible etiologic factor, especially when it includes tooth positioning beyond the labial or lingual alveolar plate, which might lead to bone dehiscences.[53] This is of particular interest, because the recipients of orthodontic treatment are often young, periodontally healthy patients, so any recessions might have considerable long-term impact for the rest of their lives. The average gingival recession among patients treated orthodontically with fixed appliances and untreated patients was assessed in the systematic review of Bollen et al,[3] and although an attempt was made to update the analysis for this chapter, the search yielded no additional studies. Reanalysis of the review's data indicated that orthodontic patients were associated with a statistically significant but clinically irrelevant amount of average gingival recession across all teeth (MD = 0.06 mm; 95% CI = −0.01 to 0.13 mm) (see Fig 11-2).

However, it must be noted that calculating the average amount of gingival recession across all sites might not be the most appropriate way to scientifically assess recessions, due to the specific pattern of gingival recessions. There is a predilection of recessions for specific intraoral regions, with about 20.0% of recessions among orthodontic patients occurring at the mandibular anterior region, compared with only 5.1% of recessions among untreated patients.[54] Also, there is usually a clustering of multiple recessions within the mouth of treated patients, as 51.4% of affected patients have one to two recessions, 40% have three to four recessions, and the remaining 8.6% have five or more recessions, with an average of three recessions per affected patient.[54]

An analysis of gingival recession development among treated and untreated patients conducted for this chapter (Fig 11-4) gives a different picture. Orthodontic treatment seems to be associated with

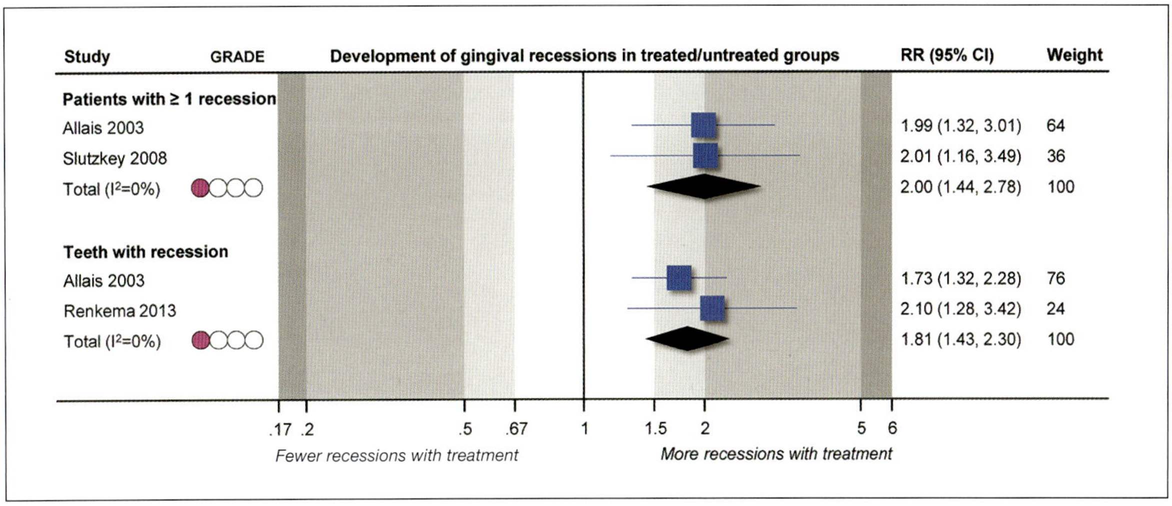

Fig 11-4 Meta-analyses of nonrandomized studies on the development of gingival recessions among treated and untreated patients. The forest plot has been enhanced with contours of effect magnitude, and the data used stems from a literature search performed solely for this chapter, including three nonrandomized studies.[54–56]

higher risk of developing at least one gingival recession, be it at the patient level (where treated patients are at twice the risk of untreated ones; RR = 2.00; 95% CI = 1.44 to 2.78) or at the tooth level (where treated teeth have an increased recession risk by 81% compared with untreated ones; RR = 1.81; 95% CI= 1.43 to 2.30). However, it is important to note that recessions were assessed in this analysis as a binary variable (recession present or absent), which leads to some loss of information, as most recessions that are clinically seen are of small magnitude. Allais and Melsen[55] reported that for the vast majority of patients, treatment-associated recessions were in the range of 0 to 2 mm and that less than 10% of the cases exhibited treatment-associated recessions greater than 2 mm. This is corroborated by Slutzkey and Levin,[56] who found that 8.4% of treated patients had recessions greater than 2 mm (compared with 0.9% of untreated patients).

Nonetheless, while orthodontic treatment might be a contributing factor to recession development, it does not necessarily lead to gingival recessions, and several patient- or treatment-related risk factors have been proposed. As such, craniofacial morphology seems to be associated with recession development, with long and narrow faces being significantly associated with increased recession risk, and greater maximum intracranial width being associated with lower recession risk.[57] Considerable changes in the inclination of mandibular incisors in Class III malocclusions, in both compensatory and decompensatory directions, also seems to be a risk factor for treatment-induced gingival recessions.[58,59] Additionally, preexisting recessions, baseline width of keratinized gingiva, gingival biotype, and visual gingival inflammation during orthodontic treatment seem to contribute significantly to the development of gingival recession during treatment.[60] Furthermore, there seems to exist a weak correlation between the amount of dental arch expansion and the development of gingival recessions,[61] although in these cases the recessions tend to occur at the first premolars that are expanded the most. On the contrary, no evidence could be found that factors like symphysis dimensions[62] and orthodontic proclination of the mandibular incisors in general[63,64] contribute to recession development. However, given the possibility of increased recession risk in orthodontic patients, orthodontists should be made aware of the risks in terms of careful risk assessment of each case prior to the commencement of treatment, sensible treatment planning, and monitoring for gingival recessions during treatment to minimize such adverse effects.

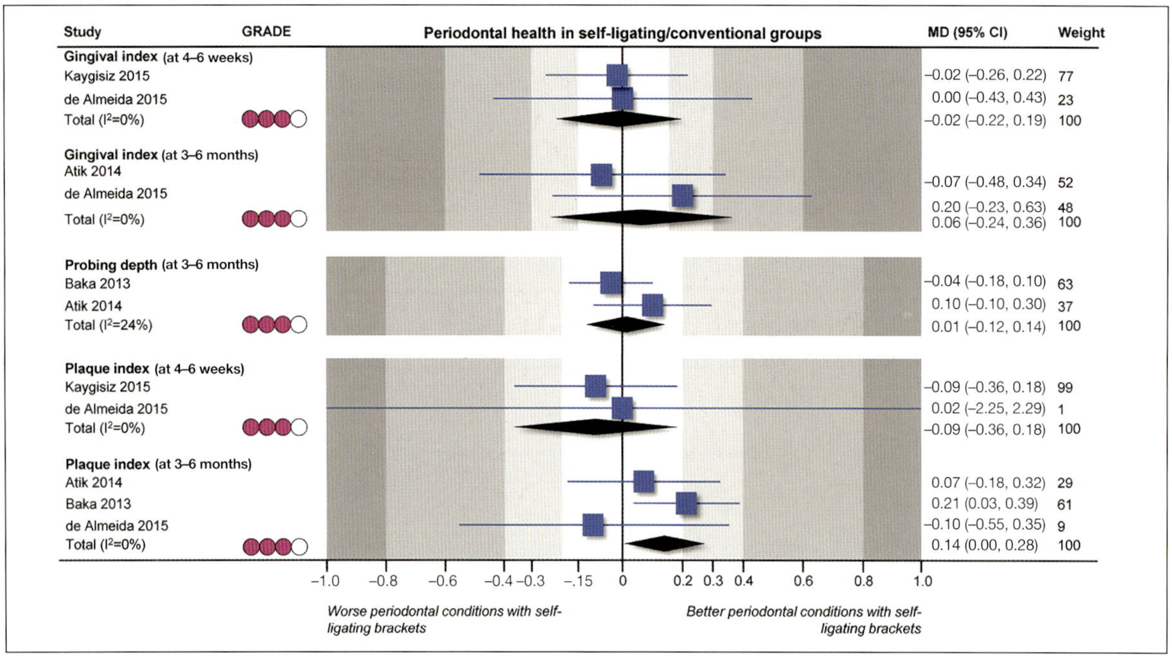

Fig 11-5 Meta-analyses of nonrandomized studies on the clinical periodontal parameters among patients treated with self-ligating or conventional brackets. The forest plot has been enhanced with contours of effect magnitude, and the data used stems from the systematic review of Arnold et al.[68]

Effect of Appliance Design on Periodontal Parameters

A wide variety of modifications to the classical orthodontic appliance have been proposed, some of which are aimed at minimizing the microbial load around the appliances and thereby alleviating the burden of orthodontic treatment on the periodontal tissues. One of the first modifications of the fixed appliance from a historical point of view was the transition from full-mouth banding to bonding of brackets, with bands now being used only for molars. It has been documented that considerable differences exist in the periodontal response to band insertion as opposed to bracket bonding. Kim et al[65] reported higher bleeding on probing at banded sites compared to bonded sites within orthodontic treatment. Shifts in the microbial composition due to orthodontic bands may be a result of decreased plaque control, but the appliances themselves may also alter the microbial composition of the mouth due to their positioning. Most commonly, this is attributed to the microbial shift around subgingivally placed orthodontic bands, especially those with subgingival excess cement, which develop red complex bacteria similar to that seen around overhanging restorations.[7] Nonetheless, Kim et al[65] found no differences between supragingival and subgingival band margins. On the contrary, van Gastel et al[26] found faster increases in probing depth, bleeding on probing, and gingival crevicular flow in bonded versus banded sites, which was attributed to orthodontic wires hindering proper hygiene.

Among the various appliances that exist in the market, the self-ligating appliances hold a prominent place,[66] based on the notion that they lack the biofilm-adsorbing elastomeric modules[67] and are therefore more hygienic. The results of a recent systematic review of randomized trials[68] were reanalyzed here (Fig 11-5) and indicated that no significant difference exists between the two bracket designs during the first 4 to 6 weeks of treatment, although at 3 to 6 months after appliance placement, patients with self-ligating brackets had significantly lower plaque indices than patients with

Table 11-1 Results of single trials from a systematic review[70] comparing lingual and labial appliances in terms of periodontal outcomes

Outcome	*Effect*	*95% CI*	*P*
Questionnaire			
Oral hygiene problems (3 months)	RR = 1.40	0.91, 2.15	.123
Oral hygiene problems: High intensity (3 months)	RR = 0.24	0.01, 5.57	.376
Food impaction (3 months)	RR = 1.25	1.03, 1.50	.022
Bleeding gingiva (3 months)	RR = 1.38	0.65, 2.93	.410
Bad taste (3 months)	RR = 1.40	0.50, 3.92	.522
Clinical			
Plaque index (1 month)	MD = −0.01	−0.14, 0.12	.879
Plaque index (2 months)	MD = 0.11	0.00, 0.22	.049
Gingival bleeding index (1 month)	MD = −0.10	−0.20, 0.00	.057
Gingival bleeding index (2 months)	MD = 0.09	−0.03, 0.21	.136
Number of new WSL per jaw (multivariable)	IRR = 0.28	0.10, 0.73	.010
Incidence of new WSL per jaw (multivariable)	OR = 0.43	0.11, 1.61	.209

IRR, incidence rate ratio; OR, odds ratio; WSL, white spot lesion.

conventional brackets (MD = 0.14; 95% CI = 0.00 to 0.28). However, despite this evidence being of moderate quality according to the GRADE approach and the results statistically significant, the effect would bear little clinical relevance. Apart from this difference in the plaque index, no significant differences could be seen between self-ligating and conventional brackets for gingival inflammation or sulcus probing depth at any time point. Additionally, a retrospective cohort study reported that there were no significant differences in marginal bone loss between self-ligating and conventional brackets measured with CBCT at first premolars, second premolars, or first molars (MDs of −0.04 mm, 0.02 mm, and 0.01 mm, respectively, with $P > .05$ for all). The same has been reported for the salivary levels of *S mutans*, where no difference was seen between the two bracket designs.[69] This indicates that self-ligating brackets cannot be advocated in terms of better periodontal effects.

Fixed appliances bonded on the palatal/lingual side of the tooth constitute another popular alternative to the classical appliance that has emerged in the last few decades, mainly due to their obvious esthetic advantage. However, a recent systematic review[70] on lingual appliances found very limited evidence on their effect on periodontal parameters, with mostly single studies informing most comparisons (Table 11-1). As such, lingual appliances were associated with a statistically significant greater difficulty in holding an adequate level of oral hygiene, which could be seen by greater chance of food impaction (RR = 1.25; 95% CI = 1.03 to 1.50) and increased plaque index (MD = 0.11; 95% CI = 0 to 0.22). However, it should be noted that even though the microbial load on the tooth or appliance surfaces seems to be greater, this had a lesser impact on enamel demineralizations, as patients with lingual appliances were less probable to develop white spot lesions than patients with labial appliances (incidence rate ratio = 0.28; 95% CI = 0.10 to 0.73). This could possibly be attributed to an increased flow of saliva on the lingual/palatal tooth surfaces, keeping the pH high.[71] Therefore, lingual appliances might be useful in reducing the effect of orthodontic treatment on enamel, but there is no evidence

Table 11-1 (cont) Results of single trials from a systematic review[70] comparing lingual and labial appliances in terms of periodontal outcomes

Outcome	*Effect*	*95% CI*	*P*
Clinical/laboratory			
Salivary flow rate (1 month)	MD = −0.12	−0.45, 0.21	.474
Salivary flow rate (2 months)	MD = −0.16	−0.73, 0.41	.579
Salivary buffering capacity (1 month)	MD = −0.30	−0.80, 0.20	.235
Salivary buffering capacity (2 months)	MD = −0.35	−0.76, 0.06	.097
S mutans high count (1 month)	RR = 1.00	0.65, 1.55	> .999
S mutans high count (3 months)	RR = 1.13	0.78, 1.63	.535
Lactobacillus high count (1 month)	RR = 2.00	0.68, 5.85	.206
Lactobacillus high count (3 months)	RR = 1.50	0.60, 3.74	.384

that they can be advocated in terms of microbial or bony changes.

Aligner treatment has been also proposed as an alternative to fixed appliances in order to reduce the periodontal burden to the patient, provided the aligners match the set treatment goals, as evidence has indicated that they might be less effective than fixed appliances.[72] Furthermore, the effect of orthodontic aligners on periodontal health has been assessed by only one randomized clinical trial reporting data from the first 3 months in treatment.[73] According to the results of that trial, patients treated with aligners seem to present statistically significantly lower plaque index (MD = −0.75; 95% CI= −1.30 to −0.20), sulcus probing depths (MD = −0.65; 95% CI = −1.12 to -0.18), and bleeding on probing (MD = −0.55; 95% CI = −0.92 to −0.18) than patients treated with fixed appliances—all of which might also be clinically relevant. Although only a single trial with 20 patients was identified, this indicates that aligner treatment might be a good alternative to minimize the consequences of orthodontic treatment to the periodontal tissues.

Posttreatment Change in Periodontal Health

Most researchers agree that any effects the orthodontic treatment might have on the periodontal conditions of the patient are related to the increased microbial load and the changes that the subgingival environment undergoes, most of which are transient. Following the removal of the orthodontic appliances, periodontal clinical parameters like the plaque index, gingival index, bleeding on probing, and pocket probing depth reduce toward pretreatment levels, although miniscule, clinically insignificant changes in periodontal clinical parameters such as probing depth[3] and attachment loss[4] remain (see Figs 11-2 and 11-3). Considerable adverse effects might be seen in only a small subset of patients.[34] The same holds true for the bacterial profile of orthodontic patients, which tends to revert back to pretreatment levels after 6 months[24] (see Fig 11-1).

Conclusion

In summary, reported adverse effects of orthodontic treatment with fixed appliances are minimal for the average patient and are mainly characterized by transient clinical and microbiologic changes mediated by the increased plaque accumulation around orthodontic appliances, the increased difficulty in exercising proper oral hygiene, and the deepening of the gingival sulcus. For most patients, awareness of the problem, oral hygiene motivation, and regular visits to the dentist to reinforce oral hygiene instructions might be adequate. There is a small subset of patients to which orthodontic treatment might confer a significant risk for irreversible periodontal destruction, and careful pretreatment consideration as well as in-treatment monitoring of factors like poor oral hygiene, active periodontal disease, and clinical attachment loss are advised.

References

1. Sadowsky C, BeGole EA. Long-term effects of orthodontic treatment on periodontal health. Am J Orthod 1981;80:156–172.
2. Polson AM, Subtelny JD, Meitner SW, et al. Long-term periodontal status after orthodontic treatment. Am J Orthod Dentofacial Orthop 1988;93:51–58.
3. Bollen AM, Cunha-Cruz J, Bakko DW, Huang GJ, Hujoel PP. The effects of orthodontic therapy on periodontal health: A systematic review of controlled evidence. J Am Dent Assoc 2008;139:413–422.
4. Papageorgiou SN, Papadelli AA, Eliades T. Effect of orthodontic treatment on periodontal clinical attachment: A systematic review and meta-analysis. Eur J Orthod 2018;40:176–194.
5. Freitas AO, Marquezan M, Nojima Mda C, Alviano DS, Maia LC. The influence of orthodontic fixed appliances on the oral microbiota: A systematic review. Dental Press J Orthod 2014;19:46–55.
6. Diamanti-Kipioti A, Gusberti FA, Lang NP. Clinical and microbiological effects of fixed orthodontic appliances. J Clin Periodontol 1987;14:326–333.
7. Huser MC, Baehni PC, Lang R. Effects of orthodontic bands on microbiologic and clinical parameters. Am J Orthod Dentofacial Orthop 1990;97:213–218.
8. van Gastel J, Quirynen M, Teughels W, Coucke W, Carels C. Influence of bracket design on microbial and periodontal parameters in vivo. J Clin Periodontol 2007;34:423–431.
9. Thornberg MJ, Riolo CS, Bayirli B, Riolo ML, Van Tubergen EA, Kulbersh R. Periodontal pathogen levels in adolescents before, during, and after fixed orthodontic appliance therapy. Am J Orthod Dentofacial Orthop 2009;135:95–98.
10. Liberati A, Altman DG, Tetzlaff J, et al. The PRISMA statement for reporting systematic reviews and meta-analyses of studies that evaluate health care interventions: Explanation and elaboration. J Clin Epidemiol 2009;62:e1–e34.
11. Veroniki AA, Jackson D, Viechtbauer W, et al. Methods to estimate the between-study variance and its uncertainty in meta-analysis. Res Synth Methods 2016;7:55–79.
12. Papageorgiou SN. Meta-analysis for orthodontists: Part II—Is all that glitters gold? J Orthod 2014;41:327–336.
13. Guyatt GH, Oxman AD, Schünemann HJ, Tugwell P, Knottnerus A. GRADE guidelines: A new series of articles in the *Journal of Clinical Epidemiology*. J Clin Epidemiol 2011;64:380–382.
14. Liu H, Sun J, Dong Y, et al. Periodontal health and relative quantity of subgingival *Porphyromonas gingivalis* during orthodontic treatment. Angle Orthod 2011;81:609–615.
15. Karkhanechi M, Chow D, Sipkin J, et al. Periodontal status of adult patients treated with fixed buccal appliances and removable aligners over one year of active orthodontic therapy. Angle Orthod 2013;83:146–151.
16. Baricevic M, Mravak-Stipetic M, Majstorovic M, Baranovic M, Baricevic D, Loncar B. Oral mucosal lesions during orthodontic treatment. Int J Paediatr Dent 2011;21:96–102.
17. Baer PN, Coccaro PJ. Gingival enlargement coincident with orthodontic therapy. J Periodontol 1964;35:436–439.
18. Atack NE, Sandy JR, Addy M. Periodontal and microbiological changes associated with the placement of orthodontic appliances. A review. J Periodontol 1996;67:78–85.
19. Rosenbloom RG, Tinanoff N. Salivary *Streptococcus mutans* levels in patients before, during, and after orthodontic treatment. Am J Orthod Dentofacial Orthop 1991;100:35–37.
20. Sinclair PM, Berry CW, Bennett CL, Israelson H. Changes in gingiva and gingival flora with bonding and banding. Angle Orthod 1987;57:271–278.
21. Ximénez-Fyvie LA, Haffajee AD, Socransky SS. Comparison of the microbiota of supra- and subgingival plaque in health and periodontitis. J Clin Periodontol 2000;27:648–657.
22. Moore WE, Moore LV. The bacteria of periodontal diseases. Periodontol 2000 1994;5:66–77.
23. Haffajee AD, Socransky SS. Microbial etiological agents of destructive periodontal diseases. Periodontol 2000 1994;5:78–111.
24. Papageorgiou SN, Xavier GM, Cobourne MT, Eliades T. Effect of orthodontic treatment on the subgingival microbiota: A systematic review and meta-analysis [epub ahead of print 20 July 2018]. Orthod Craniofac Res doi:10.1111/ocr.12237.

25. Jewtuchowicz VM, Brusca MI, Mujica MT, et al. Subgingival distribution of yeast and their antifungal susceptibility in immunocompetent subjects with and without dental devices. Acta Odontol Latinoam 2007;20:17–22.
26. van Gastel J, Quirynen M, Teughels W, Coucke W, Carels C. Longitudinal changes in microbiology and clinical periodontal variables after placement of fixed orthodontic appliances. J Periodontol 2008;79:2078–2086.
27. Naranjo AA, Triviño ML, Jaramillo A, Betancourth M, Botero JE. Changes in the subgingival microbiota and periodontal parameters before and 3 months after bracket placement. Am J Orthod Dentofacial Orthop 2006;130:275.e17–e22.
28. van Gastel J, Quirynen M, Teughels W, Coucke W, Carels C. Longitudinal changes in microbiology and clinical periodontal parameters after removal of fixed orthodontic appliances. Eur J Orthod 2011;33:15–21.
29. Gomes SC, Varela CC, da Veiga SL, Rösing CK, Oppermann RV. Periodontal conditions in subjects following orthodontic therapy. A preliminary study. Eur J Orthod 2007;29:477–481.
30. Zachrisson S, Zachrisson BU. Gingival condition associated with orthodontic treatment. Angle Orthod 1972;42:26–34.
31. Zachrisson BU. Cause and prevention of injuries to teeth and supporting structures during orthodontic treatment. Am J Orthod 1976;69:285–300.
32. Robinson PJ, Vitek RM. The relationship between gingival inflammation and resistance to probe penetration. J Periodontal Res 1979;14:239–243.
33. Melsen B, Agerbaek N, Eriksen J, Terp S. New attachment through periodontal treatment and orthodontic intrusion. Am J Orthod Dentofacial Orthop 1988;94:104–116.
34. Zachrisson BU, Alnaes L. Periodontal condition in orthodontically treated and untreated individuals. I. Loss of attachment, gingival pocket depth and clinical crown height. Angle Orthod 1973;43:402–411.
35. Corbacho de Melo MM, Cardoso MG, Faber J, Sobral A. Risk factors for periodontal changes in adult patients with banded second molars during orthodontic treatment. Angle Orthod 2012;82:224–228.
36. Bondemark L. Interdental bone changes after orthodontic treatment: A 5-year longitudinal study. Am J Orthod Dentofacial Orthop 1998;114:25–31.
37. Lund H, Gröndahl K, Gröndahl HG. Cone beam computed tomography evaluations of marginal alveolar bone before and after orthodontic treatment combined with premolar extractions. Eur J Oral Sci 2012;120:201–211.
38. Fuhrmann R. Three-dimensional interpretation of periodontal lesions and remodeling during orthodontic treatment. Part III. J Orofac Orthop 1996;57:224–237.
39. Lombardo L, Bragazzi R, Perissinotto C, Mirabella D, Siciliani G. Cone-beam computed tomography evaluation of periodontal and bone support loss in extraction cases. Prog Orthod 2013;14:29.
40. Castro LO, Castro IO, de Alencar AH, Valladares-Neto J, Estrela C. Cone beam computed tomography evaluation of distance from cementoenamel junction to alveolar crest before and after nonextraction orthodontic treatment. Angle Orthod 2016;86:543–549.
41. Jäger F, Mah JK, Bumann A. Peridental bone changes after orthodontic tooth movement with fixed appliances: A cone-beam computed tomographic study. Angle Orthod 2017;87:672–680.
42. Garlock DT, Buschang PH, Araujo EA, Behrents RG, Kim KB. Evaluation of marginal alveolar bone in the anterior mandible with pretreatment and posttreatment computed tomography in nonextraction patients. Am J Orthod Dentofacial Orthop 2016;149:192–201.
43. Litonjua LA, Andreana S, Bush PJ, Cohen RE. Tooth brushing and gingival recession. Int Dent J 2003;53:67–72.
44. Susin C, Haas AN, Oppermann RV, Haugejorden O, Albandar JM. Gingival recession: Epidemiology and risk indicators in a representative urban Brazilian population. J Periodontol 2004;75:1377–1386.
45. Smith RG. Gingival recession: Reappraisal of an enigmatic condition and new index for monitoring. J Clin Periodontol 1997;24:201–205.
46. Lawrence HP, Hunt RJ, Beck JD. Three-year root caries incidence and risk modeling in older adults in North Carolina. J Public Health Dent 1995;55:69–78.
47. Al-Wahadni A, Linden GJ. Dentine hypersensitivity in Jordanian dental attenders. A case control study. J Clin Periodontol 2002;29:688–693.
48. Löe H, Anerud A, Boysen H. The natural history of periodontal disease in man: Prevalence, severity, and extent of gingival recession. J Periodontol 1992;63:489–495.
49. Albandar JM, Streckfus CF, Adesanya MR, Winn DM. Cigar, pipe, and cigarette smoking as risk factors for periodontal disease and tooth loss. J Periodontol 2000;71:1874–1881.
50. Kassab MM, Cohen RE. The etiology and prevalence of gingival recession. J Am Dent Assoc 2003;134:220–225.
51. Rawal SY, Claman LJ, Kalmar JR, Tatakis DN. Traumatic lesions of the gingiva: A case series. J Periodontol 2004;75:762–769.
52. Levin L, Zadik Y, Becker T. Oral and dental complications of intra-oral piercing. Dent Traumatol 2005;21:341–343.
53. Wennström JL, Lindhe J, Sinclair F, Thilander B. Some periodontal tissue reactions to orthodontic tooth movement in monkeys. J Clin Periodontol 1987;14:121–129.
54. Renkema AM, Fudalej PS, Renkema AA, Abbas F, Bronkhorst E, Katsaros C. Gingival labial recessions in orthodontically treated and untreated individuals: A case-control study. J Clin Periodontol 2013;40:631–637.
55. Allais D, Melsen B. Does labial movement of lower incisors influence the level of the gingival margin? A case-control study of adult orthodontic patients. Eur J Orthod 2003;25:343–352.
56. Slutzkey S, Levin L. Gingival recession in young adults: Occurrence, severity, and relationship to past orthodontic treatment and oral piercing. Am J Orthod Dentofacial Orthop 2008;134:652–656.
57. Salti L, Holtfreter B, Pink C, et al. Estimating effects of craniofacial morphology on gingival recession and clinical attachment loss. J Clin Periodontol 2017;44:363–371.
58. Vasconcelos G, Kjellsen K, Preus H, Vandevska-Radunovic V, Hansen BF. Prevalence and severity of vestibular recession in mandibular incisors after orthodontic treatment. Angle Orthod 2012;82:42–47.

59. Johal A, Katsaros C, Kiliaridis S, et al. State of the science on controversial topics: Orthodontic therapy and gingival recession (A report of the Angle Society of Europe 2013 meeting). Prog Orthod 2013;14:16.
60. Melsen B, Allais D. Factors of importance for the development of dehiscences during labial movement of mandibular incisors: A retrospective study of adult orthodontic patients. Am J Orthod Dentofacial Orthop 2005;127:552–561.
61. Morris JW, Campbell PM, Tadlock LP, Boley J, Buschang PH. Prevalence of gingival recession after orthodontic tooth movements. Am J Orthod Dentofacial Orthop 2017;151:851–859.
62. Closs LQ, Bortolini LF, dos Santos-Pinto A, Rösing CK. Association between post-orthodontic treatment gingival margin alterations and symphysis dimensions. Acta Odontol Latinoam 2014;27:125–130.
63. Renkema AM, Fudalej PS, Renkema A, Bronkhorst E, Katsaros C. Gingival recessions and the change of inclination of mandibular incisors during orthodontic treatment. Eur J Orthod 2013;35:249–255.
64. Renkema AM, Navratilova Z, Mazurova K, Katsaros C, Fudalej PS. Gingival labial recessions and the post-treatment proclination of mandibular incisors. Eur J Orthod 2015;37:508–513.
65. Kim K, Heimisdottir K, Gebauer U, Persson GR. Clinical and microbiological findings at sites treated with orthodontic fixed appliances in adolescents. Am J Orthod Dentofacial Orthop 2010;137:223–228.
66. Papageorgiou SN, Konstantinidis I, Papadopoulou K, Jäger A, Bourauel C. Clinical effects of pre-adjusted edgewise orthodontic brackets: A systematic review and meta-analysis. Eur J Orthod 2014;36:350–363.
67. Eliades T, Eliades G, Watts DC. Structural conformation of in vitro and in vivo aged orthodontic elastomeric modules. Eur J Orthod 1999;21:649–658.
68. Arnold S, Koletsi D, Patcas R, Eliades T. The effect of bracket ligation on the periodontal status of adolescents undergoing orthodontic treatment. A systematic review and meta-analysis. J Dent 2016;54:13–24.
69. Pandis N, Papaioannou W, Kontou E, Nakou M, Makou M, Eliades T. Salivary *Streptococcus mutans* levels in patients with conventional and self-ligating brackets. Eur J Orthod 2010;32:94–99.
70. Papageorgiou SN, Gölz L, Jäger A, Eliades T, Bourauel C. Lingual vs. labial fixed orthodontic appliances: Systematic review and meta-analysis of treatment effects. Eur J Oral Sci 2016;124:105–118.
71. Britse A, Lagerlöf F. The diluting effect of saliva on the sucrose concentration in different parts of the human mouth after a mouth-rinse with sucrose. Arch Oral Biol 1987;32:755–756.
72. Papageorgiou SN, Höchli D, Eliades T. Outcomes of comprehensive fixed appliance orthodontic treatment: A systematic review with meta-analysis and methodological overview. Korean J Orthod 2017;47:401–413.
73. Levrini L, Abbate GM, Migliori F, Orrù G, Sauro S, Caprioglio A. Assessment of the periodontal health status in patients undergoing orthodontic treatment with fixed or removable appliances. A microbiological and preliminary clinical study. Cumhuriyet Dent J 2013;16:296–307.

CHAPTER 12

Orthodontic Mechanics in Patients with Periodontal Disease

Carlalberta Verna
Turi Bassarelli

The loss of supporting bone typically observed in patients with periodontal disease often leads to migration of the affected teeth and therefore changes in the occlusal stability. In order to limit the damage created by the periodontal bone loss, proper occlusal contact must be re-established (Fig 12-1). However, it is paramount to understand that **no orthodontic treatment can be performed in the presence of active periodontal disease**.[1] Moreover, in cases of functional interference with the position of the teeth, like in cases of lip catch (Fig 12-2), relapse of the orthodontic movement is certain; therefore, the cause of tooth migration (ie, loss of periodontal bone support and subsequent functional interference) should be completely eliminated prior to orthodontic treatment.[2]

Stress-Strain Distribution

The immediate consequence of orthodontic loading is a change in the stress-strain distribution in the periodontal ligament (PDL). This is associated with bending of the alveolar bone and the so-called "cone effect" (Fig 12-3). The cone effect is the result of the resolution of a force into a horizontal and a vertical component once applied to an inclined plane (eg, root surfaces and alveolar walls). Any horizontal force application will cause an extrusive component, which in a healthy situation is controlled by the supracrestal fibers. In periodontally affected teeth, however,

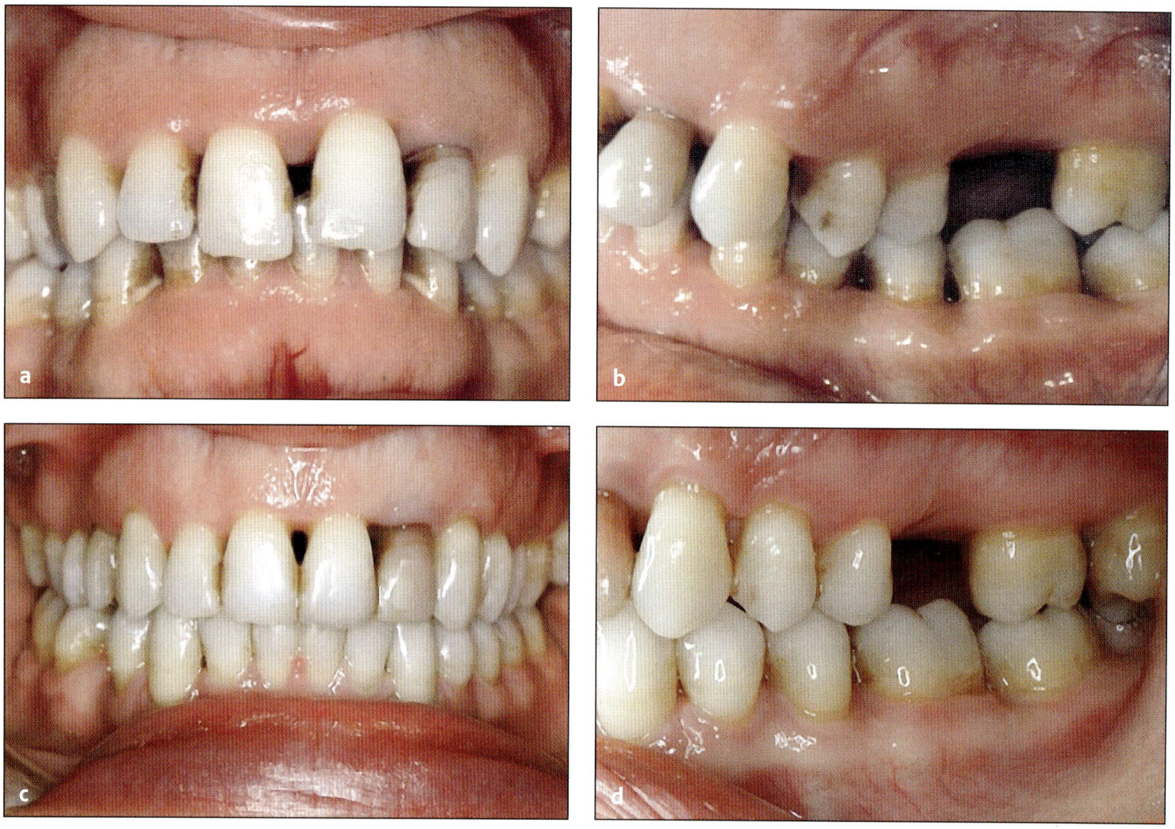

Fig 12-1 *(a and b)* Frontal and lateral intraoral views of a 48-year-old woman affected by horizontal bone loss and vertical collapse. *(c and d)* Same views 7 years after combined periodontal and orthodontic treatment. Of utmost importance is the establishment of proper occlusal contact that allows maintenance of the results by the patient.

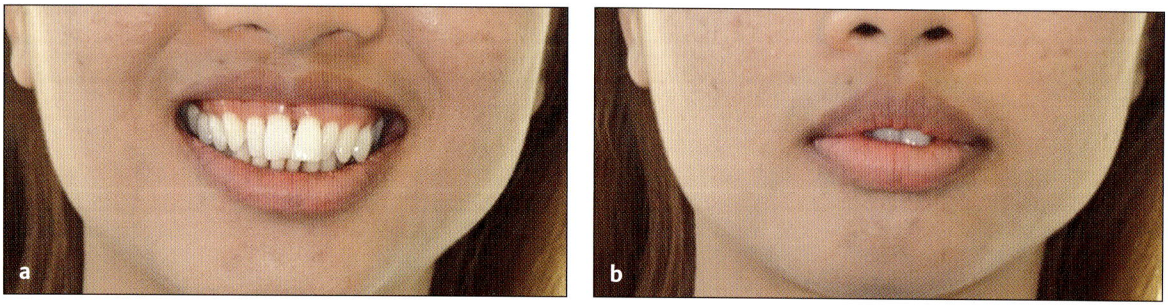

Fig 12-2 *(a and b)* The loss of periodontal support leads to tooth migration, which is further worsened by a functional interference, in this case a lip catch.

where bone support is reduced, the stresses and strains are distributed over a smaller surface area, so the resistance offered by the alveolar crest is less and the extrusive component is more pronounced.[3,4]

In patients with periodontal disease whose teeth have already extruded as a result of the condition, maximum control of the vertical movement is mandatory. From a biomechanical point of view, the use of any continuous arch technique, in which action and reaction forces are not clearly defined, must be limited. Therefore segmented arches, in which active and reactive units are clearly defined, are indicated.[5] Figure 12-4 illustrates a segmented arch approach to retract and intrude the maxillary incisors. The activation of PDL cells should be minimized in order to avoid movement in the posterior anchorage unit. To

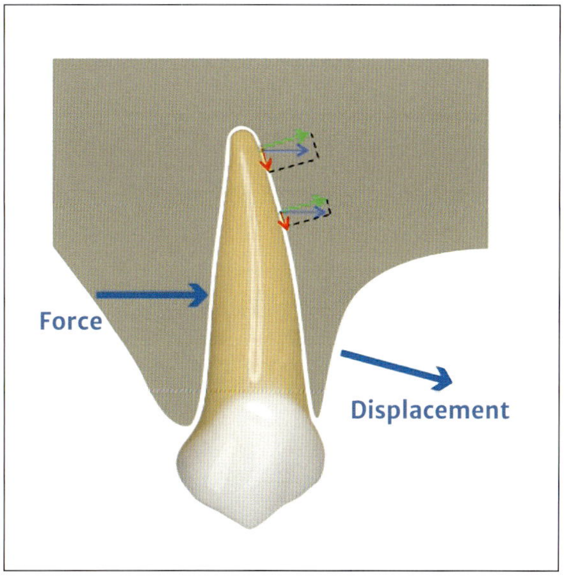

Fig 12-3 The cone effect. A horizontal force applied on an inclined plane is resolved into its normal components. In periodontally compromised teeth, the vertical component is less controlled by the supracrestal fibers, and therefore the extrusive component of a horizontal force is more visible.

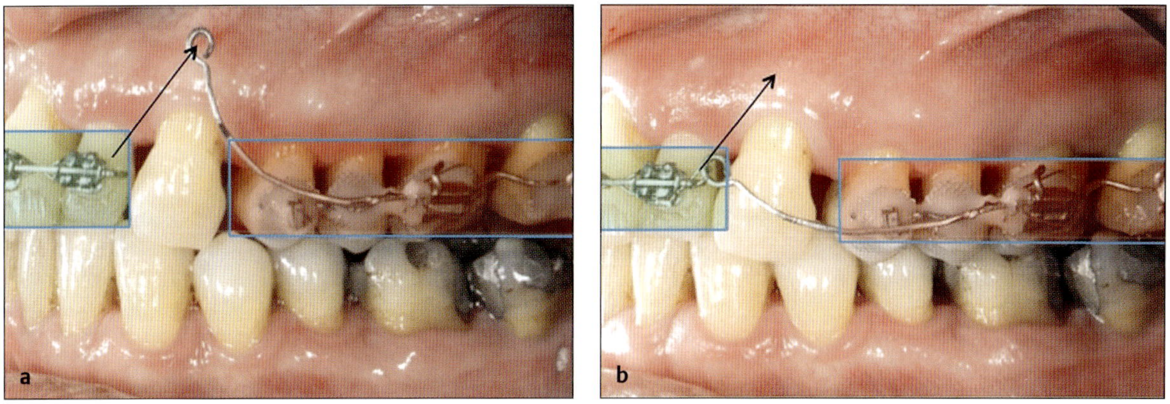

Fig 12-4 *(a and b)* Segmented arch approach to intrude the maxillary incisors. The reactive unit, the anchorage, is shaded *red*. It is achieved through the bonding of a stiff segment and by a tight interdigitation. In cases where interdigitation is not firm, occlusal composite indentation may be added. The active unit, shaded *green*, is the unit to be displaced. The displacement is performed thanks to a cantilever with a low load-deflection rate that is able to deliver low forces with sufficient springback. The 3D plan dictates the direction of the force to be applied through the cantilever.

achieve this, a stiff segment of 0.019 × 0.025–inch stainless steel (SS) wire was welded to individual meshes and passively bonded to the posterior anchor teeth *(red area)*. The active unit *(green area)* comprised the maxillary incisors, which needed to be intruded. These teeth were connected using a stiff segment of 0.019 × 0.025–inch SS wire, and the intrusion force was applied by means of a cantilever made of 0.017 × 0.025–inch titanium molybdenum alloy, which was activated to intrude the active unit along the line of action indicated by the *black arrow*.[6]

CENTER OF RESISTANCE

Tooth movement is the consequence of the application of a force, characterized by type and amount. The type of mechanics employed on teeth with reduced periodontal support is influenced by the fact that the center of resistance is displaced more apically (Fig 12-5). The clinical consequence is that any force applied at the level of the crown will result in tooth movement characterized by a larger rotational component. In other words, tipping movements are

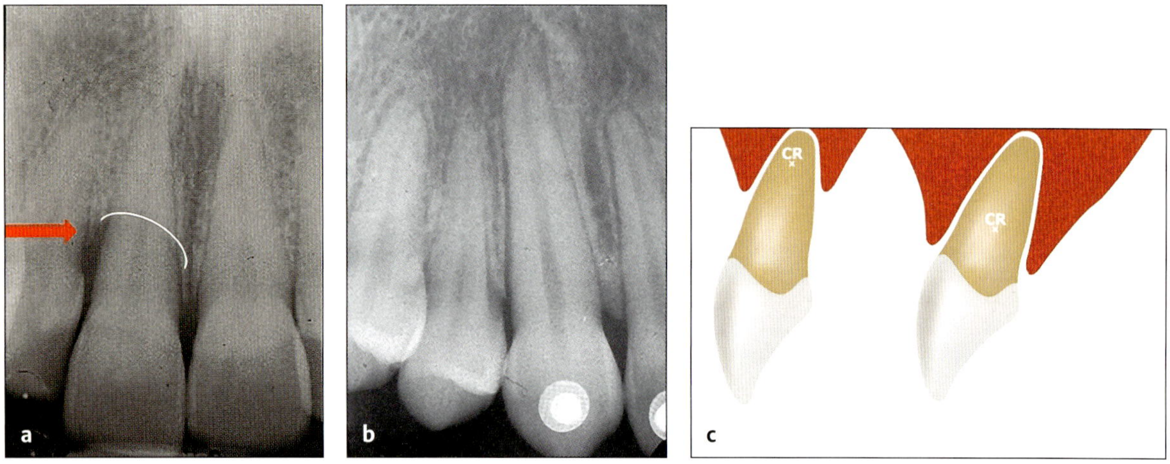

Fig 12-5 *(a to c)* Due to periodontal bone loss *(red arrow)* resulting from periodontal disease, the center of resistance (CR) of this tooth is displaced more apically. As a consequence, to obtain the same type of tooth movement as in healthy periodontal conditions, the point of force application should be displaced more apically. In other words, if the force is still applied at the level of the crown, a larger rotational component (moment) should be added.

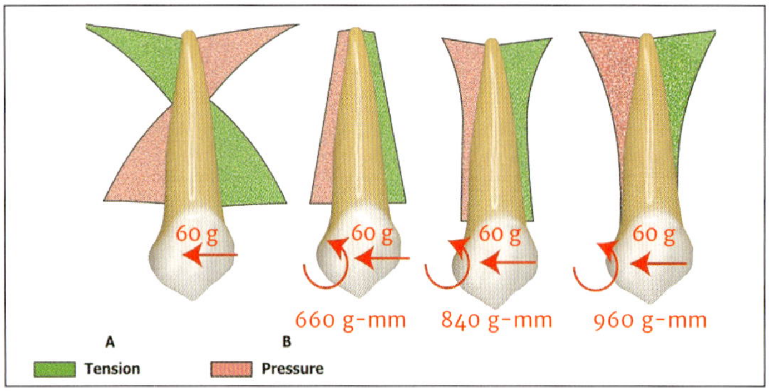

Fig 12-6 According to Nikolai,[7] the concentrations of the tensile and compressive strains are maximal in tipping movements at the apex and at the coronal level in a single tooth. The more the moment added to the force at the level of the bracket, the better the root control, until the translatory movement is achieved. In this movement, the strains are uniformly distributed, reducing the chance of the final pressure in the PDL exceeding that of the capillary vessels.

easier to achieve. The stress-strain distribution is uneven when tipping occurs, being most concentrated at the coronal and apical levels[7,8] (Fig 12-6). These high force levels may risk causing obstruction of capillary vessels, thus leading to hyalinization,[9] which has been shown to cause indirect bone resorption and root resorption.[10–12]

BONE SUPPORT

The bone support of periodontally affected teeth is often reduced not only in the vertical dimension (decreased bone height) but also in the buccolingual dimension (very thin cortical walls). When this is the case, hyalinization occurs, and indirect resorption will take place from the periosteum, further reducing the vertical height and, as a consequence, irreversibly damaging the bone support. Therefore, tooth movements on periodontally affected teeth are not recommended if the control of the root position is poor because of the high strain levels created at the level of the crown.

FORCE LEVELS

The force levels that need to be applied for specific tooth movements have always been calculated in relationship to the type of desired movement and the root surface area onto which the force has to be applied. However, in the case of periodontally

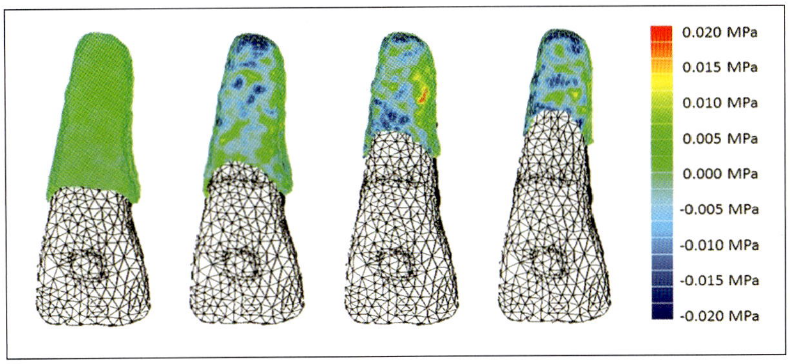

Fig 12-7 Normal stresses in the PDL of a normal central incisor and the same tooth affected by mild, moderate, and severe periodontitis respectively *(from left to right)* for an external intrusion force of 30 cN. *Red*, tensile stresses; *blue*, compressive stresses. (Result of a finite element analysis kindly supplied by G. Hauber Gameiro, M. Dalstra, and P. M. Cattaneo.)

compromised teeth, this general rule cannot be applied, and the force level has to be adjusted to take into account the amount of bone surface connected to the tooth via the remaining PDL. Figure 12-7 shows the results of a finite element study in which the same amount of force was delivered to a tooth with various simulated amounts of remaining PDL. This analysis shows that when there is a reduced PDL present, the amount of stress and strain increases. In order to avoid undesired hyalinization in periodontally compromised teeth, the amount of force must be kept as low as possible.[13] Because the minimum amount of force necessary to activate the cellular reaction has been found to be 4 g, it is possible to obtain tooth movement in periodontally compromised teeth with extremely low force levels.[14] These will vary according to the desired displacement.

Biomechanical Approach for Periodontally Compromised Patients

The biomechanical approach for periodontally compromised patients differs from that of healthy patients. The cellular activation of the PDL has to be limited as much as possible in the teeth to be moved. The force level has to be kept as low as possible, and the loads should be evenly distributed with root-controlled movements, thus keeping the moment-to-force ratios constant. In practical terms, this concept has consequences on the treatment goals and on the anchorage planning.

The treatment goals are often limited to the re-establishment of a proper interarch relationship and satisfactory esthetic and periodontal results that can be maintained.[15] Once the treatment goals are set, the biomechanical system necessary to achieve the goals has to be established.[16] First, the active and passive units must be clearly identified (see Fig 12-4). Vertical-control mechanics should be considered not only to correct the tooth position but also to control the cone effect. The PDL should be loaded in a uniform way. The types of tooth movement that ensure this loading include translation and controlled tipping (Fig 12-8). In order to achieve translation, the line of action of the force has to pass through the center of resistance of a tooth or a group of teeth. The moment should be sufficient to achieve root control and to avoid round tripping of the teeth, which happens when the force is applied at the crown level. The constancy of the moment-to-force ratio protects against round tripping, which would promote undesired cell activity, and therefore decreases treatment time. The group of teeth that needs to be displaced should be moved along a line of action that is determined during the planning of the biomechanical system. According to the different clinical situations, different lines of action may need to be planned.

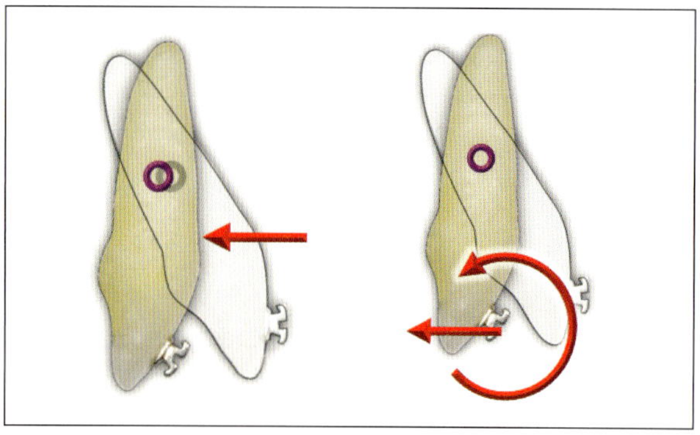

Fig 12-8 The treatment plan foresees a controlled tipping of the incisors, without round tripping. This movement can be obtained either by moving the point of application of the force more apically *(left)* or by adding a moment at the crown to counteract the tipping component of a single force application *(right)*.

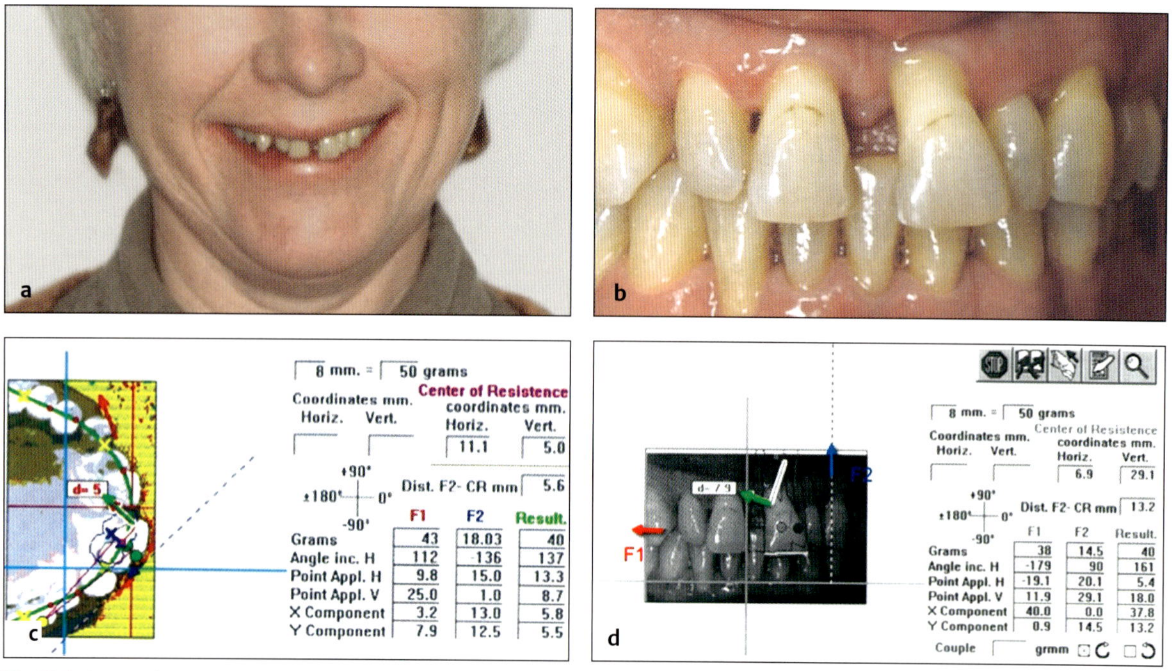

Fig 12-9 *(a and b)* Pretreatment facial and intraoral views of a 49-year-old woman concerned about losing her maxillary anterior teeth. Note the asymmetric tooth elongation and the lip catch present at rest, thus making the tooth position unstable. *(c and d)* The 3D plan was necessary to establish the proper line of action of the force. Once that is established, the next step is to find out which tools will allow the desired movement. Based on the clinical situation, the force may be applied at the crown or at a distance from the center of resistance. In some critical inclinations, the sole approach that has maximal biomechanical advantage is the lingual one. →

Figure 12-9 clarifies this situation. This 49-year-old woman was unhappy with the appearance of her smile and extremely concerned about the degeneration of her dentition; in the last few years, she had noticed a progressive vertical and sagittal movement of her maxillary anterior teeth, and she was afraid of losing them in the future (Figs 12-9a and 12-9b). 3D planning of tooth movement was carried out to establish the appropriate line of action of the force (Figs 12-9c and 12-9d). The plan relied on restricting the activation of cells to a specific area. Initially a two-cantilever system was used to intrude and mesialize the maxillary left central and lateral incisors. Once they reached the level of the contralateral incisors, all four teeth were united as a block, and further intrusion was performed. Figure 12-9c shows the line of action of the force necessary to achieve the desired movement and the two vectors necessary to obtain the desired line of action. Due to anatomical limitations, it is not possible to obtain this line

BEFORE AFTER

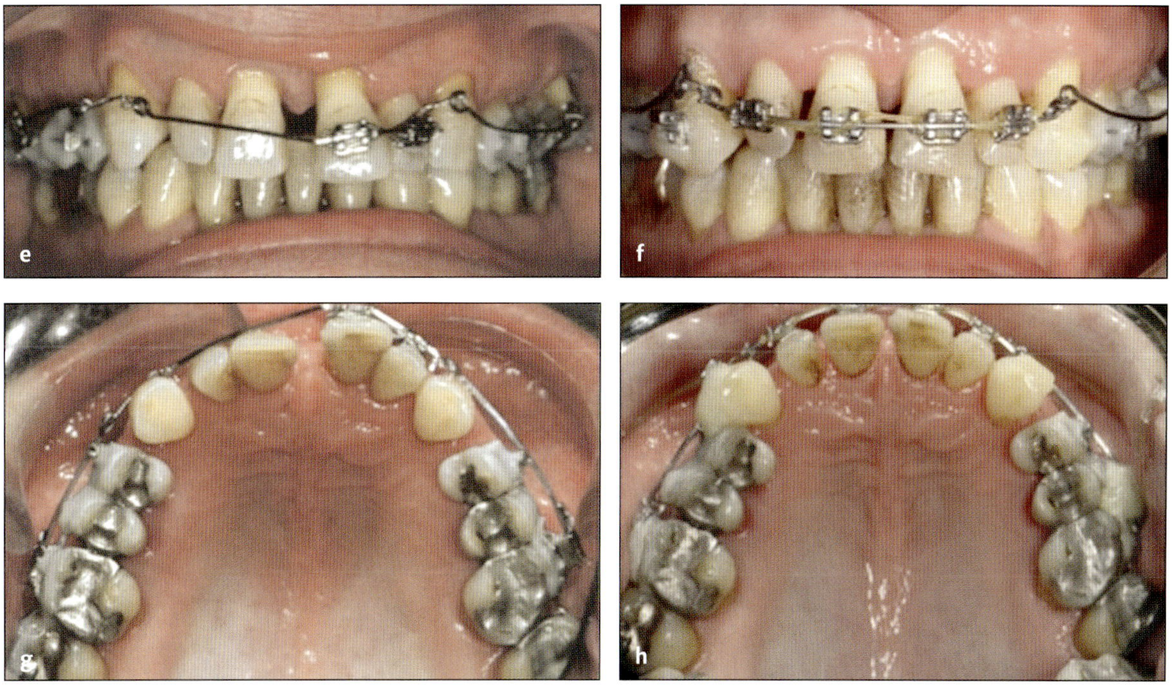

Fig 12-9 *(cont)* *(e to h)* The two-cantilever system allowed for correction of the overeruption and midline deviation in about 8 months. First the maxillary left incisors were the active unit, and once they were vertically leveled, all four maxillary incisors were further intruded and retracted. *(i)* Superimpositions showing the intrusion and retraction obtained and the midline correction without anchorage loss.

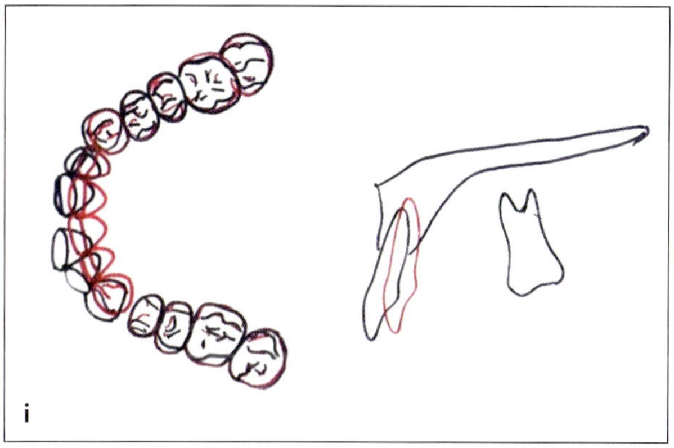

of action with a single cantilever system, so instead the force was obtained by resolving it into two vectors—one applying an intrusive and lateral force and the other an intrusive and slightly retractive force. Once the target teeth (maxillary left incisors) had been moved, the contralateral incisors were added to the anterior active unit, and the same cantilevers were then applied. The reactive unit was stabilized by stiff passive segments joined by a stiff wire.

A continuous archwire would have extruded the maxillary right central and lateral incisors, which actually required intrusion. The use of a segmented arch approach is therefore particularly indicated in teeth with a reduced periodontium, because it allows maximal control of force delivery to both the active and the reactive units (Figs 12-9e to 12-9h). In this particular case, a minimum amount of reactive extrusion was allowed because the periodontal condition of the posterior teeth was good and the facial type of the patient allowed for light extrusive forces (Fig 12-9i). The final results are shown in Figs 12-9j and 12-9k. The periapical radiographs confirmed an improved bone level after the segmental intrusion (Figs 12-9l and 12-9m).

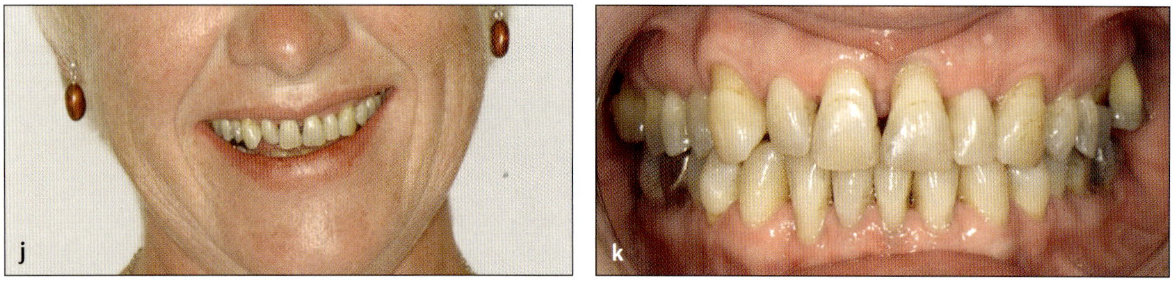

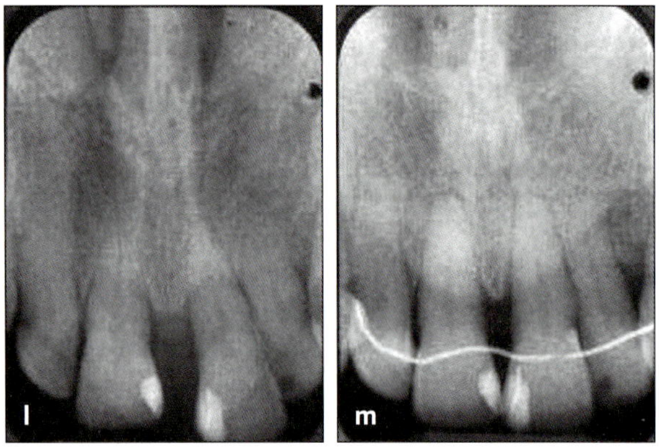

Fig 12-9 *(cont)* *(j and k)* Final results. Better smile esthetics and a proper overbite and overjet were achieved. Note the better interincisal papilla. All of these will help to facilitate periodontal health. *(l and m)* Periapical radiographs before and after treatment. After treatment, there is better bone support of the incisors, no further bone loss, and a slight root blunting.

In cases where the bone loss is particularly severe, the center of resistance moves apically, and so too should the line of action of the force. In other cases, the vertical stability of the posterior unit is more critical, and the use of absolute anchorage (ie, skeletal anchorage) is mandatory. The case presented in Fig 12-10 is a typical example of intrusion of posterior and anterior teeth in a periodontally compromised dentition. The 57-year-old woman was unhappy with her smile and worried about further degeneration of her dentition (Figs 12-10a and 12-10b). Her anterior and posterior occlusal planes were asymmetric due to loss of periodontal support together with tooth loss. After initial periodontal therapy and good maintenance, the posterior segments were asymmetrically intruded by means of two bracket-head miniscrews inserted in the buccal alveolar bone and ligated with a segment of 0.017 × 0.025–inch titanium molybdenum alloy. The anterior and posterior segments were activated by equal amounts to facilitate intrusion while avoiding additional moments on the miniscrews and thereby undermining their primary stability (Figs 12-10c to 12-10e). The use of mini-implants has tremendously improved the anchorage options in orthodontics and is especially beneficial for the treatment of periodontally compromised patients. Figures 12-10f and 12-10g show the final results of treatment.

When the maxillary anterior teeth in a periodontally compromised adult patient are proclined in combination with a deep bite and palatal impingement, the use of a straight-wire technique is not always indicated. In order to achieve a bodily movement of intrusion and retraction of the anterior teeth, the line of action of the force has to pass behind the center of resistance of these teeth, which in the case of reduced periodontium is located more apically. To avoid round tripping, intrusion and retraction must be delivered simultaneously, generating a line of action of the force passing through the center of resistance. The use of a segmented arch technique can provide the two movements simultaneously. For anatomical reasons, the ideal approach in such cases is from the lingual side, because it allows the application of the forces closer to the center of resistance of the anterior teeth. A typical example is shown in Fig 12-11. A 41-year-old man presented with a severe overjet in combination with an extremely increased overbite

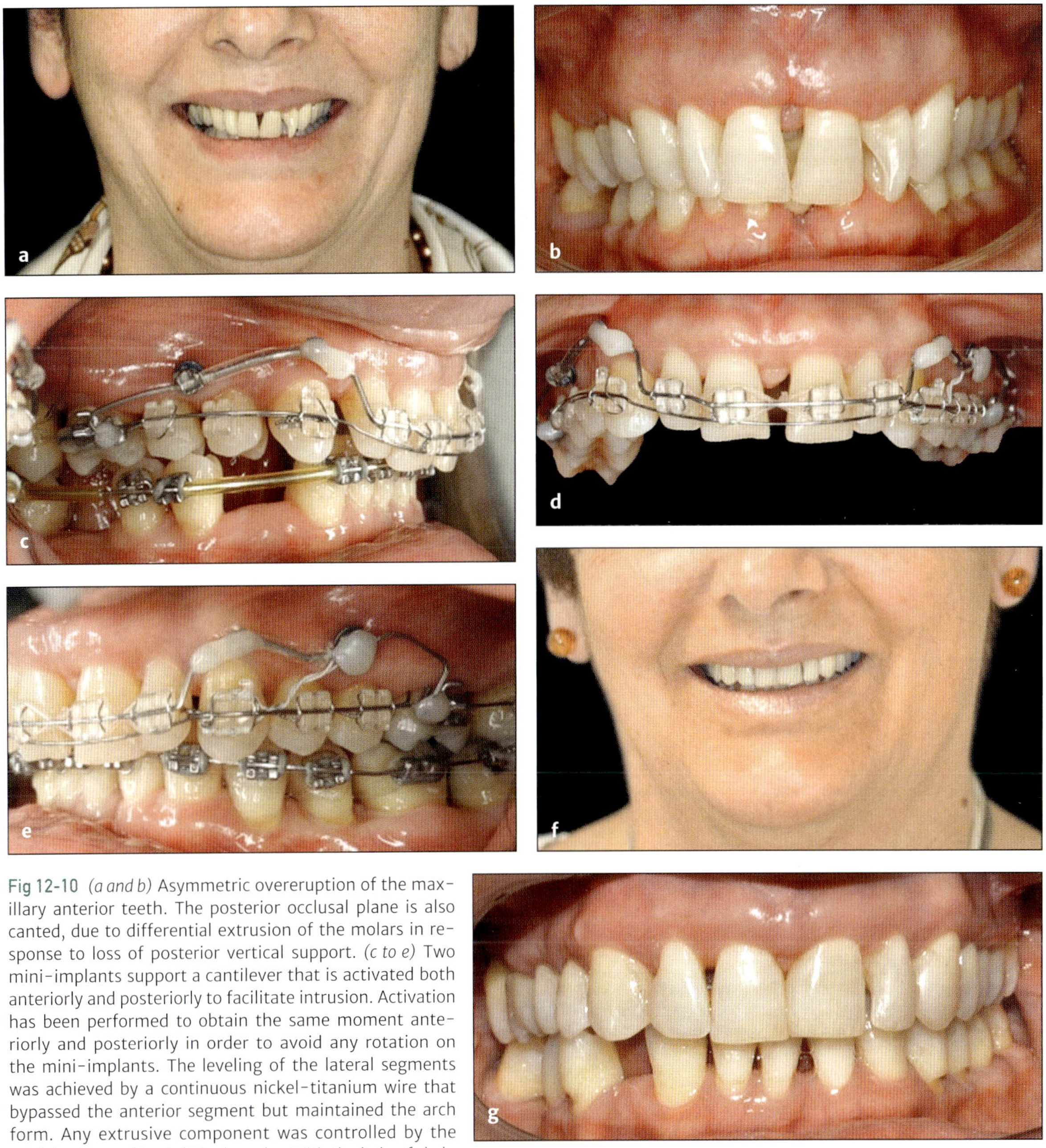

Fig 12-10 *(a and b)* Asymmetric overeruption of the maxillary anterior teeth. The posterior occlusal plane is also canted, due to differential extrusion of the molars in response to loss of posterior vertical support. *(c to e)* Two mini-implants support a cantilever that is activated both anteriorly and posteriorly to facilitate intrusion. Activation has been performed to obtain the same moment anteriorly and posteriorly in order to avoid any rotation on the mini-implants. The leveling of the lateral segments was achieved by a continuous nickel-titanium wire that bypassed the anterior segment but maintained the arch form. Any extrusive component was controlled by the mini-implants. *(f and g)* Final results. With the help of skeletal anchorage, better smile esthetics have been achieved.

and palatal impingement that required correction (Figs 12-11a to 12-11d). The correct line of action of the forces needed for intrusion and retroclination was one passing behind the center of resistance of the maxillary anterior incisors (Figs 12-11e and 12-11f).

This biomechanical system consisted of an anterior unit, or active unit, where the maxillary central incisors were connected through a palatal bonded mesh to a soldered power arm, and a posterior or passive unit (anchorage) consisting of the maxillary

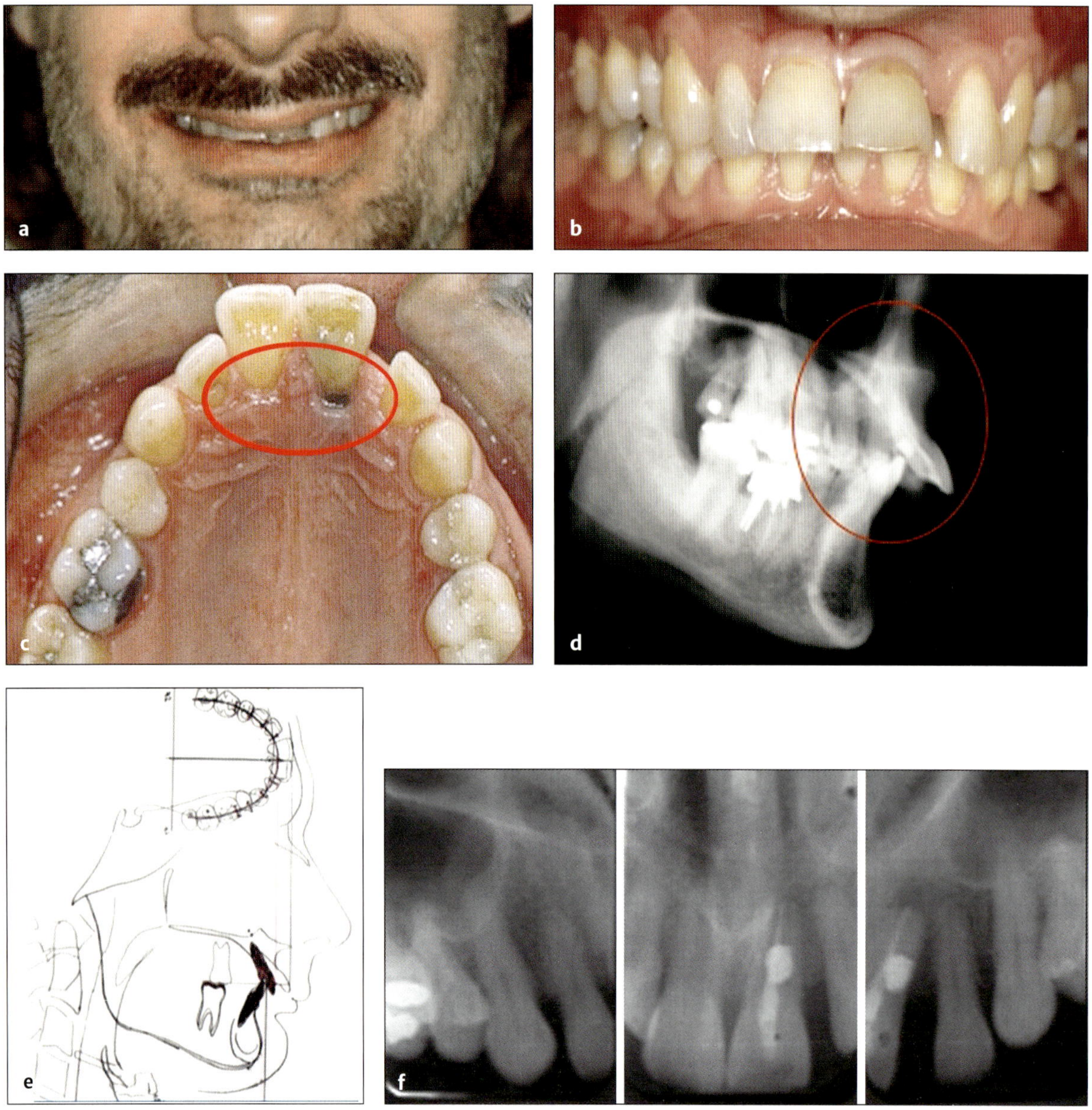

Fig 12-11 *(a to d)* A 41-year-old man presented with a skeletal and dental deep bite with palatal impingement, leading to periodontal damage. *(e and f)* The 3D visual treatment objective shows that to achieve the desired intrusive controlled tipping in this case of reduced periodontal support, the line of action of the force should pass behind the center of resistance of the anterior teeth. Therefore, application of the force on the palatal side is indicated. →

first molars connected with a transpalatal arch. The intrusive and distalizing active force was delivered by a 50-g nickel-titanium (NiTi) coil spring that connected the two units (Figs 12-11g and 12-11h). Once the two maxillary central incisors were intruded and retroclined to reach the same level as the lateral incisors, all four maxillary incisors were linked in a single anterior unit. The points of application for the intruding and distalizing forces were then moved to the buccal (Figs 12-11i to 12-11k). Two NiTi coil springs

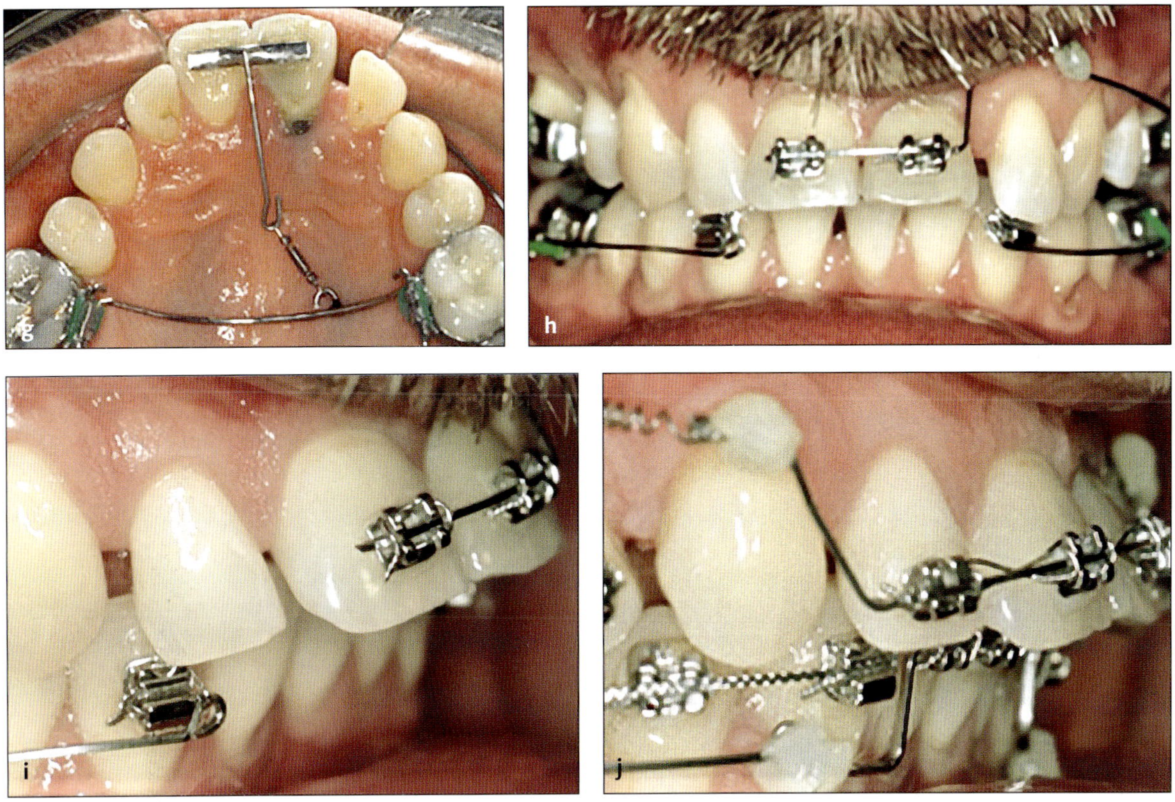

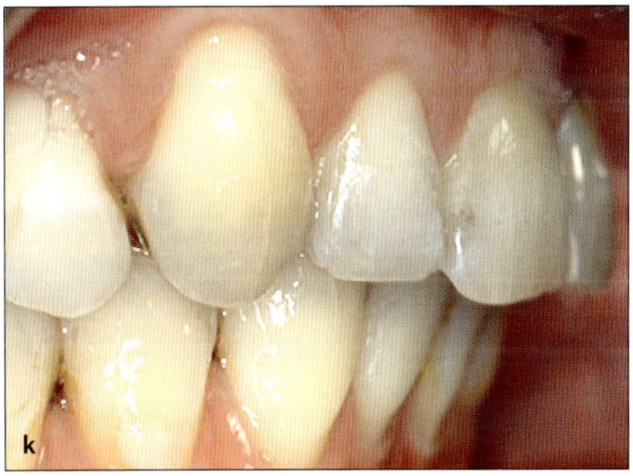

Fig 12-11 *(cont)* *(g and h)* The central incisors are solidarized through a bonded mesh and attached to a power arm that allows application of the intrusive and retractive force from the transpalatal arch. The midline shift is controlled by a cantilever activated in lateral movement and ligated at the center of resistance of the two incisors through an SS power arm. *(i and j)* Once the first intrusive and retractive movements have been performed through the lingual mechanics, the force is applied from the buccal with NiTi coil springs applied at the anterior segment through a stiff segment. *(k)* After 24 months, the desired results have been achieved.

were connected between the 0.017 × 0.025–inch SS power arms of the maxillary first molars and the two hooks at the distal end of the 0.019 × 0.025–inch SS anterior unit. Once the maxillary anterior teeth had been distalized and intruded and the spacing had been closed, a continuous 0.019 × 0.025–inch NiTi wire was placed in both arches to align and level. (Note that the leveling and alignment in these cases is not the first phase of treatment.) The finishing stage was carried out using 0.019 × 0.025–inch SS coordinated wires. The total treatment time was under 24 months, and the final result is shown in Figs 12-11l to 12-11p.

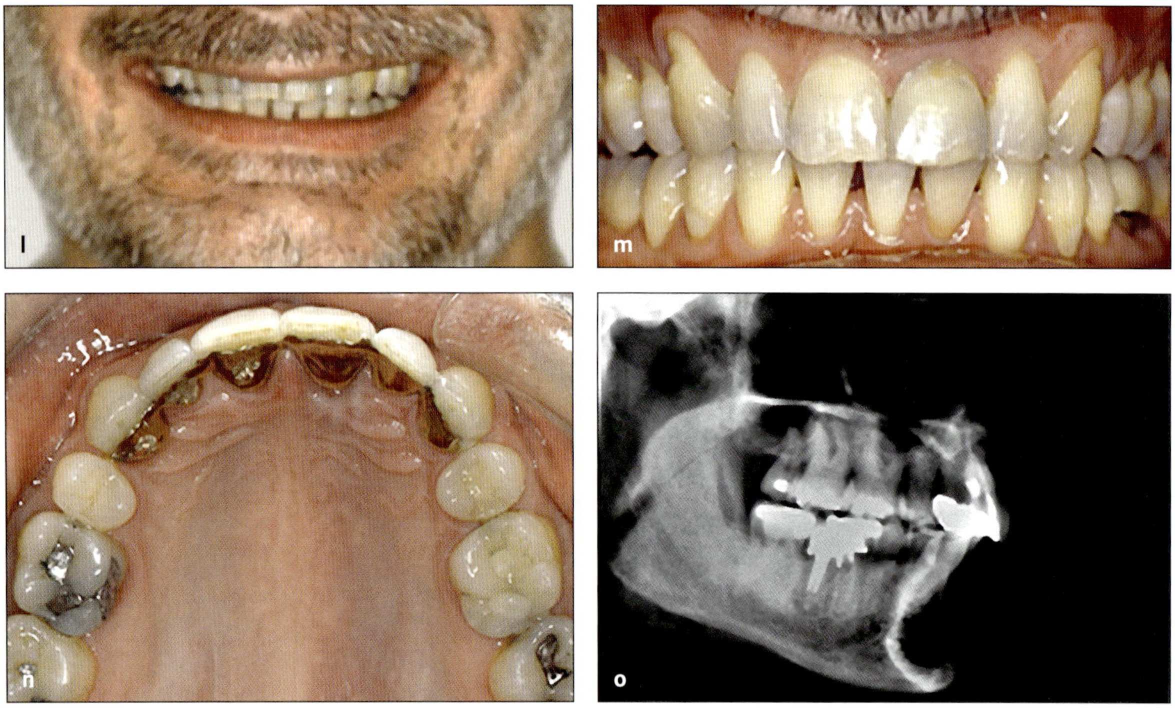

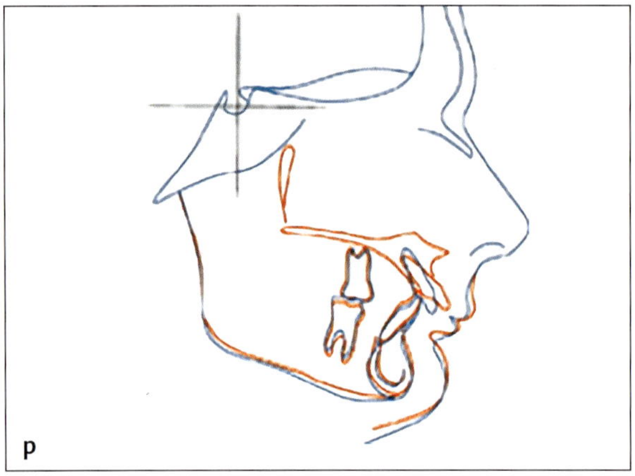

Fig 12-11 *(cont)* *(l to o)* Final results. The overjet has been normalized, and the deep bite has been corrected. The stiff lingual retainer, which will require thorough daily maintenance of oral hygiene, will ensure long-term stability. *(p)* Superimposition on the cranial base shows that the achieved tooth movements mirror the planned ones.

Conclusion

Planning the proper biomechanical system is crucial to avoid round tripping of teeth that have reduced periodontal support. These teeth must be loaded in the most effective way, using the lowest force levels possible, in order to achieve the treatment goal.

References

1. Ericsson I, Thilander B, Lindhe J, Okamoto H. The effect of orthodontic tilting movements on the periodontal tissues of infected and non-infected dentitions in dogs. J Clin Periodontol 1997;4:278–293.
2. Melsen B, Agerbaek N. Orthodontics as an adjunct to rehabilitation. Periodontol 2000 1994;4:148–159.
3. Cattaneo PM, Dalstra M, Melsen B. Moment-to-force ratio, center of rotation, and force level: A finite element study predicting their interdependency for simulated orthodontic loading regimens. Am J Orthod Dentofacial Orthop 2008;133:681–689.

4. Fiorelli G, Melsen B (eds). Biomechanics in Orthodontics. Available at http://www.ortho-biomechanics.com/en/. Accessed 6 April 2018.
5. Burstone CJ. The mechanics of the segmented arch techniques. Angle Orthod 1966;36:99–120.
6. Shroff B, Lindauer SJ, Burstone CJ, Leiss JB. Segmented approach to simultaneous intrusion and space closure: Biomechanics of the three-piece base arch appliance. Am J Orthod Dentofacial Orthop 1995;107:136–143.
7. Nikolai RJ. Bioengineering Analysis of Orthodontic Mechanics. Philadelphia: Lea & Febiger, 1985.
8. Verna C. Biology of tooth movement. In: Fiorelli G, Melsen B (eds). Biomechanics in Orthodontics. Available at http://www.ortho-biomechanics.com/en/. Accessed 6 April 2018.
9. Reitan K. Evaluation of orthodontic forces as related to histologic and mechanical factors. SSO Schweiz Monatsschr Zahnheilkd 1970;80:579–596.
10. Baron R. Remodeling of alveolar bone in spontaneous and induced tooth displacement [in French]. Rev Orthop Dento Faciale 1975;9:309–325.
11. Brudvik P, Rygh P. Root resorption beneath the main hyalinized zone. Eur J Orthod 1994;16:249–263.
12. Roscoe MG, Meira JB, Cattaneo PM. Association of orthodontic force system and root resorption: A systematic review. Am J Orthod Dentofacial Orthop 2015;147:610–626.
13. Sanders NL. Evidence-based care in orthodontics and periodontics: A review of the literature. J Am Dent Assoc 1999;130:521–527.
14. Weinstein S, Haack DC, Morris LY, Snyder BB, Attaway HE. On an equilibrium theory of tooth position. Angle Orthod 1963;33:1–26.
15. Melsen B. Potential adult orthodontic patients: Who are they? In: Melsen B (ed). Adult Orthodontics. Chichester, UK: Blackwell, 2014:1–11.
16. Melsen B, Fiorelli G. Treatment Planning: The 3D VTO. In: Melsen B (ed). Adult Orthodontics. Chichester, UK: Blackwell, 2012:64–76.

CHAPTER 13

Orthodontic Treatment in Patients with Severe Periodontal Disease

Tali Chackartchi
Stella Chaushu
Ayala Stabholz

Periodontitis is a progressive, infectious, multifactorial, inflammatory disease. Its pathogenesis involves pathogenic microorganisms, harbored in a dental biofilm, that trigger an excessive defense reaction of the host (host response). This host-bacterial interaction, along with bone and connective tissue metabolism and genetic factors, which vary among individuals, will result in some cases in periodontal attachment and bone loss.[1]

The 1999 World Workshop on Classification of Periodontal Diseases and Conditions identified three types of periodontal disease based on specific etiologic formulation: chronic periodontitis, aggressive periodontitis, and periodontitis as a manifestation of systemic disease.[2] Periodontal considerations in patients undergoing orthodontic treatment can be divided into two age groups: *(1)* children, adolescents, and young adults (under 30 years) and *(2)* adult patients (30 years and over).

Periodontal Considerations in Children, Adolescents, and Young Adults Undergoing Orthodontic Treatment

Orthodontic treatment is commonly performed in young individuals, mostly driven by functional and esthetic demands. The orthodontist and the treating team continuously struggle with compromised oral hygiene and the resulting gingival inflammation

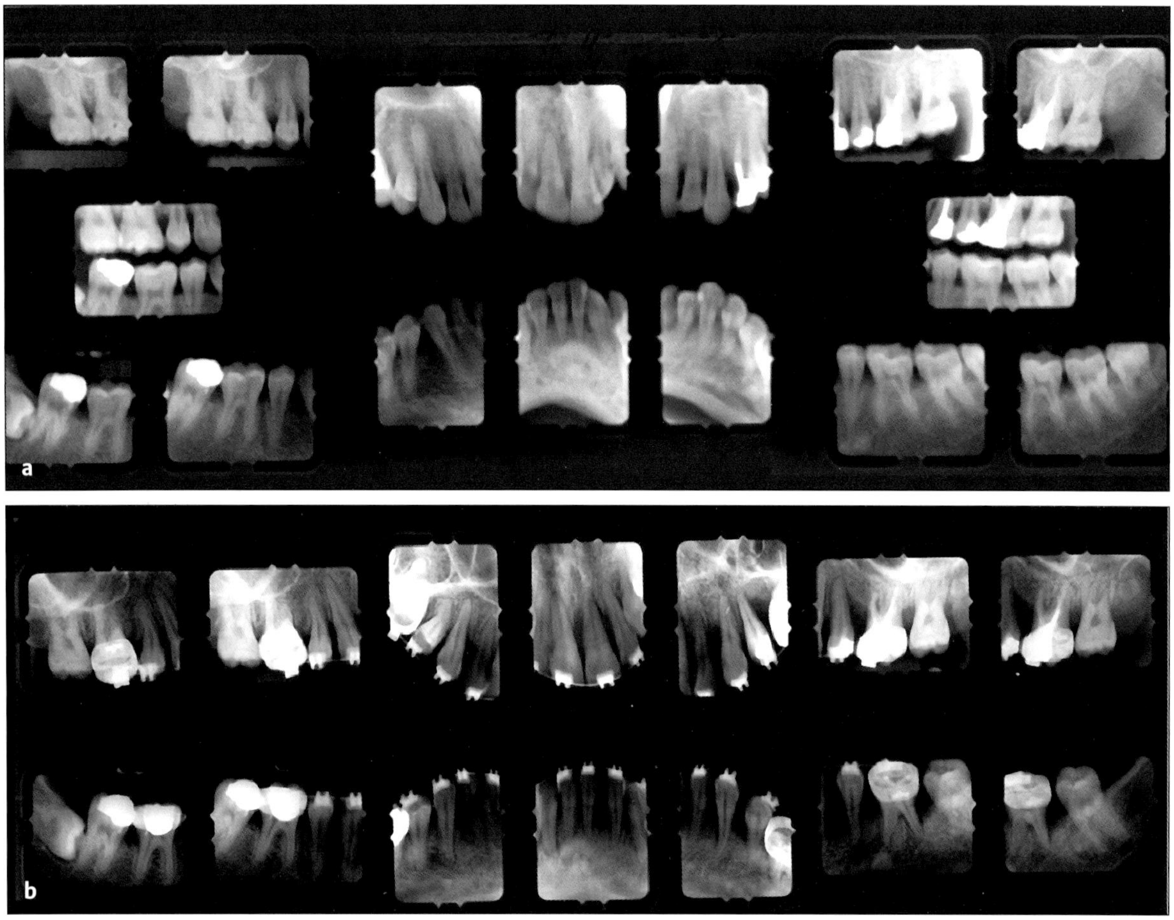

Fig 13-1 *(a)* A 22-year-old patient presented with no periodontal disease or signs of bone resorption at initial examination. *(b)* Two years after administration of orthodontic treatment, a marked periodontal breakdown was recorded.

(gingivitis) in these young patients. Luckily, periodontal diseases are less prevalent among this age group. However, when present, they are often characterized by rapid bone loss.

While chronic periodontitis has been described among adolescents and young adults,[3] the most frequently diagnosed form of periodontitis that affects young individuals is aggressive periodontitis (AP), mainly in its localized form.[4,5] AP is an uncommon and often severe periodontal disease, primarily characterized by the rapid loss of supporting bone and attachment.[6] Oral microorganisms that are present in biofilms are known to contribute to the onset of the disease. For example, *Aggregatibacter actinomycetemcomitans*, a periodontal pathogen, is closely associated with AP.[7–10] The generalized form of AP is characterized by interproximal attachment loss affecting at least three permanent teeth other than the first molars and the incisors.[2] Although most clinicians would agree that AP is clinically distinct, the clinical features distinguishing between generalized chronic periodontitis and generalized AP remain obscure.[11]

Poorly controlled AP can result in rapid and irreversible progression of the existing disease.[12] Therefore, the application of orthodontic forces in patients suffering from AP requires special attention and consideration[13] before, during, and after orthodontic treatment (Fig 13-1; see also Figs 13-3a and 13-3b). Several reports of successful orthodontic treatment in patients with localized AP[14–16] and generalized AP[17] have been described in the literature.

The main periodontal challenge in adolescents and young adults who are starting orthodontic treatment is early diagnosis of any periodontal pathology

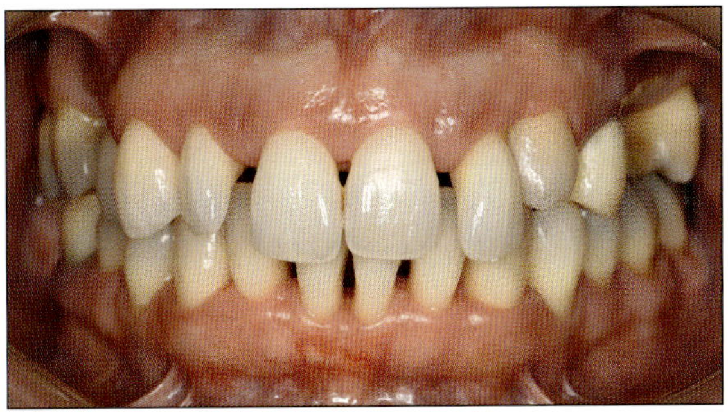

Fig 13-2 Flared and widely spaced anterior teeth resulting from severe periodontitis.

before the commencement of tooth movement. The average age of onset for AP is about the same as the average age for starting orthodontic treatment. Therefore, the orthodontist is often the first or the only clinician to diagnose any abnormal periodontium either clinically or radiographically during the initial examination. When periodontal disease develops during tooth movement, again the orthodontist will likely be the first clinician to diagnose it.[18,19]

Periodontal bone loss observed in young adults could be associated with an undiagnosed existing periodontal disease or could be an initial expression of chronic periodontitis, which would be expressed as initial bone loss mainly at the molars.

Periodontal Considerations in Adult Patients Undergoing Orthodontic Treatment

The prevalence of severe periodontal disease increases gradually with age, showing a steep increase during the fourth and fifth decades of life and reaching its peak at around 38 years of age.[20] No significant differences in prevalence or incidence of severe periodontal disease were found between men and women.[21]

One of the main complaints of adults affected by severe periodontitis is impaired anterior esthetics due to tooth migration, characterized by flared and spaced anterior teeth accompanied by rotation and overeruption (Fig 13-2). Dental migration associated with periodontal tissue breakdown is defined as pathologic tooth migration. According to Brunsvold,[13] pathologic tooth migration has been found to have a prevalence of about 30% to 55% and is statistically associated with clinical attachment loss, bone loss, tooth loss, and gingival inflammation. Because periodontitis is frequently a painless and asymptomatic disease, many of the affected adults do not seek treatment until esthetic disturbances evolve. As a result, the adult patient's esthetic needs motivate him or her to reach available solutions that include orthodontic as well as periodontal treatment.[13]

Recently, orthodontists are being challenged with an increased demand for treatment by adult patients, some with moderate to advanced periodontitis, which poses a unique challenge.[22,23] Orthodontic treatment of adult patients differs in many aspects from that of adolescent patients. One major aspect to be considered is the reduced cellular activity in older patients, which slows the rate of orthodontic tooth movement compared with younger patients.[24,25]

Orthodontic Movement of Periodontally Involved Teeth

It is well established that orthodontic tooth movement by itself does not induce periodontal bone loss or convert transient gingivitis into destructive periodontitis.[26–28] Findings by Garat et al[29] and Geraci et al[30] even suggest that orthodontic movement of periodontally compromised teeth can increase alveolar bone volume and allow periodontal reattachment if inflammation is under control.

The movement of teeth with reduced but healthy periodontium has been studied in both animal and human studies,[31–33] which confirmed that in the absence of inflammation, the periodontal attachment is not damaged. However, in the presence of plaque-induced inflammation, orthodontic forces cause uncontrolled periodontal attachment loss.[17,18,34]

Orthodontic tooth movement occurs in response to mechanical force application and involves the remodeling of the periodontal ligament and alveolar bone.[35] Tissue changes are regulated and maintained by an aseptic acute inflammatory response characterized by the release of proinflammatory mediators.[35–38] Clinical studies have shown high levels of cytokines and chemokines in gingival crevicular fluid during orthodontic therapy.[37,39,40] Therefore, orthodontic forces can aggravate periodontal destruction by intensifying periodontal inflammation with the aseptic acute inflammatory response initiated by orthodontic tooth movement.[41] These molecular changes described are associated with an increase in inflammatory cells and vascularity, which consequently lead to increased bone resorption.[42] This could explain why orthodontic forces applied in the presence of periodontal disease might accelerate periodontal breakdown.[34,43] In a rat model, it was observed that orthodontic force application in the presence of active periodontitis accelerated the inflammatory processes within the periodontium, together with reinforced osteoclastogenesis, and subsequently escalated dental root resorption as well as periodontal bone loss. At the same time, however, the periodontal inflammation facilitated faster orthodontic tooth movement.[44]

Under these conditions of periodontal disease and hyperocclusal forces, the changes in the subgingival microbiologic environment caused by orthodontic devices might contribute to the aggravation of the periodontal disease.[45,46] Orthodontic tooth movement will lead to enlargement of the space between the tooth and its socket. This anatomical change will enable supragingival plaque to migrate to a more apical position, leading eventually to a rapid deepening of periodontal pockets and loss of bone support,[32] which will further facilitate the formation of angular bony pockets.[32]

Some orthodontic tooth movements are considered quite risky to the periodontium. Intrusion and bodily movements can cause conversion of the supragingival plaque into subgingival plaque, resulting in intrabony pocket formation when uncontrolled periodontal inflammation exists or in the absence of good patient oral hygiene control.[31–34] On the other hand, orthodontic tooth movement implemented in the presence of reduced but healthy periodontal tissues with good patient compliance using light continuous forces will not induce detrimental effects on the periodontal tissue level.[47]

Periodontal Treatment Prior to Orthodontic Tooth Movement

DATA COLLECTION, DIAGNOSIS, AND PERIODONTAL MONITORING

Tooth movement in individuals with untreated periodontitis can be detrimental to the periodontium; therefore, it is of utmost importance to identify those who are at risk of developing periodontitis or aggravating an existing periodontal condition before starting any orthodontic intervention. Orthodontic treatment in children and adolescents is usually performed at ages that parallel those of the onset of AP. Therefore, it is very important to carefully monitor the periodontal status of each patient before and during orthodontic treatment.

In children, adolescents, and young adults

It is recommended to collect periodontal baseline data before starting any orthodontic treatment. This includes periodontal pocket depth measurements of all permanent first molars and incisors as well as dental radiographs including vertical bitewings and maxillary and mandibular anterior periapical radiographs. If the clinical periodontal data raise suspicions of any deviation from normal, a full-mouth set of periapical radiographs is indicated (see Figs 13-3a to 13-3d).

In cases of dental crowding, root prominence (especially in mandibular anterior teeth), or a planned orthodontic expansion of the dental arch, computed tomography scans should be considered for 3D inspection of root position within the bony arch to prevent future mucogingival complications.

In adults

Prior to orthodontic treatment, the patient should undergo a comprehensive dental examination including a systemic and medical history, full periodontal examination, a full series of periapical radiographs, and oral examination.

When considering the treatment of adult patients with periodontal disease, it is essential to obtain a detailed medical and drug history. Adult patients often present with medical conditions or take multiple medications that might affect their periodontal and/or orthodontic therapy. To ensure a positive response to periodontal therapy, smokers should be advised to cease smoking, and diabetic patients should reach an acceptable glycemic control. An accurate drug history should also be obtained. There are several drugs frequently consumed by adults that might affect the cells that are targeted by the orthodontic forces during tooth movement:

- *Nonsteroidal anti-inflammatory drugs (NSAIDs):* NSAIDs affect the sequence of tooth movement by reducing the associated inflammatory and bone-resorptive processes. Newer generations of anti-inflammatory drugs such as nabumetone have also been shown to reduce the amount of root resorption that coincides with intrusive orthodontic forces without affecting the speed of tooth movement.[22]
- *Tricyclic antidepressants:* These drugs, such as amitriptyline and benzodiazepines, may cause xerostomia that could negatively affect the proper maintenance of oral hygiene, which is crucial for treatment success.
- *Chronic use of inhalers with steroids:* Steroid inhalers can induce oral candidiasis and xerostomia. Appropriate measures should be implemented in these patients, such as the use of topical antifungal agents and salivary substitutes, before and during orthodontic treatment.
- *Medication for osteoporosis:* Osteoporosis drugs, such as bisphosphonates, selective estrogen receptor modulators, and calcitonin, might interfere with bone remodeling, which in turn could affect the orthodontic treatment.
- *Medication for rheumatoid arthritis or other chronic inflammatory conditions:* Therapy aims to block the catabolic cytokine production responsible for the damage to soft tissues and bones (tumor necrosis factor or interleukin antagonists). These immune-modulatory agents might also inhibit orthodontic tooth movement.
- *Drugs that are associated with gingival hyperplasia such as phenytoin (for seizure disorders), calcium channel blockers (antihypertension), or cyclosporine A (for organ transplant patients):* These drugs induce gingival hyperplasia and might therefore impair certain orthodontic mechanics as well as the practice of proper oral hygiene, negatively affecting periodontal health.
- *Chemotherapy with busulfan/cyclophosphamide within the previous 2 years*: These drugs are known to damage the precursor cells involved in bone-remodeling processes.

A thorough periodontal evaluation should be performed before the initiation of orthodontic tooth movement. Such an evaluation should include a full-mouth recording of inflammation and bacterial biofilm scores and a full-mouth periodontal chart including probing depths, furcation involvements, mucogingival abnormalities, and tooth mobility. In case of any deviation from a healthy periodontium (see Figs 13-4a and 13-4b), periodontal treatment must be first performed. In addition to the clinical examination, a full series of periapical radiographs should be obtained and evaluated (see Fig 13-4d). The panoramic views that are routinely obtained before orthodontic treatment are not accurate or detailed enough for an adequate periodontal evaluation.

Assessment of the entire dentition should be performed as well and treatment delivered accordingly.

PERIODONTAL CAUSE-RELATED THERAPY

The first stage of periodontal treatment should include periodontal cause-related therapy.[48] Orthodontic instruments challenge daily oral hygiene and will pose a risk for periodontal deterioration. Therefore, cause-related therapy should be performed with the utmost care to achieve optimal plaque and bleeding scores (see Figs 13-4e to 13-4g).

The patient's compliance with acceptable oral hygiene practice as well as the clinical periodontal parameters should be recorded just before starting orthodontic tooth movement. The presence of shallow probing depths (≤ 4 mm), minimal plaque accumulation, and minimal bleeding on probing should be confirmed before beginning orthodontic treatment.

PERIODONTAL SURGERY

After the completion of periodontal cause-related therapy, residual periodontal pockets (≥ 5 mm) may still be present. These periodontal pockets are generally the result of alveolar bone resorption and carry an increased risk for further periodontal deterioration, which might eventually lead to tooth loss.[49] These pockets serve as niches for bacterial biofilm accumulation, which may be detrimental during movement of the affected tooth. Therefore, any periodontal pockets deeper than 5 mm should be further treated to make sure that all etiologic risk factors of periodontal breakdown are eliminated and residual inflammation eradicated,[50] especially if intrusion or retroclination movements are to be considered.

There are two types of preorthodontic periodontal surgical procedures to consider:

1. *Access flap periodontal surgery*, designed to improve access for the control and removal of plaque, calculus, and infected cementum from deep bone defects and periodontal pockets. Wide defects are easier to access for an efficient removal of granulation tissue and root debridement.
2. *Regenerative periodontal surgery*, designed to restore damaged tissues and reconstruct lost supporting tissues, namely alveolar bone, root cementum, and periodontal ligament bony defects amenable for regeneration.

When planning regenerative surgery in collaboration with orthodontic intervention, the dilemma that arises is the proper sequence of treatment: Should regenerative surgery be performed before or after orthodontic tooth movement?

Despite the risks involved in orthodontic tooth movements in the presence of inflammation, some clinicians are in favor of orthodontic tooth movement immediately after initial preparation, even in the presence of severe periodontal disease. Their clinical justification is that moving the roots closer to one another can narrow the defect and thus facilitate better prognosis of regenerative treatment. Improving tooth position in early treatment stages can also improve patient compliance, helping patients realize the functional and esthetic advantages of treatment.[51]

A different clinical approach aims for completion of periodontal cause-related therapy and periodontal surgery before initiation of orthodontic tooth movement. The rationale for this approach is that periodontal therapy will reduce the risk for periodontal deterioration during orthodontic tooth movement and therefore ensure better results in regenerative treatment as well as improved esthetics. Data from animal histologic studies support this clinical approach. In fact, when the periodontal inflammation is properly controlled, a sequential orthodontic tooth movement can contribute to periodontal improvement, encouraging the formation of new periodontal attachment following open flap debridement along with orthodontic treatment.[30,52] Moreover, open flap debridement associated with orthodontic tooth movement may result in formation of a new connective tissue attachment coronally to the deepest point of root instrumentation when intrusive tooth movement is performed.[52] Another study showed that it was possible to rebuild lost periodontal support in three-wall defects in conjunction with bodily tooth movement.[30]

Periodontal regeneration can be achieved by a number of surgical procedures using various biologic agents: bone grafting materials (with autografts, allogeneic bone grafts, or bone mineral matrix), barrier membranes (resorbable or nonresorbable), and the application of enamel matrix derivative (EMDs). All of these techniques, alone or in combination, seem to be effective in the treatment of periodontal intrabony defects—that is, angular bony defects with inflamed connective tissues and dentogingival epithelium located apical to the crest of bone.[53]

The positive effect of regenerative procedures on bone level can facilitate soft tissue adaptation or more favorable dental contour, reducing the size of black triangles, and when approximating roots during orthodontic treatment, reconstruction of interdental papillae may be expected.[54,55] Orthodontic approximation of the roots and crowns will narrow the interdental papillae. If orthodontic root approximation is performed prior to periodontal surgery, it will compromise blood supply to the tip of the papilla and the surgical handling of interdental soft tissues. This could impair the efficacy of soft tissue coverage over the regenerated lesion, the stability of the blood clot, and ultimately healing.

Periodontal Regenerative Procedures Around Teeth Planned to Be Orthodontically Moved

Periodontal regenerative procedures are performed in an attempt to regenerate the lost supporting tissues. Most regenerative procedures use bone or bone substitutes in combination with membrane coverage or the application of EMD. It is up to clinicians to decide which combination of materials to use based on their experience and professional judgment. Each material and protocol has its advantages and disadvantages, which might affect the future orthodontic rate or outcome. For example, it has been shown that bone substitute interferes with bone-modeling and bone-remodeling processes.[56] The tooth movement rate is influenced by the density of the alveolar bone, and thus identical orthodontic forces will translate to different rates of tooth movement depending on the surrounding bone. As a result, orthodontic tooth movement is slower in sites with bone substitute remnants.[57,58]

BONE SUBSTITUTES

Autogenous bone is recognized as the gold standard for bone grafts thanks to the viability of transferable osteogenic cells; however, it requires a second surgery at the donor site. Consequently, various allogeneic, xenogeneic, and synthetic bone grafts have been suggested as a replacement for autogenous bone grafts.

Despite the fact that bone substitutes hinder bone remodeling, Araújo et al[59] showed that orthodontic tooth movement in the presence of xenogeneic bone grafts could be carried out with no complications. The graft material was partially resorbed on the pressure side, enhanced by the osteoclastic activity, with no signs of resorption on the tension side.

Similar observations were also made by da Silva et al.[60] To evaluate the effect of orthodontic movement following regenerative treatment, they implanted xenogeneic grafts into furcation defects in four mongrel dogs. The procedure was followed by orthodontic treatment once the healing process was complete. The test group underwent orthodontic tooth movement of the second premolars, while the premolars in the control group remained unmoved. They found no statistically significant differences between the two groups in the amount of newly developed bone and no signs of root resorption. Comparable results were reported with the use of synthetic biomaterials and bioglasses in rats.[61,62]

Deproteinized bovine bone mineral (DBBM; Bio-Oss, Geistlich) can be used as a graft material to augment an alveolar ridge defect.[63] In an animal study on five beagle dogs,[59] teeth were orthodontically moved into an area previously augmented with DBBM. No adverse effects were reported, and the bone substitute was mostly degraded and eliminated. The positive outcomes of this combined treatment were confirmed in several clinical case reports,[64] some with surgical re-entry.[65,66] However, because DBBM degrades very slowly and induces certain immune responses and fibrous encapsulation during healing,[67] its effect on future tooth movement is currently being investigated in the authors' laboratory.

Synthetic materials such as BoneCeramic (Straumann), which consists of 60% hydroxyapatite and 40% β-tricalcium phosphate, were also suggested as bone substitutes to be used in regenerative procedures. After grafting, the β-tricalcium phosphate is rapidly resorbed and completely replaced by regenerated bone.[68] The slowly resorbed hydroxyapatite serves as a useful matrix scaffold for the ingrowth of new blood vessels and for the attachment of bone-forming cells.[69] If the graft material is completely resorbed, the entire volume can be expected to be replaced by natural bone.[70] While it has been suggested that this synthetic bone substitute slows orthodontic tooth movement, it was found to have better osteoconductive potential and to induce less root resorption compared with DBBM and naturally recovered extraction sites.[71]

Uneventful results have also been demonstrated for orthodontic movements in teeth previously treated with EMD in both experimental studies[72] and human clinical case reports.[73]

GUIDED TISSUE REGENERATION

Guided tissue regeneration (GTR) requires the use of a barrier membrane (eg, a collagen membrane) either alone or together with a bone graft. Collagen membranes are designed to effectively prevent the ingrowth of soft tissues and are resorbed within a few weeks. Therefore, they may affect tooth movement.

Diedrich[72] conducted a series of experimental studies demonstrating that in the presence of both resorbable and nonresorbable barrier membranes, periodontal regeneration was achieved. Subsequent orthodontic treatment did not affect the gain of newly created periodontal structures.

Lee et al[74] used DBBM and a resorbable collagen membrane during orthodontic buccal tipping in dogs. They concluded that the application of a native (eg non-crosslinked) collagen membrane in an augmented corticotomy using DBBM might stimulate periodontal tissue re-establishment and that the collagen membrane could control the formation of mesenchymal matrix, facilitating the formation of an even bone surface.

Orthodontic Treatment After Periodontal Surgery

At present, there is no treatment protocol that points to an optimal timing for commencing orthodontic tooth movement following periodontal surgery. The authors' treatment protocols are based on clinical experience and biologic rationale.

In the case of access flap periodontal surgery, there is no need to wait for healing before beginning orthodontic treatment. In fact, in 1981 Harold Frost first described the regional accelerated phenomenon (RAP). RAP is a complex physiologic process caused by the combination of a significantly accelerated bone turnover rate and reduced regional bone density following hard and soft tissue injury. RAP usually occurs within about 10 days after surgery and can be sustained for up to 4 months.[75,76] With this method, immediate initiation of orthodontic treatment after flap elevation will accelerate the expected tooth movement.

In the case of regenerative periodontal surgery, initiation of orthodontic tooth movement might influence the regenerative result. Periodontists are mainly concerned about bone graft stability and root surface coverage during the initial stages of wound healing, since from periodontal and wound healing points of view, these are key factors to a successful regenerative outcome.[77,78] Based on the authors' clinical experience and established biologic principles, if using a resorbable membrane, it is advised that tooth movement not be initiated until the membrane has begun to resorb, as the soft tissues above the regenerated site are not yet mature until this has occurred. Initiating orthodontic tooth movement too soon will accelerate the resorption of the collagen membrane and impair the regenerative outcome.

Animal and clinical studies initiating orthodontic tooth movement at different time frames after regenerative surgery report successful results. Re et al[65] performed GTR of a circumferential bony defect at the palatal side of the central incisor using a combination of DBBM and a fibrin-fibronectin sealing system. Orthodontic tooth movement toward the palatal defect started 10 days after surgery, and in a re-entry surgery performed 6 months later, positive outcomes of the combined GTR and orthodontic treatment were seen. A human study conducted by Attia et al[79] found that orthodontic tooth movement toward the bone graft immediately after GTR resulted in more clinical attachment level gain 1 year after surgery. A study by Ahn et al[80] on beagle dogs found that orthodontic tooth movement initiated either immediately after grafting the alveolar bony defect with a DBBM graft or 2 weeks after surgery without a bone graft achieved better bone mineral density compared with orthodontic tooth movement initiated 12 weeks after surgery. Araújo et al[59] used DBBM to fill a bony defect 3 months before moving a tooth into the edentulous ridge. They observed that the grafting material degraded and was eventually eliminated during tooth movement. Their study shows that starting tooth movement 3 to 6 months after surgery does not adversely affect the regenerative process.

Orthodontic Tooth Movement Toward an Edentulous Ridge

One of the challenges facing orthodontists who treat adult patients is the maintenance or creation of an acceptable mesiodistal space for a missing tooth or teeth in order to accommodate an implant-supported prosthesis. In other cases, the treatment plan will include tooth movement to close the space created by tooth extraction. Tooth extraction is always followed by horizontal and vertical bone resorption,[81,82] subsequently limiting tooth movement into the narrow edentulous ridge. An edentulous alveolar ridge where a tooth has been missing for several years will become narrow and in some cases will comprise two cortical plates only (corticalized). Studies show that this may substantially limit tooth movement into the edentulous ridge by inhibiting bone resorption in the compression side.[83]

Goldberg and Turley[84] studied the periodontal changes associated with orthodontic space closure of an edentulous maxillary first molar area in adults. With a space closure averaging 5.3 mm, the resulting vertical bone loss averaged 1.2 mm in the second molar and 0.6 mm in the second premolar, with 60% of the teeth showing ≤ 1.5 mm of bone loss. Although space closure can be considered a potential solution in the absence of the permanent first molar, attachment loss and space reopening can be common complications.

Another consideration in orthodontic tooth movement into a narrow ridge is the risk of root exposure. There are cases in which orthodontic tooth movement will not be feasible without re-establishment of the alveolar width with bone grafts prior to tooth movement.[85] To alleviate alveolar ridge resorption and regenerate alveolar bone in the defects, bone grafts can be placed in the extraction sites immediately after tooth extraction. To avoid root exposure, Mayer et al[86] suggested performing guided bone regeneration in the edentulous area 6 months before moving a tooth into the atrophic alveolar ridge.

Coordinated periodontal and orthodontic treatment in adult patients can be useful in cases of tooth movement into an edentulous corticated ridge. If these patients require interdisciplinary dental therapy involving orthodontic treatment and regenerative surgery, coordinating surgery with tooth movement will take advantage of RAP[75] and increase the rate of tooth movement for a limited period of time, thus compensating for the reduced rate of movement resulting from age-related atrophy and corticalization of the alveolar ridge where teeth have been missing for a long time.

Periodontal Maintenance During Orthodontic Treatment

HEALTHY PATIENTS

In children and adolescents, if no signs of periodontal disease are detected at the initial examination, orthodontic treatment can be initiated following intensive oral hygiene instructions and dietary education. During treatment, the orthodontist is responsible for monitoring the oral hygiene status at each recall appointment. Adolescents have been shown to suffer from more severe gingivitis than adults during orthodontic treatment.[87] Professional checkup visits by the dental hygienist are usually performed every 3 months, but their frequency should be increased in specific cases in which there are objective impediments to proper oral hygiene maintenance. The particular aims of the dental hygienist are to *(1)* debride the sulcular areas of plaque pathogens that accumulate due to the presence of orthodontic appliances, *(2)* to motivate the patient by reinforcing the importance of maintaining good oral hygiene, and *(3)* to instruct the patient how to efficiently use adjunctive plaque-control measures such as interproximal brushes, single-tuft toothbrushes, and antibacterial and fluoride mouthwashes. In general, powered toothbrushes may promote gingival health better than manual toothbrushes, especially in orthodontic patients.[88]

In adults, the situation is more complex due to the common presence of restorations, such as crowns, partial dentures, implants, and deep interproximal restorations, which increase plaque accumulation and the risk of deterioration of a periodontal disease (see Fig 13-5). Many adult patients already suffer from initial alveolar bone loss, which can be exacerbated by supra- and subgingival plaque accumulation. Therefore, as already mentioned, a thorough dental and periodontal examination should be performed before initiating orthodontic treatment. The orthodontist should be able to recognize faulty restorations and refer the patient to the prosthodontist for their replacement. In the case of healthy periodontium, adult patients should adhere to a similar maintenance protocol as adolescents, including professional cleaning every 3 months. These intervals should decrease in cases with multiple restorations. When lingual appliances are used, visits to the dental hygienist should also be more frequent (at least once every 2 months), due to the increased difficulty in brushing an appliance situated on the lingual side of the teeth. Maintenance visits will also include periodic evaluation of periodontal pockets to recognize initial signs of attachment loss. If not otherwise indicated, vertical bitewing radiographs and periapical radiographs of anterior teeth should be taken every 6 months. The orthodontist should coordinate with the prosthodontist to ensure that caries development will not be overlooked.

PERIODONTALLY COMPROMISED PATIENTS

In periodontally compromised patients, it is the orthodontist's responsibility to screen the preliminary status of the patient, make a preliminary diagnosis, and refer the patient to a periodontist for a full periodontal examination and treatment. The orthodontist should be aware of AP in young patients, which can present not only before orthodontic therapy but also during and after active treatment. In these cases, the orthodontist should immediately involve a periodontist. The periodontist is responsible for performing a full periodontal charting and a full-mouth radiographic survey before initiation of the orthodontic treatment. Orthodontic tooth movement should not be initiated until the periodontal disease is controlled, the inflammation is reduced, and the patient proves he or she is able to comply with meticulous oral hygiene measures. During orthodontic tooth movement, the periodontal status should be closely monitored by the periodontist so that he or she is able to recognize initial signs of periodontal deterioration and adjust the periodontal and orthodontic treatment accordingly. Orthodontic tooth movements should be discontinued if the patient is not cooperating and maintaining proper oral hygiene.

In general, professional cleaning should be administered every 1 to 3 months. Its frequency should be increased when additional patient risk factors are present (eg, smoking, diabetes) and in cases of advanced or aggressive periodontal disease. Periodontal examination (full periodontal charting) should be performed every 3 to 6 months (see Fig 13-30). When an increase in periodontal probing depth or bleeding scores is detected, orthodontic tooth movement should be paused until periodontal stability is achieved. If not otherwise indicated, vertical bitewing radiographs and periapical radiographs of anterior teeth should be performed every 6 months.

In periodontally compromised patients, it is advisable to use the least plaque-accumulative orthodontic appliances in order to facilitate optimal hygiene performance for the patient. Bracket design may significantly affect bacterial accumulation and gingival inflammation. In this context, self-ligating brackets or wire ligatures rather than elastomeric ligatures have been shown to perform better.[89] Orthodontic bands should be avoided, especially on teeth treated by regenerative means. It has been demonstrated that in cases where orthodontic bands were used on anchorage teeth, the prevalence of putative periodontopathogens increased.[90] Clear aligners are superior to fixed appliances with regard to oral hygiene, as they can be removed and are not plaque retentive. Patients treated with clear aligners have been shown to have better periodontal health during orthodontic treatment than patients treated with fixed appliances.[91] Retainers also need to be selected with oral hygiene in mind.

Cases

Figures 13-3 to 13-5 illustrate orthodontic treatment in patients with severe periodontal disease.

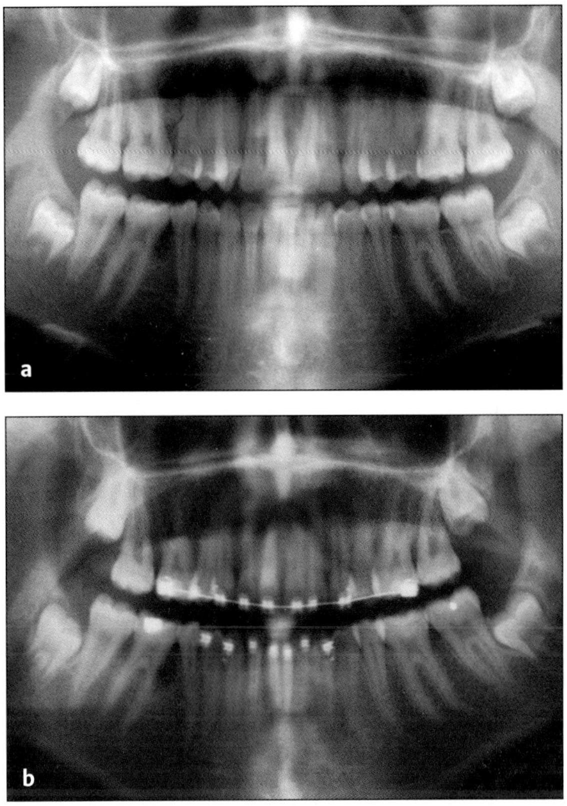

Fig 13-3 A 15-year-old girl with localized AP presented with periodontal deterioration that occurred during orthodontic treatment. *(a)* Panoramic radiograph before orthodontic treatment. There is undiagnosed bone loss around the right first molars and around the maxillary lateral and central incisors. *(b)* Significant periodontal deterioration was observed during orthodontic treatment. Orthodontic treatment was stopped at that point, and the patient was referred for periodontal consultation. →

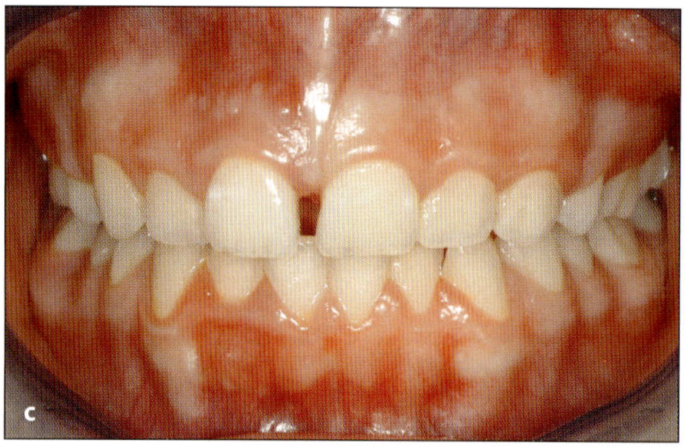

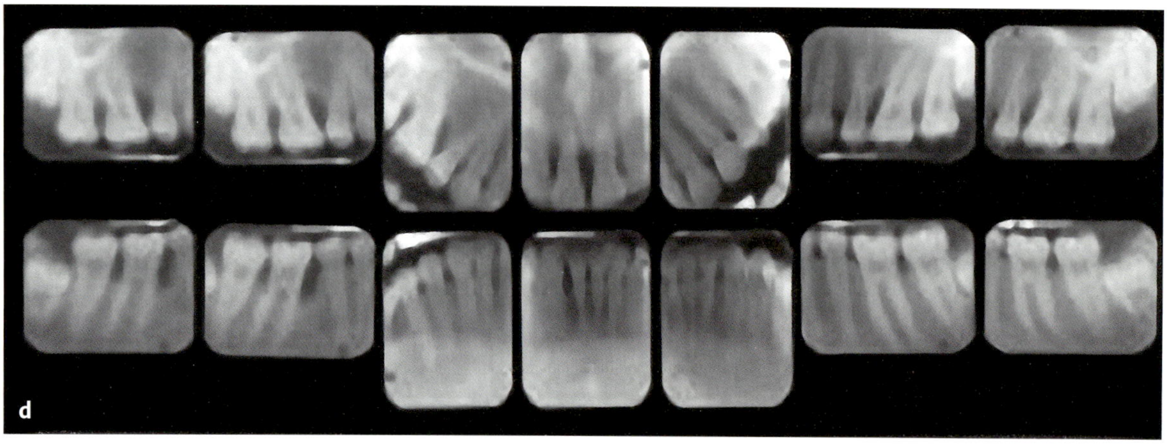

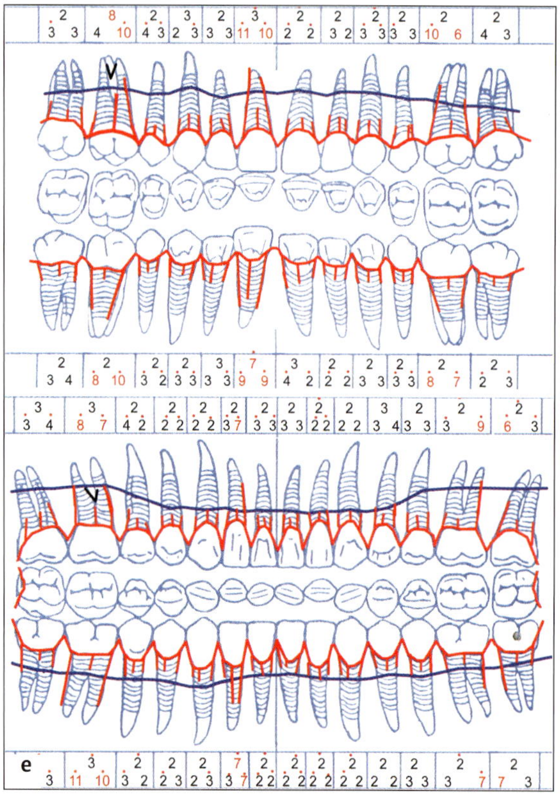

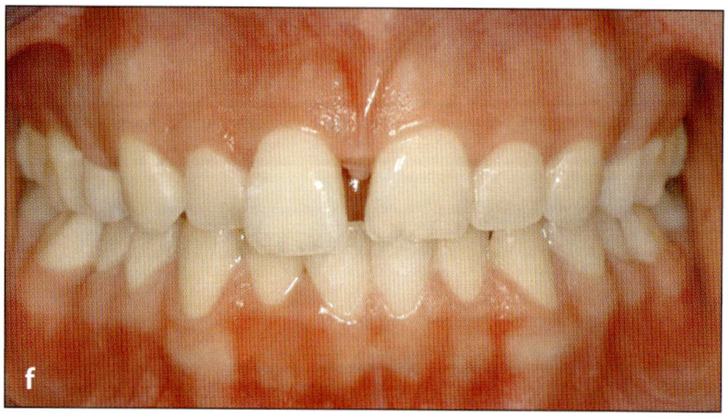

Fig 13-3 *(cont)* *(c and d)* Clinical view and periapical radiographs at the beginning of periodontal treatment. *(e)* Initial periodontal chart. *(f)* Clinical view at re-evaluation following anti-infective periodontal treatment. Note the migration of the maxillary right central incisor.

→

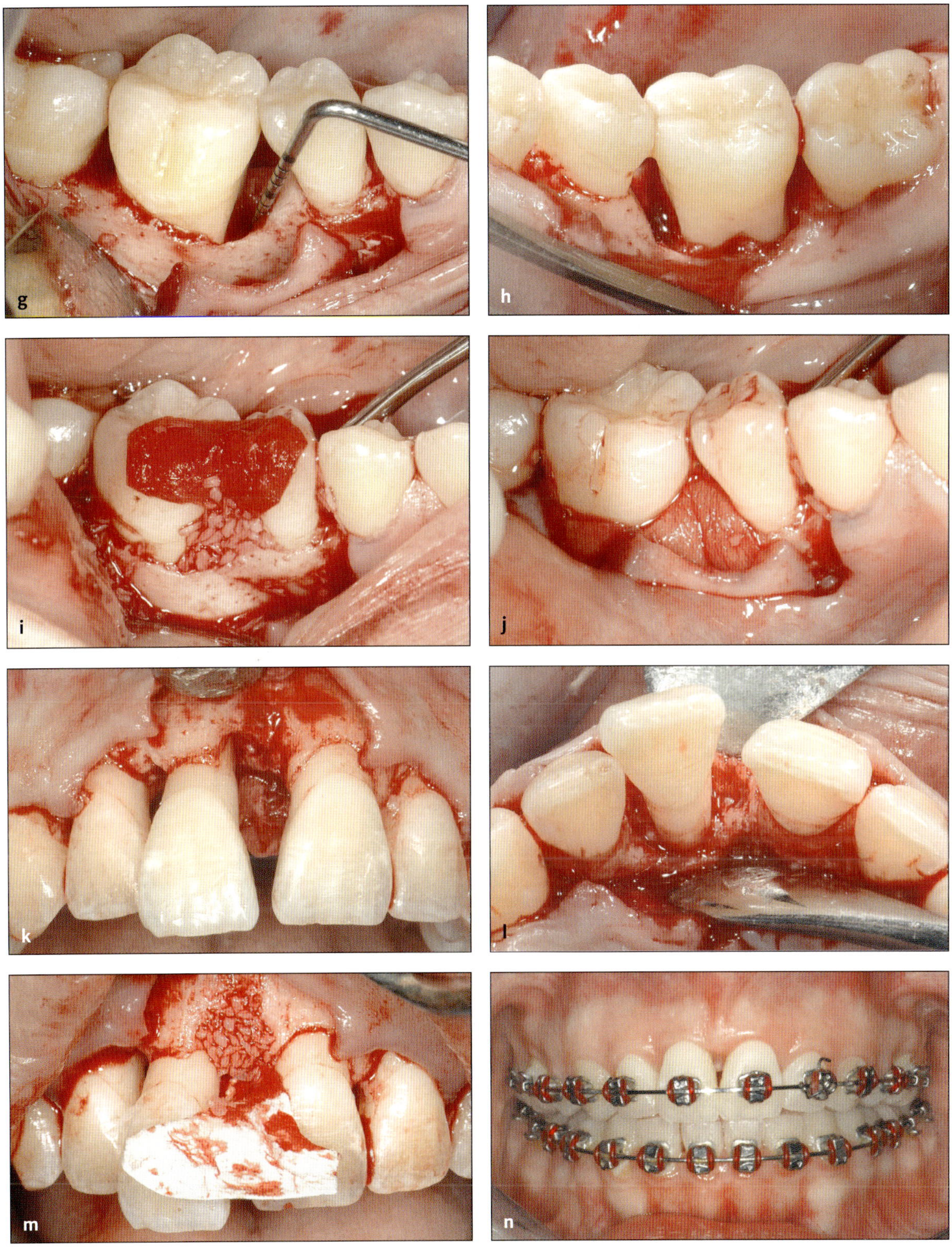

Fig 13-3 *(cont)* *(g to m)* Surgical treatment included regeneration of intrabony lesions by particulate bone allograft and resorbable collagen membrane. *(n)* Orthodontic tooth movement was initiated 8 months after the completion of periodontal surgeries. The maintenance program included supragingival professional tooth cleaning every month.

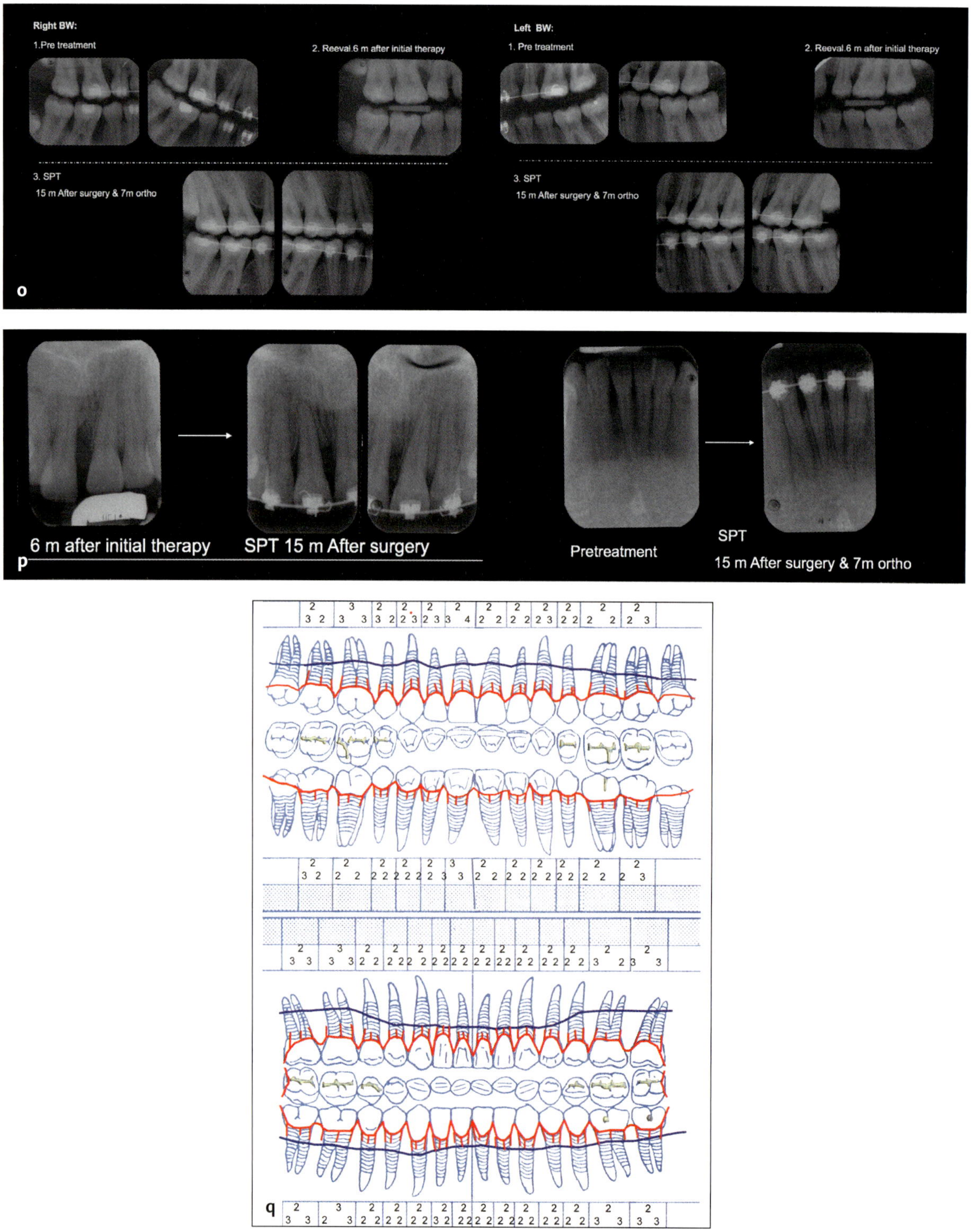

Fig 13-3 *(cont)* *(o)* Periapical radiographs taken before treatment, 6 months after initial therapy, and 15 months after periodontal surgery. *(p)* Radiographs showing alveolar bone growth after periodontal surgery and supportive periodontal therapy (SPT). *(q)* Periodontal data registered at the end of orthodontic tooth movement. (Case treated by Drs Tali Chackartchi, Ayala Stabholz, and Stella Chaushu.)

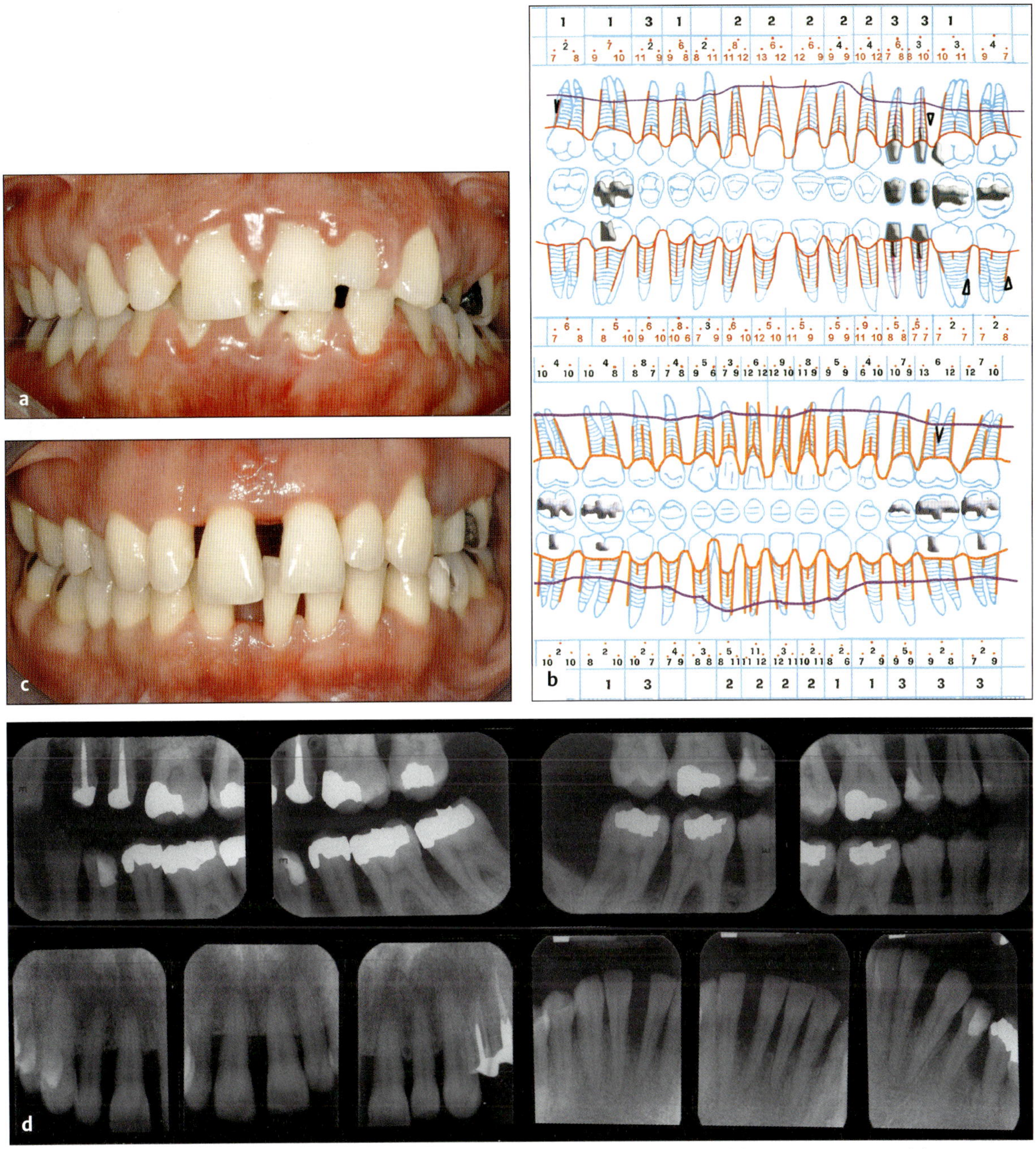

Fig 13-4 A 28-year-old woman who was 8 weeks pregnant presented with generalized AP. *(a)* Initial clinical view. *(b)* Preoperative periodontal chart showing deep pockets. Due to her pregnancy, no radiographs were taken. *(c)* Clinical view after periodontal anti-infective therapy. *(d)* Full-mouth radiographs were taken after delivery.

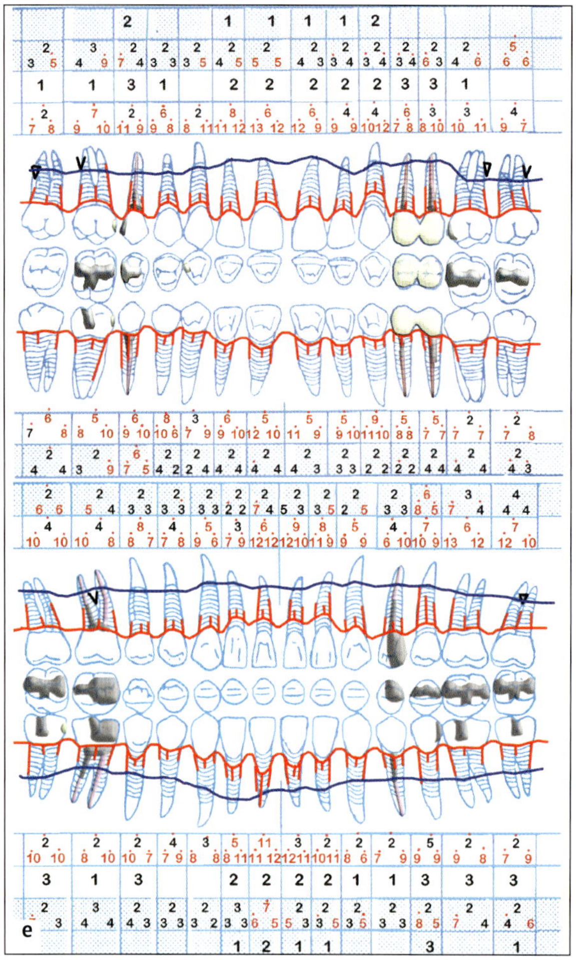

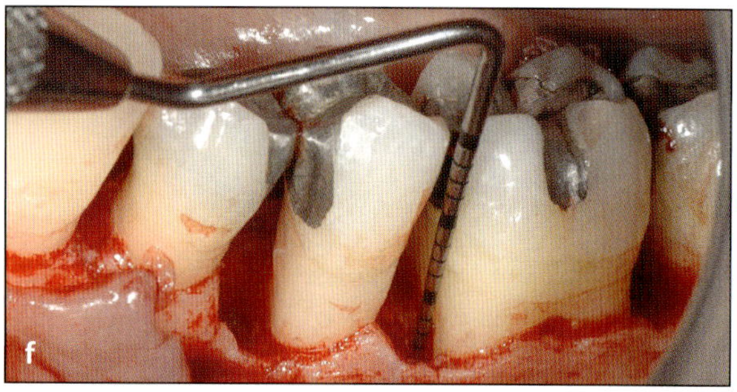

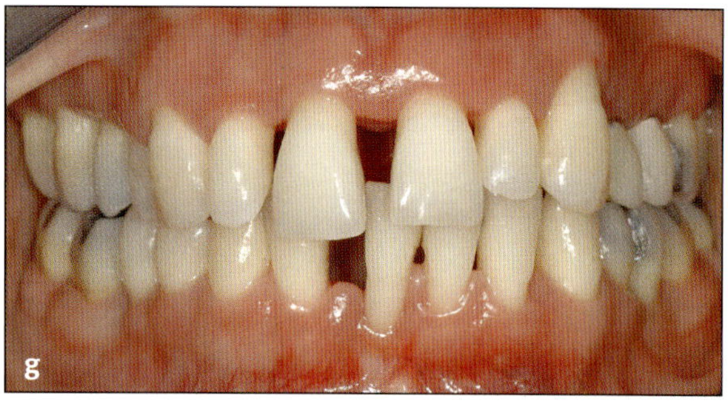

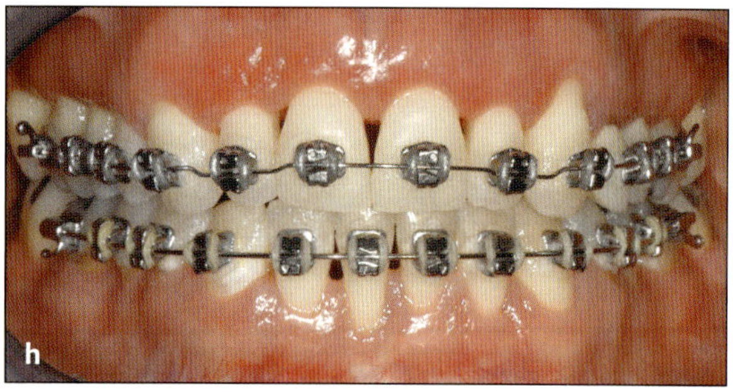

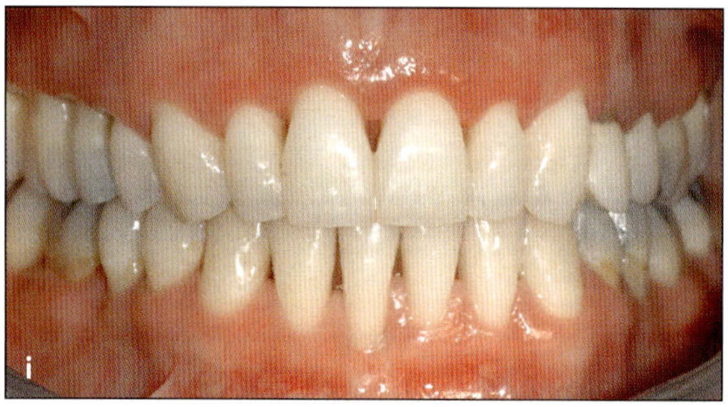

Fig 13-4 *(cont)* *(e)* Periodontal chart at re-evaluation. *(f)* Surgical clinical view shows reverse bone architecture with shallow intrabony defects. *(g)* Clinical view on completion of active periodontal treatment. *(h)* Orthodontic treatment is initiated once the periodontal disease is controlled. *(i)* Final clinical view.

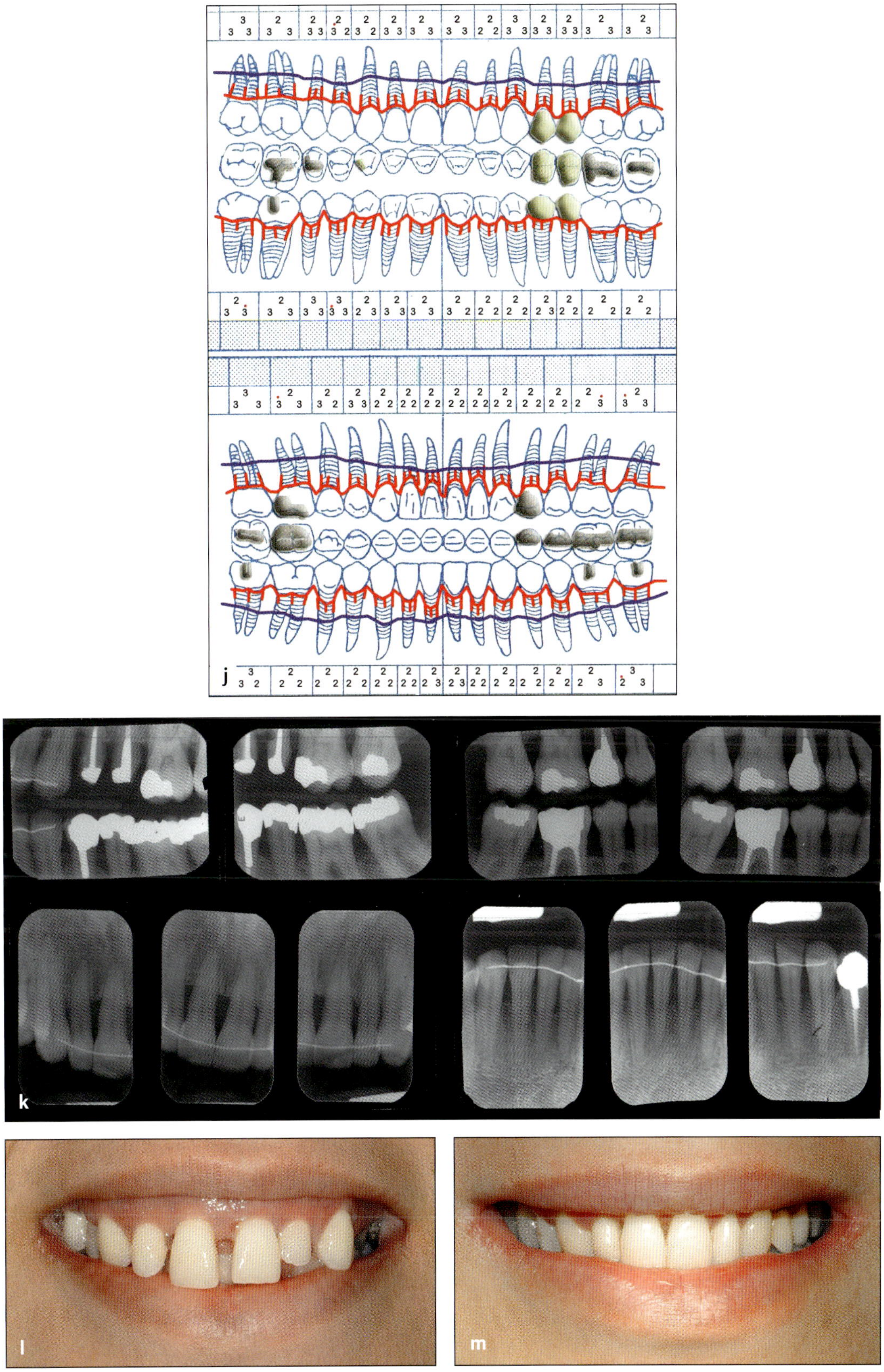

Fig 13-4 *(cont)* *(j)* Final periodontal chart. *(k)* Final radiographs. *(l and m)* Comparison of smiles before and after orthodontic treatment. (Case treated by Drs Tali Chackartchi, Ayala Stabholz, and Adrian Becker.)

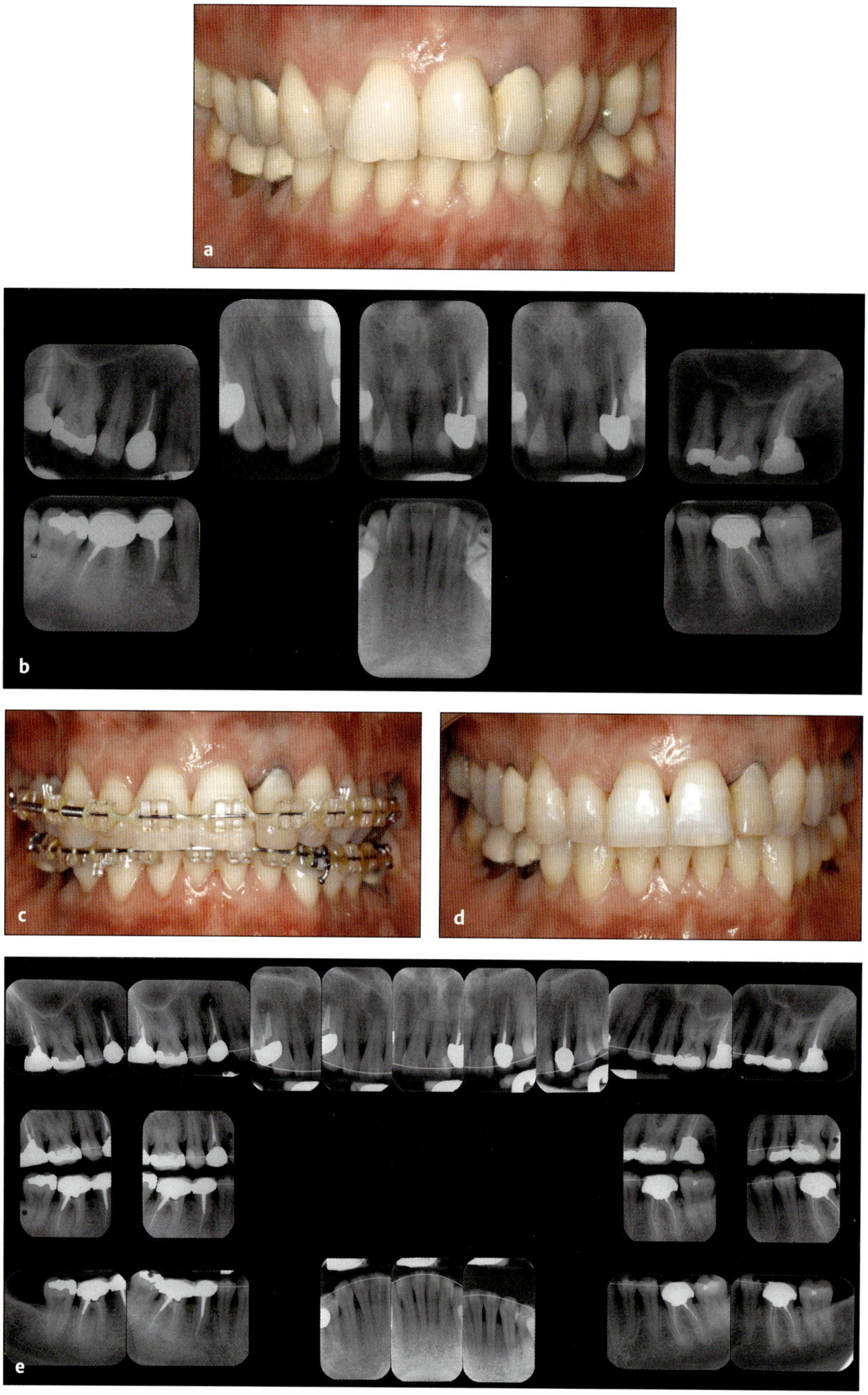

Fig 13-5 A 43-year-old woman with chronic periodontitis wanted orthodontic treatment to improve her facial esthetics. *(a)* Initial clinical view showing multiple restorations. *(b)* Initial radiographs. *(c)* Orthodontic tooth movement was initiated only after controlling the periodontal inflammation. *(d)* Final clinical view. *(e)* Final radiographs. (Case treated by Drs Tali Chackartchi and Stella Chaushu.)

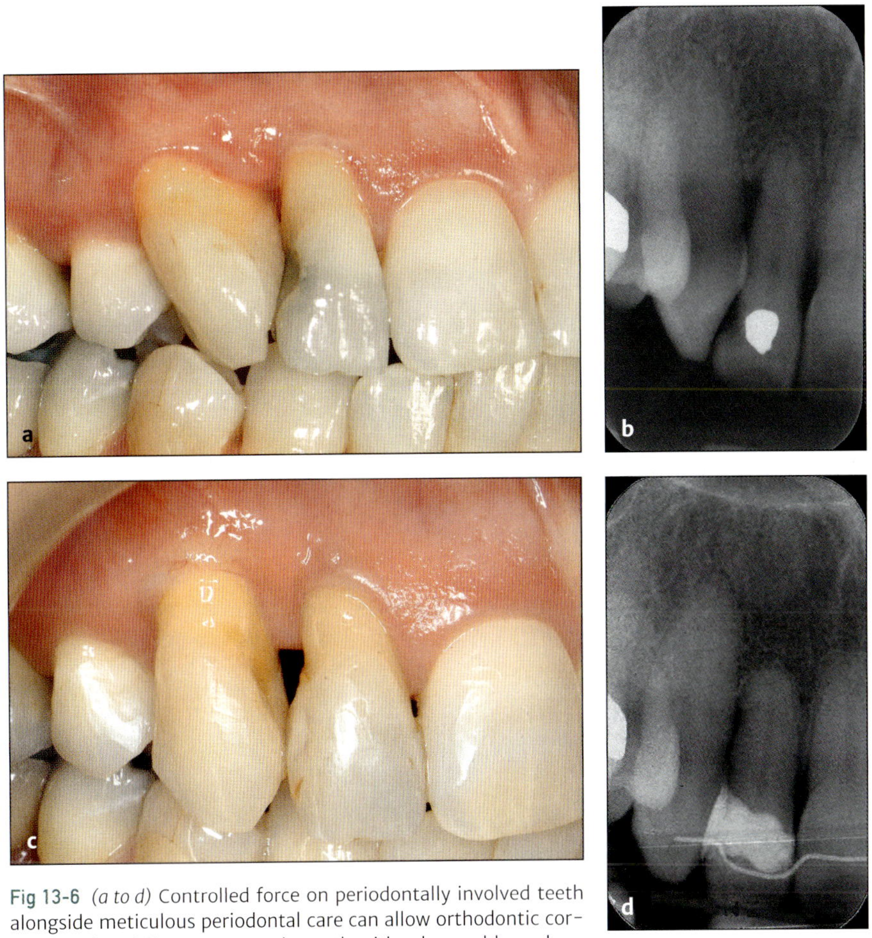

Fig 13-6 *(a to d)* Controlled force on periodontally involved teeth alongside meticulous periodontal care can allow orthodontic correction of malalignment even in teeth with advanced bone loss. (Case treated by Drs Tali Chackartchi and Ruth Gleis.)

Conclusion

An integrated treatment combining appropriate orthodontic and periodontal therapies has been shown to be effective in patients with periodontal disease undergoing orthodontic treatment. Under such conditions, long-term stable treatment outcomes are expected in most treated cases (Fig 13-6). The key for obtaining therapeutic success is that orthodontic treatment should only be performed on a periodontally healthy dentition, and this health condition should be well maintained throughout the orthodontic treatment until appliances are removed. Unfortunately, because we are treating living, variable subjects, we cannot ensure that all cases will show the same results, but the literature and the authors' clinical experience confirm that complicated perio-ortho cases can result in successful outcomes. Close monitoring is a key factor for successful treatment, allowing any points of deterioration to be identified and treated to get the periodontal health back on track.

References

1. Page RC, Kornman KS. The pathogenesis of human periodontitis: An introduction. Periodontol 2000 1997;14:9–11.
2. Armitage GC. Periodontal diagnoses and classification of periodontal diseases. Periodontol 2000 2004;34:9–21.
3. Bimstein E. Periodontal health and disease in children and adolescents. Pediatr Clin North Am 1991;38:1183–1207.
4. Kronauer E, Borsa G, Lang NP. Prevalence of incipient juvenile periodontitis at age 16 years in Switzerland. J Clin Periodontol 1986;13:103–108.
5. Clerehugh V, Lennon MA, Worthington HV. 5-year results of a longitudinal study of early periodontitis in 14- to 19-year-old adolescents. J Clin Periodontol 1990;17:702–708.
6. Parameter on chronic periodontitis with advanced loss of periodontal support [editorial]. American Academy of Periodontology. J Periodontol 2000;71:856–858.
7. Newman MG, Socransky SS, Savitt ED, Propas DA, Crawford A. Studies of the microbiology of periodontosis. J Periodontol 1976;47:373–379.
8. Mandell RL, Socransky SS. A selective medium for *Actinobacillus actinomycetemcomitans* and the incidence of the organism in juvenile periodontitis. J Periodontol 1981;52:593–598.
9. Bragd L, Dahlén G, Wikström M, Slots J. The capability of *Actinobacillus actinomycetemcomitans*, *Bacteroides gingivalis* and *Bacteroides intermedius* to indicate progressive periodontitis; A retrospective study. J Clin Periodontol 1987;14:95–99.
10. Tonetti MS, Mombelli A. Early-onset periodontitis. Ann Periodontol 1999;4:39–53.
11. Armitage GC. Development of a classification system for periodontal diseases and conditions. Ann Periodontol 1999;4:1–6.
12. Thilander B. Infrabony pockets and reduced alveolar bone height in relation to orthodontic therapy. Semin Orthod 1996;2:55–61.
13. Brunsvold MA. Pathologic tooth migration. J Periodontol 2005;76:859–866.
14. Okada K, Yamashiro T, Tenshin S, Takano-Yamamoto T. Orthodontic treatment for a patient with Pierre-Robin sequence complicated by juvenile periodontitis. Cleft Palate Craniofac J 2000;37:318–324.
15. Maeda S, Maeda Y, Ono Y, Nakamura K, Sasaki T. Interdisciplinary treatment of a patient with severe pathologic tooth migration caused by localized aggressive periodontitis. Am J Orthod Dentofacial Orthop 2005;127:374–384.
16. Passanezi E, Janson M, Janson G, Sant'Anna AP, de Freitas MR, Henriques JF. Interdisciplinary treatment of localized juvenile periodontitis: A new perspective to an old problem. Am J Orthod Dentofacial Orthop 2007;131:268–276.
17. Ishihara Y, Tomikawa K, Deguchi T, et al. Interdisciplinary orthodontic treatment for a patient with generalized aggressive periodontitis: Assessment of IgG antibodies to identify type of periodontitis and correct timing of treatment. Am J Orthod Dentofacial Orthop 2015;147:766–780.
18. Mathews DP, Kokich VG. Managing treatment for the orthodontic patient with periodontal problems. Semin Orthod 1997;3:21–38.
19. Kokich VG. Don't start without the charting. Am J Orthod Dentofacial Orthop 2011;139:S14.
20. Kassebaum NJ, Bernabé E, Dahiya M, Bhandari B, Murray CJ, Marcenes W. Global burden of severe periodontitis in 1990-2010: A systematic review and meta-regression. J Dent Res 2014;93:1045–1053.
21. Kassebaum NJ, Bernabé E, Dahiya M, Bhandari B, Murray CJ, Marcenes W. Global burden of severe tooth loss: A systematic review and meta-analysis. J Dent Res 2014;93:20S–28S.
22. Krishnan V, Davidovitch Z. The effect of drugs on orthodontic tooth movement. Orthod Craniofac Res 2006;9:163–171.
23. Gkantidis N, Christou P, Topouzelis N. The orthodontic-periodontic interrelationship in integrated treatment challenges: A systematic review. J Oral Rehabil 2010;37:377–390.
24. Bridges T, King G, Mohammed A. The effect of age on tooth movement and mineral density in the alveolar tissues of the rat. Am J Orthod Dentofacial Orthop 1988;93:245–250.
25. Bagga D. Adult orthodontics versus adolescent orthodontics: An overview. J Oral Health Comm Dent 2010;4:42–47.
26. Alstad S, Zachrisson BU. Longitudinal study of periodontal condition associated with orthodontic treatment in adolescents. Am J Orthod 1979;76:277–286.
27. Boyd RL, Leggott PJ, Quinn RS, Eakle WS, Chambers D. Periodontal implications of orthodontic treatment in adults with reduced or normal periodontal tissues versus those of adolescents. Am J Orthod Dentofacial Orthop 1989;96:191–198.
28. Ong G. Periodontal disease and tooth loss. Int Dent J 1998;48:233–238.
29. Garat JA, Gordillo ME, Ubios AM. Bone response to different strength orthodontic forces in animals with periodontitis. J Periodontal Res 2005;40:441–445.
30. Geraci TF, Nevins M, Crossetti HW, Drizen K, Ruben MP. Reattachment of the periodontium after tooth movement into an osseous defect in a monkey. 1. Int J Periodontics Restorative Dent 1990;10:184–197.
31. Lindhe J, Svanberg G. Influence of trauma from occlusion on progression of experimental periodontitis in the beagle dog. J Clin Periodontol 1974;1:3–14.
32. Ericsson I, Thilander B, Lindhe J, Okamoto H. The effect of orthodontic tilting movements on the periodontal tissues of infected and non-infected dentitions in dogs. J Clin Periodontol 1977;4:278–293.
33. Re S, Corrente G, Abundo R, Cardaropoli D. Orthodontic treatment in periodontally compromised patients: 12-year report. Int J Periodontics Restorative Dent 2000;20:31–39.
34. Wennström JL, Stokland BL, Nyman S, Thilander B. Periodontal tissue response to orthodontic movement of teeth with infrabony pockets. Am J Orthod Dentofacial Orthop 1993;103:313–319.
35. Krishnan V, Davidovitch Z. On a path to unfolding the biological mechanisms of orthodontic tooth movement. J Dent Res 2009;88:597–608.

36. Ren Y, Maltha JC, Van't Hof MA, Von Den Hoff JW, Kuijpers-Jagtman AM, Zhang D. Cytokine levels in crevicular fluid are less responsive to orthodontic force in adults than in juveniles. J Clin Periodontol 2002;29:757–762.
37. Bletsa A, Berggreen E, Brudvik P. Interleukin-1α and tumor necrosis factor-α expression during the early phases of orthodontic tooth movement in rats. Eur J Oral Sci 2006;114:423–429.
38. Krishnan V, Davidovitch Z. Cellular, molecular, and tissue-level reactions to orthodontic force. Am J Orthod Dentofacial Orthop 2006;129:469.e1–32.
39. Uematsu S, Mogi M, Deguchi T. Increase of transforming growth factor-β 1 in gingival crevicular fluid during human orthodontic tooth movement. Arch Oral Biol 1996;41:1091–1095.
40. Ren Y, Vissink A. Cytokines in crevicular fluid and orthodontic tooth movement. Eur J Oral Sci 2008;116:89–97.
41. Nogueira AVB, de Souza J, de Molon RS, et al. HMGB1 localization during experimental periodontitis. Mediators Inflamm 2014;2014:816320.
42. Nogueira AV, de Molon RS, Nokhbehsaim M, Deschner J, Cirelli JA. Contribution of biomechanical forces to inflammation-induced bone resorption. J Clin Periodontol 2017;44:31–41.
43. Harrel SK, Nunn ME. The effect of occlusal discrepancies on periodontitis. II. Relationship of occlusal treatment to the progression of periodontal disease. J Periodontol 2001;72:495–505.
44. Kirschneck C, Fanghänel J, Wahlmann U, Wolf M, Roldán JC, Proff P. Interactive effects of periodontitis and orthodontic tooth movement on dental root resorption, tooth movement velocity and alveolar bone loss in a rat model. Ann Anat 2017;210:32–43.
45. Sallum EJ, Nouer DF, Klein MI, et al. Clinical and microbiologic changes after removal of orthodontic appliances. Am J Orthod Dentofacial Orthop 2004;126:363–366.
46. Lee SM, Yoo SY, Kim HS, et al. Prevalence of putative periodontopathogens in subgingival dental plaques from gingivitis lesions in Korean orthodontic patients. J Microbiol 2005;43:260–265.
47. Corrente G, Abundo R, Re S, Cardaropoli D, Cardaropoli G. Orthodontic movement into infrabony defects in patients with advanced periodontal disease: A clinical and radiological study. J Periodontol 2003;74:1104–1109.
48. Axelsson P, Lindhe J. The significance of maintenance care in the treatment of periodontal disease. J Clin Periodontol 1981;8:281–294.
49. Papapanou PN, Wennström JL. The angular bony defect as indicator of further alveolar bone loss. J Clin Periodontol 1991;18:317–322.
50. Caffesse RG, Sweeney PL, Smith BA. Scaling and root planing with and without periodontal flap surgery. J Clin Periodontol 1986;13:205–210.
51. Tsitoura E, Tucker R, Suvan J, Laurell L, Cortellini P, Tonetti M. Baseline radiographic defect angle of the intrabony defect as a prognostic indicator in regenerative periodontal surgery with enamel matrix derivative. J Clin Periodontol 2004;31:643–647.
52. Melsen B, Agerbaek N, Eriksen J, Terp S. New attachment through periodontal treatment and orthodontic intrusion. Am J Orthod Dentofacial Orthop 1988;94:104–116.
53. Sculean A, Nikolidakis D, Nikou G, Ivanovic A, Chapple IL, Stavropoulos A. Biomaterials for promoting periodontal regeneration in human intrabony defects: A systematic review. Periodontol 2000 2015;68:182–216.
54. Cardaropoli D, Re S, Corrente G, Abundo R. Reconstruction of the maxillary midline papilla following a combined orthodontic-periodontic treatment in adult periodontal patients. J Clin Periodontol 2004;31:79–84.
55. Cardaropoli D, Re S. Interdental papilla augmentation procedure following orthodontic treatment in a periodontal patient. J Periodontol 2005;76:655–661.
56. Stavropoulos A, Kostopoulos L, Mardas N, Randel Nyengaard J, Karring T. Deproteinized bovine bone used as an adjunct to guided bone augmentation: An experimental study in the rat. Clin Implant Dent Relat Res 2001;3:156–165.
57. Deguchi T, Takano-Yamamoto T, Yabuuchi T, Ando R, Roberts WE, Garetto LP. Histomorphometric evaluation of alveolar bone turnover between the maxilla and the mandible during experimental tooth movement in dogs. Am J Orthod Dentofacial Orthop 2008;133:889–897.
58. Sidiropoulou-Chatzigiannis S, Kourtidou M, Tsalikis L. The effect of osteoporosis on periodontal status, alveolar bone and orthodontic tooth movement. A literature review. J Int Acad Periodontol 2007;9:77–84.
59. Araújo MG, Carmagnola D, Berglundh T, Thilander B, Lindhe J. Orthodontic movement in bone defects augmented with Bio-Oss. An experimental study in dogs. J Clin Periodontol 2001;28:73–80.
60. da Silva VC, Cirelli CC, Ribeiro FS, Costa MR, Comelli Lia RC, Cirelli JA. Orthodontic movement after periodontal regeneration of class II furcation: A pilot study in dogs. J Clin Periodontol 2006;33:440–448.
61. Hossain MZ, Kyomen S, Tanne K. Biologic responses of autogenous bone and beta-tricalcium phosphate ceramics transplanted into bone defects to orthodontic forces. Cleft Palate Craniofac J 1996;33:277–283.
62. Kawamoto T, Motohashi N, Kitamura A, et al. A histological study on experimental tooth movement into bone induced by recombinant human bone morphogenetic protein-2 in beagle dogs. Cleft Palate Craniofac J 2002;39:439–448.
63. Norton MR, Odell EW, Thompson ID, Cook RJ. Efficacy of bovine bone mineral for alveolar augmentation: A human histologic study. Clin Oral Implants Res 2003;14:775–783.
64. Cardaropoli D. Orthodontics for the adult periodontal patient: First or second choice treatment? Prog Orthod 2009;10:88–96.
65. Re S, Corrente G, Abundo R, Cardaropoli D. Orthodontic movement into bone defects augmented with bovine bone mineral and fibrin sealer: A reentry case report. Int J Periodontics Restorative Dent 2002;22:138–145.
66. Cardaropoli D, Re S, Manuzzi W, Gaveglio L, Cardaropoli G. Bio-Oss collagen and orthodontic movement for the treatment of infrabony defects in the esthetic zone. Int J Periodontics Restorative Dent 2006;26:553–559.
67. Artzi Z, Tal H, Dayan D. Porous bovine bone mineral in healing of human extraction sockets. Part 1: Histomorphometric evaluations at 9 months. J Periodontol 2000;71:1015–1023.

68. Piattelli A, Scarano A, Mangano C. Clinical and histologic aspects of biphasic calcium phosphate ceramic (BCP) used in connection with implant placement. Biomaterials 1996;17:1767–1770.
69. Cordaro L, Bosshardt DD, Palattella P, Rao W, Serino G, Chiapasco M. Maxillary sinus grafting with Bio-Oss or Straumann BoneCeramic: Histomorphometric results from a randomized controlled multicenter clinical trial. Clin Oral Implants Res 2008;19:796–803.
70. Mardas N, Chadha V, Donos N. Alveolar ridge preservation with guided bone regeneration and a synthetic bone substitute or a bovine-derived xenograft: A randomized, controlled clinical trial. Clin Oral Implants Res 2010;21:688–698.
71. Ru N, Liu SS, Bai Y, Li S, Liu Y, Wei X. BoneCeramic graft regenerates alveolar defects but slows orthodontic tooth movement with less root resorption. Am J Orthod Dentofacial Orthop 2016;149:523–532.
72. Diedrich PR. Guided tissue regeneration associated with orthodontic therapy. Semin Orthod 1996;2:39–45.
73. Ogihara S, Wang HL. Periodontal regeneration with or without limited orthodontics for the treatment of 2- or 3-wall infrabony defects. J Periodontol 2010;81:1734–1742.
74. Lee DY, Ahn HW, Herr Y, Kwon YH, Kim SH, Kim EC. Periodontal responses to augmented corticotomy with collagen membrane application during orthodontic buccal tipping in dogs. Biomed Res Int 2014;2014:873–918.
75. Yaffe A, Fine N, Binderman I. Regional accelerated phenomenon in the mandible following mucoperiosteal flap surgery. J Periodontol 1994;65:79–83.
76. Frost HM. The biology of fracture healing. An overview for clinicians. Part II. Clin Orthop Relat Res 1989;(248):294–309.
77. Wikesjö UM, Crigger M, Nilvéus R, Selvig KA. Early healing events at the dentin-connective tissue interface. Light and transmission electron microscopy observations. J Periodontol 1991;62:5–14.
78. Haney JM, Nilvéus RE, McMillan PJ, Wikesjö UM. Periodontal repair in dogs: Expanded polytetrafluoroethylene barrier membranes support wound stabilization and enhance bone regeneration. J Periodontol 1993;64:883–890.
79. Attia MS, Shoreibah EA, Ibrahim SA, Nassar HA. Regenerative therapy of osseous defects combined with orthodontic tooth movement. J Int Acad Periodontol 2012;14:17–25.
80. Ahn HW, Ohe JY, Lee SH, Park YG, Kim SJ. Timing of force application affects the rate of tooth movement into surgical alveolar defects with grafts in beagles. Am J Orthod Dentofacial Orthop 2014;145:486–495.
81. Tan WL, Wong TL, Wong MC, Lang NP. A systematic review of post-extractional alveolar hard and soft tissue dimensional changes in humans. Clin Oral Implants Res 2012;23(suppl 5):1–21.
82. Araújo MG, Silva CO, Misawa M, Sukekava F. Alveolar socket healing: What can we learn? Periodontol 2000 2015;68:122–134.
83. Graber LW, Vanarsdall RL, Vig KWL. Orthodontics: Current Principles & Techniques. Philadelphia: Elsevier/Mosby, 2012.
84. Goldberg D, Turley PK. Orthodontic space closure of the edentulous maxillary first molar area in adults. Int J Adult Orthodon Orthognath Surg 1989;4:255–266.
85. Kaminishi R, Davis WH, Hochwald D, Berger R, Davis C. Reconstruction of alveolar width for orthodontic tooth movement: A case report. Am J Orthod 1986;89:342–345.
86. Mayer T, Basdra EK, Komposch G, Staehle HJ. Localized alveolar ridge augmentation before orthodontic treatment. A case report. Int J Oral Maxillofac Surg 1994;23:226–228.
87. Kudirkaite I, Lopatiene K, Zubiene J, Saldunaite K. Age and gender influence on oral hygiene among adolescents with fixed orthodontic appliances. Stomatologija 2016;18:61–65.
88. Al Makhmari SA, Kaklamanos EG, Athanasiou AE. Short-term and long-term effectiveness of powered toothbrushes in promoting periodontal health during orthodontic treatment: A systematic review and meta-analysis. Am J Orthod Dentofacial Orthop 2017;152:753–766.e7.
89. Alves de Souza R, Borges de Araújo Magnani MB, Nouer DF, et al. Periodontal and microbiologic evaluation of 2 methods of archwire ligation: Ligature wires and elastomeric rings. Am J Orthod Dentofacial Orthop 2008;134:506–512.
90. Mártha K, Lőrinczi L, Bică C, Gyergyay R, Petcu B, Lazăr L. Assessment of periodontopathogens in subgingival biofilm of banded and bonded molars in early phase of fixed orthodontic treatment. Acta Microbiol Immunol Hung 2016;63:103–113.
91. Azaripour A, Weusmann J, Mahmoodi B, et al. Braces versus Invisalign: Gingival parameters and patients' satisfaction during treatment: A cross-sectional study. BMC Oral Health 2015;15:69.

INDEX

Page references followed by "f" denote figures; those followed by "t" denote tables; and those followed by "b" denote boxes.

A

Access flap periodontal surgery, 194, 196
Acellular afibrillar cementum, 72, 72f, 73t
Acellular extrinsic fiber cementum, 72, 73t
Acquired pellicle
  biomaterial surface properties effect on formation of, 49–51, 50f–51f
  cementum, 50
  enamel
    biomaterial surface properties effect on formation of, 49–50
    definition of, 27, 38
  formation of, 49, 51f
  functions of, 49
  microbial colonization of, 51
  structure of, 49
Activator protein 1, 3
Adhesins, 28
Adolescents
  aggressive periodontitis in, 190–191
  data collection, diagnosis, and periodontal monitoring in, 192–193
  periodontal considerations in, 189–191
Age. *See also* Adolescents; Children; Young adults.
  bone affected by, 16–19
  gingival recessions and, 79
  orthodontic tooth movement affected by, 21
  osteoporosis associated with, 16–19
  periodontal disease prevalence affected by, 191
  periodontal ligament affected by, 19–20, 20f
  periodontal tissues affected by, 3
Aggregatibacter actinomycetemcomitans, 162, 190
Aggressive periodontitis, 190–191, 203f
Aligner treatment, 170, 199
Alkaline phosphatase, 8, 20
Altered active eruption, 115
Altered passive eruption, 115
Alveolar bone
  anatomy of, 4, 73–74, 74f
  bundle bone of, 74, 74f
  cells of, 4
  compact bone versus, 4
  composition of, 4, 73–74
  cortical bone, 73
  lamina dura of, 4
  masticatory forces on, 4, 10
  mechanical stress on, 3
  periodontal ligament effect on, 9
  remodeling of, 10
  resorption of, 10f
  thickness of, 74
Alveolar bone proper, 4, 73
Alveolar crest
  description of, 74
  gingival margin and, average distance between, 109
Alveolar mucosa, 139
Alveolar ridge
  augmentation surgery for, 144f
  edentulous, 197
  resorption of, 197
Anchorage, for impacted maxillary canines, 149–150, 150f–151f
Antiseptics, 54
Apically positioned flap, for labially impacted maxillary canines, 138, 140f, 143–145, 144f–145f
Attached gingiva, 75, 95, 97, 115, 139
Autogenous free gingival grafting, 95

B

Bacteria. *See also* Biofilms; Plaque.
  adherence of, 27
  bonding material effects on accumulation of, 39–40
  bracket accumulation of, 36f, 36–38
  colonization of, 27–28
  ligation effects on accumulation of, 38–39, 39f
  microbiologic analysis of, 63
  orthodontic treatment effects on, 162–163
  periodontopathogenic, 38, 163f
  supragingival tooth surface colonization of, 35
Bands, orthodontic. *See* Orthodontic bands.
Basic multicellular unit, 5f, 5–6
Basic periodontal examination, 61–62
ß-tricalcium phosphate, 196
Biofilms. *See also* Bacteria.
  adsorption of, 43
  bioadhesive activity of, 44
  biomaterial accumulation of, 43–44, 49
  bonding material effects on accumulation of, 39–40
  bracket effects on, 30
  Candida albicans in, 29
  definition of, 27, 33–34
  formation of, 27, 28f
  lactobacilli in, 29
  ligation effects on accumulation of, 38–39, 39f
  maturation of, 44
  microbial diversity in, 28, 34
  oral disease and, 28–29
  periodontopathogen formation of, 38
  plaque. *See* Plaque.
Biologic width, 109, 111
Biomaterials
  biofilm accumulation on, 43–44, 49
  saliva-coated, 49
  substrate definition, 44–45
  substrate modification, 45–47, 46f–47f
  surface of
    acquired pellicle formation affected by, 49–51, 50f–51f
    calculus formation affected by, 53–54
    cell attachment and organization on, 47–49
    interactions occurring at, 46f
    plaque formation affected by, 51f–52f, 51–53
    properties of, 44–49, 45f
    protein adsorption on, 46–47, 47f
    roughness of, 45, 48, 51
    stains affected by, 53–54
    texture of, 45
    thermal mobility of, 45
    water monolayer, 45–46
  wear debris, 48
Bisphosphonates, 18, 193
Bleeding on probing, 59, 61–62
BMPs. *See* Bone morphogenetic proteins.
Bone
  aging effects on, 16–19
  biology of, 5–7
  bisphosphonates' effect on, 18
  formation of
    osteoblasts in, 12
    signal transduction pathways in, 12–14
  resorption of, 14. *See also* Root resorption.
Bone loss
  marginal, 165–166
  periodontal disease as cause of, 175, 176f, 178f
Bone morphogenetic proteins, 5–6

Bone remodeling
  control of, 3, 10
  cycle of, 6
  definition of, 5
  neurotransmitters in, 15
Bone remodeling unit, 5
Bone sounding, 115, 117f
Bone substitutes, 195–196
Bony dehiscences, 79, 94, 101
BoP. *See* Bleeding on probing.
BPE. *See* Basic periodontal examination.
Brackets
  biofilm formation affected by, 30
  gingival index in patients with, 36
  materials for, 38, 38f
  plaque accumulation, 36f, 36–38, 38f, 199
  self-ligating, 38–39, 168f, 168–169, 199
Bundle bone, 74, 74f
Busulfan/cyclophosphamide, 193

C

CAL. *See* Clinical attachment level.
Calculus, 53–54
Candida albicans, 29
Canines, impacted maxillary. *See* Impacted maxillary canines.
Case studies
  orthodontic treatment in periodontal diseases, 199f–207f
  periodontal therapy, 64–68, 64f–68f
Cause-related therapy, 60, 194
CBCT. *See* Cone beam computed tomography.
CEJ. *See* Cementoenamel junction.
Cell(s). *See also specific cell.*
  biomaterial surface attachment and organization of, 47–49
  periodontal ligament, 3, 8–9, 72, 179
Cell-adhesion molecules, 3
Cellular intrinsic fiber cementum, 72, 73t
Cellular mixed stratified cementum, 72, 73t
Cement(s)
  glass-ionomer. *See* Glass-ionomer cements.
  plaque bacteria affected by, 40
Cementoenamel junction, 71, 110
Cementum, 71–72, 72f
Center of resistance, 177–178, 178f
Cetylpyridinium chloride, 40
Chemotherapy, 193
Children
  data collection, diagnosis, and periodontal monitoring in, 192–193
  periodontal considerations in, 189–191
Chronic periodontitis, 37, 206f
Cigarette smoking, 60
Clark's rule, 122
Cleidocranial dysplasia, 7, 8f
Clinical attachment level, 62
Clinical attachment loss, 164
Closed eruption
  for labially impacted maxillary canines, 145–147, 146f
  for palatally impacted maxillary canines, 148, 149f
Collagen fibers, 4, 9
Compact bone, 4
Cone beam computed tomography
  impacted maxillary canine applications of
    conventional radiographs, 123
    crown and root morphology, 124–125
    depth of impaction, 127–129, 128f–129f
    ectopic growth, 131, 132f
    proximity of impacted teeth to roots of adjacent teeth, 125, 126f
    3D orientation, 125–127, 126f
    3D simulation of tooth movement, 129, 131f
  mucogingival junction on, 139–141, 140f–141f
  rapid palatal expansion, 102
Cone effect, 175, 177f, 179
Connective tissue grafts, 82, 83f–84f, 85, 95
Continuous arch technique, 176
Core-binding factor subunit α1, 7, 12
Coronally advanced envelope technique, 83, 85
Coronally advanced flap, 83, 83f, 85
Corrective phase, of periodontal therapy, 61
Cortical bone, 16, 73
Crown lengthening, surgical
  adjacent teeth considerations, 110
  biologic width, 109, 111
  bone removal, 111, 112f–113f
  crown-to-root ratio, 110
  esthetic
    concerns regarding, 110–111
    gummy smile treated with, 114–116, 116f–117f
  free gingival margin after, 113
  gingival overgrowth treated with, 108f
  indications for, 107, 107b
  interocclusal space and, 110
  minimum dimensional requirements, 109–110
  pretreatment planning of, 109–111, 118
  root trunk anatomy, 110
  summary of, 118
  technique for, 111–113, 112f
  wound healing after, dimensional changes during, 113–114
Crown-to-root ratio, 110
Cytokines. *See also specific cytokine.*
  in bone resorption, 14
  definition of, 5, 14
  during orthodontic treatment, 192
  osteoclast activity regulated by, 3

D

DBBM. *See* Deproteinized bovine bone mineral.
Deep bite, 184f, 186f
Dental adhesives, 39
Dental alloys, extrinsic staining of, 54
Dental caries
  bacteria that cause, 36
  plaque in, 34
Dental hygienist, 198
Denture polymers, stains on, 54
Deproteinized bovine bone mineral, 195–197
Dicalcium phosphate dihydrate, 53
Digital Imaging and Communications in Medicine, 103
Dimethylaminohexadecyl methacrylate, 30
Disuse osteoporosis, 17
Drug history, 193
Dysbiosis, 29, 34

E

Ecological plaque hypothesis, 34
Edentulous ridge, 197
Elastic ligatures, 38–39, 39f
Enamel demineralization, 36, 36f, 40
Enamel matrix derivative, 82, 195
Epithelial cell rests of Malassez, 72
ERK1/2, 17
Esthetic crown lengthening
  concerns regarding, 110–111
  gummy smile treated with, 114–116, 116f–117f

F

Family history, 60
Fibroblasts, periodontal ligament
  aging effects on, 19, 20f
  description of, 3–4, 8–9
  mechanical stimulation of, 11
  senescence of, 20

Focal adhesions, 12
Force
  controlled, 207f
  masticatory, 4, 10
  for orthodontic tooth movement, 177–179, 192
Foreign-body granulomatous reactions, 48
Free gingiva, 74–75
Free gingival margin
  location of, 114
  after surgical crown lengthening, 113
Furcation involvement, 62
Fusobacterium nucleatum, 36–37

G

Genetic theory, of impacted maxillary canines, 122
Gingiva
  anatomy of, 74–75, 75f
  attached, 75, 95, 97, 115
  biotypes of, 76f, 76–77, 93, 103
  cluster analysis of, 76
  connective tissue of, 75
  drug-induced hyperplasia of, 193
  enlargement of, 162–164
  inflammation of, 40, 109
  junctional epithelium of, 75
  oral gingival epithelium of, 75, 75f
  oral sulcular epithelium of, 75, 75f
  overgrowth of, 108f
  phenotype of, 76–77, 93, 94f
  probe transparency through, 76f, 77
  recession of. *See* Gingival recession.
  thick-flat, 76, 76f, 93, 94f, 142f
  thickness of, 77
  thin-scalloped, 76f, 76–77, 93, 94f, 97, 142f
Gingival augmentation, 94–95
Gingival bleeding index, 163
Gingival index, 163
Gingival recession
  age and, 79
  bony dehiscences as risk factor for, 94
  causative pathogenic factors for, 80
  classification of, 78f, 78–79, 83f–87f
  craniofacial morphology and, 167
  definition of, 78, 93
  etiology of, 79–80
  gingival augmentation for, 94–95
  gingival biotypes associated with, 77
  gingival phenotype as risk factor for, 93, 94f
  incisor proclination as source of, 94, 97
  lingual retainer as cause of, 80–81
  in mandibular teeth, 93
  in maxillary teeth, 93
  mechanical trauma as cause of, 94
  Miller classification of, 78, 78f, 83f–87f
  orthodontic tooth movement and, 80–81, 94, 166–167, 167f–168f
  pathogenesis of, 93–94
  periodontal disease as cause of, 94, 166
  plaque accumulation as cause of, 80
  predisposing pathogenic factors for, 79
  prevalence of, 79, 93, 166
  risk factors for, 167
  root coverage treatment of
    connective tissue graft for, 82, 83f–84f, 85
    coronally advanced envelope technique for, 83, 85
    coronally advanced flap for, 83, 83f, 85
    esthetic outcome after, factors that affect, 85, 88
    flap procedures, 82–85, 83f–85f
    goals for, 82
    grafts for, 82
    indications for, 81–82
    laterally closed tunnel for, 83, 83f
    laterally sliding flap for, 82
    modified coronally advanced tunnel for, 83, 84f–87f
    outcomes of, 82f
  traumatic tooth brushing as cause of, 94
Gingivectomy
  description of, 111, 115
  labially impacted maxillary canines treated with, 141–143, 142f–143f
Gingivoplasty, 115
Glass-ionomer cements
  antimicrobial effect of, 39–40
  pellicle formation and, 51
Grafts
  connective tissue, 82, 83f–84f, 85, 95
  orthodontic treatment and, 95–97
Ground substance, 4, 9
Growth factors, 6
GTPases, 3, 12
GTR. *See* Guided tissue regeneration.
Guidance theory, of impacted maxillary canines, 122
Guided bone regeneration, 103
Guided tissue regeneration, 196–197
Gummy smile
  clinical conditions associated with, 115t
  esthetic crown lengthening for, 114–116, 116f–117f

H

Haas expander, 99, 100f
Haversian canal, 74
Hyrax expander, 99, 100f

I

Impacted maxillary canines
  bonding of the attachment, 143, 145, 146f, 147
  buccally, 123f, 126f–127f, 134f, 145f
  classification of, 133–136, 133f–136f
  cone beam computed tomography applications in. *See* Cone beam computed tomography.
  crown of, 124–125, 136
  depth of impaction of, 127–129, 128f–129f
  diagnosis of, 122–124
  enlarged follicles associated with, 128–129, 129f
  etiology of, 122
  genetic theory of, 122
  guidance theory of, 122
  illustration of, 130f
  intra-arch space for, 129, 131f, 136, 149
  labial impaction
    apically positioned flap for, 138, 140f, 143–145, 144f–145f
    closed eruption for, 145–147, 146f
    description of, 138–139
    gingivectomy/excision for, 141–143, 142f–143f
    mucogingival junction, 139–141, 140f–141f
    nickel-titanium wire for, 152–153, 153f–154f
  maxillary arch length deficiency, 122
  orthodontic treatment of
    anchorage in, 149–150, 150f–151f
    description of, 137
    force activation, 151–1652
    intra-arch space for, 129, 131f, 136, 149
    3D simulation of tooth movement in, 129, 131f
  overretained primary canines with, 154, 156f
  palatal expansion for, 129, 131f, 136

palatally, 134f, 137, 138f, 147–148, 148f, 151f–153f, 154, 155f–156f
panoramic radiograph of, 122, 123f–124f
positioning of, 125
prevalence of, 121
preventive intervention for, 136–137
proximity of, to roots of adjacent teeth, 125, 126f
root morphology of, 124–125, 125f
surgical treatment of, 137
teeth adjacent to
root resorption in, 133
roots, proximity of impacted teeth to, 125, 126f
temporary anchorage devices for, 137, 150, 150f
3D simulation of tooth movement, 129, 131f
3D-guided classification of, 133–136, 133f–136f
type A, 135f, 135–137, 146, 149, 151
type B, 136, 136f
Incisors
maxillary, 177f
proclination of, 94, 97
tipping of, 180f
Inflammation
gingival, 40, 109
in tooth movement, 15–16
Integrins, 3, 12
Interleukin-1, 14
Interocclusal space, 110
Interproximal periodontal bone loss, 103
Iodide quaternary ammonium methacryloxy silicate, 30

J

Junctional epithelium, 75

K

KPG index, 133

L

Labial impaction, of maxillary canines
apically positioned flap for, 138, 140f, 143–145, 144f–145f
closed eruption for, 145–147, 146f
description of, 138–139
gingivectomy/excision for, 141–143, 142f–143f
mucogingival junction, 139–141, 140f–141f
nickel-titanium wire for, 152–153, 153f–154f
Lactobacilli, 29–30
Lamina dura, 4
Laterally closed tunnel, 83, 83f
Laterally sliding flap, 82
Lectins, 28
Ligatures
bacteria accumulation on, 38–39, 39f
elastic, 38–39, 39f
Lingual retainer, 80–81
Lining cells, of alveolar bone, 4
Lipoproteins, 47

M

Maintenance phase, of periodontal therapy, 61
Mandibular osteonecrosis, 18f
Marginal bone loss, 165–166
Marginal periodontium, 74
Masticatory forces, on alveolar bone, 4, 10
Masticatory mucosa, 139
Matrix metalloproteinases, 13
Maxillary arch length deficiency, 122
Maxillary canines
development of, 121–122
ectopic growth of, 131, 132f, 149
impacted. *See* Impacted maxillary canines.
overretained primary, extraction of, 154, 156f
palatally displaced, 122
Maxillary incisors, 177f
Maxillary transverse deficiency, 131, 132f
MCAT. *See* Modified coronally advanced tunnel.
Mechanical stimulation
bone mass quantity increased using, 19
inflammatory responses to, 15
osteoporosis and, 17
of periodontal ligament fibroblasts, 11
signal transduction pathways affected by, 13, 13f
Medical history, 193
Menopause, osteoporosis at, 17
Mesenchymal stem cells, 5
Mesenchymal stromal cells, 9
Metaphyseal dysplasia, 7
Methodologic heterogeneity, 96–97
MGJ. *See* Mucogingival junction.
Microbiologic analysis, 63
Microorganisms. *See* Bacteria.
Miller classification, of gingival recessions, 78, 78f
Mini-implants, 182, 183f
Mitogen-activated protein kinases, 3, 12
MMPs. *See* Matrix metalloproteinases.
Modified apically positioned flap, 144
Modified coronally advanced tunnel, 83, 84f–87f
Mouthrinses, 54
Mucogingival junction
cone beam computed tomography of, 139–141, 140f–141f
description of, 74, 75f
labially impacted maxillary canines and, 139–141, 140f–141f
Mucoperiosteal flap, 116

N

Neurotransmitters, 15
NF-κß. *See* Nuclear factor κß.
Nickel-titanium coil springs, 184f, 184–185
Nonspecific plaque hypothesis, 34
Nonsteroidal anti-inflammatory drugs, 193
NSAIDs. *See* Nonsteroidal anti-inflammatory drugs.
Nuclear factor κß, 15–16

O

Octacalcium phosphate, 53
OPG. *See* Osteoprotegerin.
Oral diseases
biofilms and, 28–29
orthodontic treatment and, 35–37
polymicrobial synergy and dysbiosis model for, 34
risk evaluation for, 40
Oral gingival epithelium, 75, 75f
Oral hygiene
monitoring of, 198
orthodontic treatment effects on, 163
patient instruction in, 40
self-ligating brackets' effect on, 39
Oral sulcular epithelium, 75, 75f
Orthodontic appliances
adverse effects of, 171
design of, 168–170
labial, 169t–170t
lingual, 169t–170t
periodontal outcomes of, 169t
periodontal tissue affected by, 33, 161–171
Orthodontic bands
in periodontally compromised patients, 199
plaque accumulation on, 36
Orthodontic tooth movement. *See also* Orthodontic treatment.
adverse effects of, 171
aging effects on, 21
biology of, 4–9
bisphosphonates' effect on, 18–19
bone remodeling and, 3
in edentulous ridge, 197

force involved in, 177–179, 192
gingival recessions and, 80–81, 94
grafting and, 95–97
inflammation's role in, 15–16
microbiologic changes caused by, 162–163
molecular level of, 10–12
oral diseases and, 35–37
periodontal ligament involvement in, 10
periodontal treatment prior to, 192–195
in periodontally compromised patients, 191–192
plaque biofilm affected by, 35, 35f, 40
rate of, 195
tipping movements, 178, 178f
tissue changes associated with, 192
Orthodontic treatment. *See also* Orthodontic tooth movement.
in aggressive periodontitis, 190
comprehensive dental examination before, 193
keys to success of, 207
marginal bone loss caused by, 165–166
periodontal health after, 170
periodontal maintenance during, 198–199
periodontium affected by, 163–165, 164f–165f
Osteoblast(s)
aging of, 16
in basic multicellular unit, 6
in bone formation, 12, 16
definition of, 4
origins of, 5
osteoid degradation by, 14
Osteoblast-specific cis-acting element 2, 12
Osteocalcin, 4, 6, 8
Osteoclasts
cytokines and, 3
definition of, 4
histologic appearance of, 6f
Osteocytes, 4
Osteogenic signaling pathways, 6
Osteonecrosis, bisphosphonate-associated, 18, 18f
Osteonectin, 4, 6
Osteoporosis, 16–19, 17f–18f, 193
Osteoprotegerin, 3, 14, 15f, 19
Osteoprotegerin-Fc fusion protein, 14
Osterix, 6
Overbite, 182f
Oxytalan fibers, 72

P

Palatal expansion
for impacted maxillary canines, 129, 131f, 136
rapid. *See* Rapid palatal expansion.
slow, 100
Palatally impacted maxillary canines, 134f, 137, 138f, 147–148, 148f, 151f–153f, 154, 155f–156f
Paramidpalatal line, 155f
Pathologic tooth migration, 191
Patient history, 60
PDL. *See* Periodontal ligament.
Pellicle. *See* Acquired pellicle.
Periapical radiographs, 192
Periodontal attachment loss, 133
Periodontal biotype, 76, 76f
Periodontal charting, 62–63, 66f–68f, 198
Periodontal diseases. *See also* Periodontitis.
age-related increases in, 191
bleeding on probing associated with, 59
bone loss associated with, 175, 176f, 178f, 190
description of, 59
gingival recession caused by, 94
orthodontic treatment case studies, 199f–207f
smoking as risk factor for, 60
tooth extrusion associated with, 176, 176f
Periodontal examination
basic, 61–62
bleeding on probing, 62
case presentation of, 64–68, 64f–68f
clinical attachment level, 62
furcation involvement, 62
microbiologic analysis in, 63
periodontal charting, 62–63, 66f–68f, 198
in periodontally compromised patients, 199
photographic status, 63
plaque index, 63
pretherapeutic single-tooth prognosis, 63
probing pocket depth, 62
radiographic assessment, 63
study casts, 63
tooth mobility, 63
Periodontal ligament
age-related changes in, 19–20, 20f
alveolar bone affected by, 9
anatomy of, 7, 72, 73f
cells of, 3, 8–9, 72, 179
collagen fibers of, 7, 8f, 9, 72, 73f
fibroblasts. *See* Fibroblasts, periodontal ligament.
functions of, 72
histology of, 6f, 7–8, 8f
mechanical properties of, 10
stress-strain distribution. *See* Stress-strain distribution.
Periodontal phenotype, 79, 103
Periodontal pockets, 194
Periodontal regeneration, 195–196
Periodontal surgery
postorthodontic, 196–197
preorthodontic, 194–195
Periodontal therapy
case presentation of, 64–68, 64f–68f
cause-related therapy, 60
corrective phase of, 61
goals for, 60
initial phase of, 60–61
maintenance phase of, 61
before orthodontic tooth movement, 192–195
patient history in, 60, 193
phases of, 59–61
systemic phase of, 60
Periodontal tissues. *See also* Periodontium.
aging effects on, 3
orthodontic treatment/appliance effects on, 33, 161–171
Periodontally compromised patients
biomechanical approach for, 179–185, 180f–186f
orthodontic tooth movement in, 191–192
periodontal maintenance in, 198–199
Periodontitis. *See also* Periodontal diseases.
aggressive, 190–191, 203f
anterior esthetics affected by, 191, 191f
chronic, 206f
diagnosis of, 59
pathogenesis of, 189
signs of, 60
tooth maintenance in patients with, 69
tooth migration associated with, 191
Periodontium
alveolar bone of. *See* Alveolar bone.
anatomy of, 71
gingiva of. *See* Gingiva.
health of, after orthodontic treatment, 170
marginal, 74
orthodontic treatment effects on, 163–165, 164f–165f
periodontal ligament of. *See* Periodontal ligament.
phenotype of, 79, 103
root cementum, 71–72, 72f
Periodontopathogenic bacteria, 38, 163f
Photographic status, 63
Plaque
accumulation of
bonding material effects on, 39–40

on brackets, 36f, 36–38, 38f, 199
gingival recession caused by, 80
ligation effects on, 38–39, 39f
on orthodontic bands, 36
biomaterials' effect on formation of, 51f–52f, 51–53
calcification of, 53
composition of, 34
in dental caries, 34
description of, 33–35
development of, 49
factors that affect, 37–40
growth and maturation of, 34
orthodontic therapy effects on quantity of, 35, 35f, 40
self-performed control of, 61
subgingival, 192
supragingival, 192
Plaque index, 63
Pocket probing depth. *See* Probing pocket depth.
Polycystin-1, 12–13
Polycystin-2, 13
Porphyromonas gingivalis, 37
Posterior occlusal plane, 183f
PPD. *See* Probing pocket depth.
Preosteoblasts, 9
Prevotella intermedia, 37, 162
PRISMA guidelines, 161
Probing pocket depth, 60, 62, 163–164
Prostaglandin E2, 18
Protein adsorption, on biomaterial surface, 46–47, 47f

R

Radiographic assessment, 63
Randomized clinical trials, 161
RANKL, 3, 14, 15f, 19
RAP. *See* Regional accelerated phenomenon.
Rapid palatal expansion
age-appropriate use of, 101
bone loss after, 103
cone beam computed tomography of, 102
contraindications for, 101
dehiscence formation after, 101–102
devices for, 99–100, 100f
Haas expander for, 99, 100f
Hyrax expander for, 99, 100f
indications for, 100–101
for palatally displaced maxillary canines, 131
problems associated with, 101–102
recession after, 101–102
root resorption after, 102–103
slow palatal expansion versus, 101
surgically assisted, 99–100, 100f
temporary anchorage devices, 100f, 150
Receptor activator of nuclear factor κß ligand. *See* RANKL.
Regenerative periodontal surgery, 194, 196–197
Regional accelerated phenomenon, 196
Resin composites, staining of, 54
Resorbable collagen membrane, 196, 201f
Restorative materials
calculus formation on, 53
plaque retention capacity of, 51
Retainers, 80–81, 199
Rheumatoid arthritis, 193
Root cementum, 71–72, 72f
Root resorption
bisphosphonates' effect on, 19
impacted maxillary canines as risk factor for, 133
interproximal periodontal bone loss after, 103
after rapid palatal expansion, 102–103
Root trunk anatomy, 110
RPE. *See* Rapid palatal expansion.
Runt-related transcription factor-2, 3, 6–7, 12, 20
Runx2. *See* Runt-related transcription factor-2.

S

Saliva-coated biomaterials, 49
Salivary glycoproteins, 27–28
SARPE. *See* Surgically assisted rapid palatal expansion.
Sclerostin, 17
Segmented arch approach, 176, 177f, 182
Self-ligating brackets, 38–39, 168f, 168–169, 199
Sharpey fibers, 9, 9f, 72, 74
Signal transduction pathways
in bone formation, 12–14
description of, 10–11
mechanical stress effects on, 13f
Signaling pathways, 3
Slow palatal expansion, 100
Smile
esthetic zone in, 114
gummy, 114–116, 116f–117f
Smoking, 60
Soft tissue pedicle graft, 143
SPE. *See* Slow palatal expansion.
Specific plaque hypothesis, 34
Staining, 54
Staphylococcus aureus, 30
Steroid inhalers, 193
Stipples, 75
Streptococcus mutans, 29–30, 36, 39
Stress-strain distribution
bone support, 178
center of resistance, 177–178, 178f
cone effect, 175, 177f, 179
force levels, 178–179
orthodontic loading effects on, 175
Study casts, 63
Surgical lengthening of crown. *See* Crown lengthening, surgical.
Surgically assisted rapid palatal expansion, 99–101, 100f

T

Tannerella forsythia, 37, 162
Temporary anchorage devices, 100f, 150, 150f
TGF-ß. *See* Transforming growth factor ß.
Thick-flat gingiva, 76, 76f
Thick-scalloped gingiva, 76
Thin-scalloped gingiva, 76, 76f
Tipping movements, 178, 178f
Tooth migration, 191
Tooth mobility, 63
Tooth movement. *See* Orthodontic tooth movement.
Trabeculae, 4, 74
Transcription factors
clinical deformities caused by mutation in, 7, 7t
polycystin-1, 12–13
Runt-related transcription factor-2, 3, 6–7, 12
Transforming growth factor ß, 6
Transverse skeletal discrepancy, 102, 149
Tricyclic antidepressants, 193
Two-cantilever system, 181f

U

Undifferentiated mesenchymal cells, 8, 13

V

Volkmann's canals, 74
Vroman effect, 47

W

Wnt/ß-catenin pathway, 19
World Workshop on the Classification of Periodontal and Peri-Implant Diseases, 77, 79, 189

Y

Young adults
aggressive periodontitis in, 190–191
data collection, diagnosis, and periodontal monitoring in, 192–193